Sex, Love & Health

A Self-Help Health Guide to Love & Sex

BRIGITTE MARS

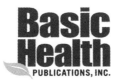

Basic Health
PUBLICATIONS, INC.

The information contained in this book is based upon the research and personal and professional experiences of the author. It is not intended as a substitute for consulting with your physician or other health care provider. Any attempt to diagnose and treat an illness should be done under the direction of a health care professional.

The publisher does not advocate the use of any particular health care protocol but believes the information in this book should be available to the public. The publisher and author are not responsible for any adverse effects or consequences resulting from the use of the suggestions, preparations, or procedures discussed in this book. Should the reader have any questions concerning the appropriateness of any procedures or preparation mentioned, the author and the publisher strongly suggest consulting a professional health care advisor.

Basic Health Publications, Inc.
8200 Boulevard East
North Bergen, NJ 07047
1-201-868-8336

Library of Congress Cataloging-in-Publication Data
Mars, Brigitte.
   Sex, love, & health : a self-help guide to love and sex / by Brigitte Mars.
      p. cm.
Includes bibliographical references and index.
   ISBN 1-59120-026-1
1. Hygiene, Sexual. 2. Sex instruction. 3. Sexual disorders—
Alternative treatment. I.Title: Sex, love, and health. II. Title.
RA788 M336   2002
613.9—dc21
                                                    2002015520

Editor: Nancy Ringer
Typesetter/Book design: Gary A. Rosenberg
Cover design: Mike Stromberg

Printed in the United States of America

10   9   8   7   6   5   4   3   2   1

Contents

To Tom Pfeiffer,
Eternal beloved.
You are forever my hero!

I met you one cold January night.
You gave me a ride home.
You had a mandala on your Jeep.
I took it as a sign
You were meant to keep.
And keep you did
And keep you well
It's been heaven.
It's been a bit of hell.
We've endured
We've delight
Weave our love
We walk in light.
Thank you for saving me
Believing in me
Asking me
your bride to be.
Thank you Tom
Om
Home
Shalom
We go on!
DNA strands
Sharing a destiny.
Why even our angels are friends!
Through universe journey
what the future may bring
This has been more than a fling
Thank you for
your
kiss of bliss.
Namaste.

THE HEART CHAKRA: COMPASSION
Scarlet

Can you float through the universe of your body . . .
And not lose your way¿
Flow with fire-blood through each tissued corridor¿
Can you let your heart pump you down long red tunnels¿
Stream into cell chambers¿
Love with your heart¿
Let your heart become central pump-house
For all human feeling . . . pulse for all love . . .
Beat for all sorrow . . . throb for all pain . . .
Thud for all joy . . . beat for all humankind . . .
Burst . . . bleed . . . into warm compassion
Flowing . . . flowing . . . pulsing . . . out . . . out

Life
Scarlet
Drum

—DR. TIMOTHY LEARY, *THE PSYCHEDELIC PRAYERS*

THE SEX CHAKRA: FUSION
Rainbow

Can you float through the universe of your body
and not lose your way¿
Lie quietly engulfed in the slippery union of male and female¿
Warm wet dance of generation¿
Endless ecstasies of couples¿
Offer your stamen trembling in the meadow
for the electric penetration of pollen While birds sing¿
Writhe together on the river bank While birds sing¿
Can you coil serpentine While birds sing¿
Become two cells merging¿
Slide together in molecule embrace¿
Can you . . . lose . . . all fusing
rainbow

—DR. TIMOTHY LEARY, *THE PSYCHEDELIC PRAYERS*

Acknowledgments

A heartfelt thank-you to my publisher, Norman Goldfind, for his integrity, years of experience, and belief in this project. Thanks also to my editor, skilled and wise, Nancy Ringer. I was truly blessed to be able to work with you again.

Tom Pfeiffer, beloved husband for over a quarter of a century, none of this would be possible without you. You were so brave to take on a young single mother and love her children as your own. I love you forever and find you beautiful and wise.

My daughters—Sunflower Sparkle Mars, firstborn, always bright, child delight, and awakener of my heart, and Rainbeau Harmony Mars, child of fortune and constant source of inspiration—how I love you both!

Thanks to my teachers on the path of healing sexuality: Light and Bryan Miller, Charles and Caroline Muir, and Margo Anand and Annie Sprinkle.

I am so grateful for my raw inspirations: Juliano, David Wolfe, and Victoria and Igor Boutenko.

Many thanks to the Garlic Queens: Rosemary Gladstar, Mindy Green, Diana DeLuca, Kathi Keville, Beth Baugh, Sara Katz, Cascade Anderson Geller, Pam Montgomery, Jane Bothwell, and Chanchal Cabrerra. Herb sisters in my life, you are beloved! Susun Weed, Jeannine Parvati Baker, and Amanda McQuade Crawford, you inspire! And thanks to the eternal flower child author Alicia Bay Laurel.

Thanks to Tamara Kerner, dearest friend, secret sharer, and feng shui mistress. To Laura Lamun for joy, laughter, and song. To Debra Saint Claire for adventure. To the late Rosemary Woodruff Leary—do you know how you inspired my life? To Alana Cini—there has never been a friend like you! To

Feather Jones, herbal visionary and founder of the Rocky Mountain Center of Botanical Studies. To friends and celestial artisans Bob Venosa and Martina Hoffmann. To Steve McIntosh and Tehya Jai, always on the path of truth, beauty, and goodness. To Mo and Jennifer Siegel for Wednesday night study groups.

Matthew Becker, herbalist extraordinaire, you always comfort and heal with your kindness and wisdom. Thanks to herbalists William LeSassier, Michael and Lesley Tierra, L.Ac., A.H.G, Christopher Hobbs, L.Ac., A.H.G., Roy Upton, Herbal Ed Smith, David Winston, David Hoffmann, Win Smith, L.Ac., James Green, Paul Bergner, N.D., and the late Terence McKenna. Dr. Andrew Lange, I appreciate your expertise in homeopathy, and Premarose, your knowledge of midwifery. Thanks to Robyn Klein for her help with pharmacognosy and to George Tuffy for his assistance with the art. Thanks to Farida Sharan, Director of the School of Natural Medicine. Much gratitude to Dr. Jia Gottlieb for his knowledge of medicine, and great thanks to Dr. Ann Mattson for her ob/gynecological and holistic medicine wisdom.

Thank you friends who show up for First Friday salons, raw potlucks, spiritual discourse, and herbal fun.

I am grateful for *The Urantia Book*, which has answered so many of my questions about life on Earth and beyond.

Thank you, Universal Father and Mother Spirit. Thank you for this beautiful planet, for the gift of love that heals, and for the passion that makes life worthwhile. Blessed be!

Introduction

Warm greetings! Sex, love, and health—it's what most of us have spent our lives searching for, although not necessarily in that order. My friends, the search may not stop here, but it is my hope that this book will help you on your way.

Sex is an extraordinary form of communication between two people. When sex is joyous, body, mind, and spirit bond together as one. In its highest form, sex leads to a transcendent, mystical experience and simple, total bliss. How do you bring that kind of joy to sex? Tend your relationship as if it were a garden. Treat your body as if it were a temple. And practice making love as if it were a sacred adventure.

My intention with this book is to stimulate new thinking on ways to make love more beautiful, sex more pleasurable, health more vibrant, and relationships more connected. Of course, there is no single approach to sex, love, and health that will work for everyone. You'll find here a broad range of ideas, drawn from many different cultures, theories, and schools of medicine. Take some of these leads and follow their paths. Accept the healing that works for you, and walk your own path toward fulfillment.

Having a lover is truly one of life's great blessings. Cherish this gift. Heal and be healed by each other. Let go of patterns that no longer serve. Honor the aspects of god and goddess that dwell in each of us. Celebrate love, and celebrate life!

May you radiate love to all corners of the universe. Many blessings!

Part 1

The Healing Power
of Love and Sex

1

Sexual Energy

n the Hindu tradition, sex is said to stimulate *kundalini,* the dormant energy or life force that lies coiled at the base of the spine. When awakened, kundalini floods up the spinal column to the brain, where it can stimulate a higher state of consciousness and bring enlightenment.

Of course, as you're probably thinking, not all sex could be described as a journey toward enlightenment. But you must admit that sometimes, every once in a while, just maybe, you find that spark of energy. That sense of losing yourself and finding yourself all at once. That feeling of having touched Spirit. That sense of "wow."

Sex can be a potent energizer of physical and emotional health, relationships, and the soul. Here's how.

SEX BUILDS HEALTH, HEALTH BUILDS SEX

The brain, controller of hormones, neurotransmitters, and other physiological compounds, is the ultimate sexual organ. Things that improve brain function generally improve sex, too, and vice versa. Brain function and sexual activity are natural cohorts; after all, the most basic human drive is to procreate. Sex stimulates the brain to release all sorts of chemicals, ranging from feel-good endorphins to libido-boosting dehydroepiandrosterone (DHEA). It lifts the spirits, stimulates the immune system, boosts circulation, lowers cholesterol levels, gets creative juices flowing, and much, much more.

Sex is aerobic exercise, but it's much more fun than riding a stationary bike. When you are making love, your heart rate increases, your muscles get a workout, your cardiovascular system gets pumping, and *chi* (life force) moves through the vital organs. And you burn about 100 calories a session!

In men, sex can help clear a backed-up prostate gland. For women, sex can help regulate menstrual cycles and improve many of the symptoms associated with premenstrual syndrome. By increasing estrogen levels, sex can also help protect menopausal women from heart disease and bone loss and keep vaginal tissues moist and healthy. For both genders, sex can help relieve pain by stimulating the release of cortisone and endorphins.

During orgasm there is an intense discharge of electrical energy in the limbic cortex or "hind brain." An arousing of emotions and relaying of nerve messages relieves tension and promotes psychological well-being. Orgasm relaxes the muscles and leads brain waves into an alpha state that encourages dreaming and creativity, or sometimes a theta, or deep sleep, state that leaves you feeling powerfully energized when you awaken.

Good sex both requires and builds good health. Good health enables us to be open to our loving nature, which in turn helps us to have fit bodies and love in our hearts. A couple can take the path toward good health—good life practices, a healthy diet, and a healthy attitude toward sex—together as they interweave their lives.

GOOD SEX ENCOURAGES A HEALTHY RELATIONSHIP

Good sex cannot be thought of as an orgasm rating on a scale of one to ten. Good sex is, rather, a healthy attitude toward sex. Enjoy each other. Let sex be a true making of love. And respect that you won't always have equal sexual needs. With a healthy attitude, you can still be compatible.

Sexual energy is like the changing moon. No matter how great the relationship is, libido will ebb and flow, often in response to powerful stressors such as work pressure, financial problems, and concerns about children. Of course, the stressor that dampens libido in your partner may not have the same effect on you. Establish the right in your relationship to say no—kindly and lovingly—to sex. Allow room for sex that is filled, not with lust, but with gentleness, love, caring, and release. Realize that sometimes it's okay for one person to just "go for it" and meet his or her needs without worrying about his or her lover. Accept masturbation, with or without the support of your partner, as a pleasurable means of sexual release in a time when your lover is just not feeling up to it.

When sex offers myriad ways to express love and support for a partner, no matter how strongly or flatly libido is felt at a particular moment, it becomes the building block for a strong relationship.

STRONG RELATIONSHIPS ARE GIFTS OF LOVE

If you want to do something wonderful for your children, your community, and humanity, focus on building a good relationship with your partner. So few of us were blessed with healthy relationship role models. Our road toward a relationship has been paved with trial and error. We've journeyed long and far in search of the meaning of love, and we've made mistakes—some that we regret, and some that we appreciate—as we've tried to negotiate the mountains and quagmires that stand in front of a good relationship. With luck, we've learned what it takes. That lesson is the most important tool we can give to our children. Our love is a gift to the world, exposing beneath our rough edges the gleaming gems of human existence.

2

A Quick Lesson in Vocabulary

he grand design of the human body is a truly wondrous mandala, filled with patterns of multiplicity. Men and women mirror and complement each other, their bodies reflecting the dance of creation. We find that even the reproductive systems, where it seems that the differences between male and female are truly made manifest, are patterned from the same mold. In scientific terms, male and female bodies are filled with homologues—structures or tissues of common origin. The penis develops from the same tissue that produces the clitoris. Both the penis and the clitoris have a glans (head). Testicles and ovaries are homologues, as are the labia majora and the scrotum. Cowper's glands are the male equivalent of the female Bartholin's glands. The list goes on and on.

Our incredible biological complexity is a sacred miracle, evidence, perhaps, of that Greater Mystery that people of different faiths (but similar beliefs) have argued and fought over for centuries. Awareness of and appreciation for the physiological beauty of the human body seems to have been lost from modern culture. Perhaps we have been jaded by waves of technological ingenuity. Perhaps we have become bewitched by our own ability to untangle biological processes, trading in our wonder and awe in favor of decoding DNA and rewriting the genetic code. Perhaps we have given in to the often-preached moralities that link sexuality to base, unnatural desires rather than giving in to beauty and awe.

The bone at the base of the spine is called the sacrum. Its name has its roots in the Latin *sacer*. The term reflects the high honor that sexual union once had. Let us restore that sense of sacredness in sexuality. Let us investi-

The Message of Posture

During the experience   Observe your body
Mandala of the Universe
Observe your body   Of ancient design
Holy temple of consciousness
Observe its structured wonders
Skin, hair, tissue   vein   muscle   net of nerve

Observe its message
Does it merge or does it strain⸮
Does it rest serene on sacred ground⸮
Or tilt, propped up by wire and sticks⸮
On tiptoe one cannot stand for long
Tension retards the flow
Observe the mandala of
your body.

—Dr. Timothy Leary, *The Psychedelic Prayers*

gate and test and research and learn all we can about human anatomy and physiology, but let us not forget to honor the sheer marvel of it all. Let us love each other with a sense of gratefulness for being here, on this planet, in this body, capable of love, sex, soulful union, and shimmering pleasure.

FEMALE ANATOMY

Bartholin's glands (bar'-thə-lənz). Two glands, comparable to the male Cowper's glands, that lie one to each side in the lower part of the vagina. They secrete a lubricating mucus.

Cervix (sər'-viks). The narrow, outer end of the uterus. It is about two inches wide and three inches long. The visible portion is only about a half-inch. It is shaped like an upside-down pear. The cervix is somewhat sensitive to pleasure when stimulated.

Clitoral hood (kli'-tə-rəl). The flap of skin that covers and protects the clitoris. Also called the *prepuce.*

Clitoris (kli'-tə-rəs). From the Greco-Latin *clavis,* meaning "key." The sole human organ whose only function is to give pleasure! The clitoris is a small shaft of tissue that is rich in nerve endings (it has about as many as the

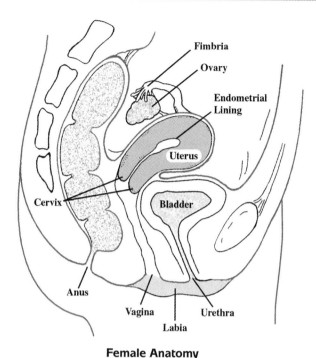

Female Anatomy

penis) and blood vessels; it is almost twice as sensitive as the vagina. It is hidden under a "hood" of skin at the top of the vagina. When stimulated, it fills with blood, throbs, becomes sensitive, and moves out from under the hood. Like an iceberg, the visible part of the clitoris is only its tip; a larger mass of clitoral tissue is buried inside the body.

Corpus luteum (kor'-pəs lü'-tē-əme). A mass of progesterone-secreting endocrine tissue that forms from the ruptured follicle in the ovary immediately after ovulation.

Endometrium (en-dō-mē'-trē-əm). A blood- and nutrient-rich membrane that forms as the lining of the uterus as part of the fertility cycle. If fertilization occurs, the fertilized egg implants in the endometrium. If fertilization does not occur, part of the endometrium is shed during the menses.

Fallopian tube (fə-lō'-pē-ən). A passageway that transports eggs from an ovary to the uterus. There is one fallopian tube for each ovary. Egg fertilization usually occurs within them.

Follicle (fǎ'-li-kəl). One of millions of vesicles containing a germ cell, or egg, in the ovaries.

G spot. Spongy tissue containing a collection of blood vessels, glands, ducts, and nerve endings surrounding the urethra; it's said to be a source of great arousal for women. It may be easiest to find after a woman's orgasm when it is already somewhat enlarged and sensitive.

Hymen (hī'-mən). Membrane that partially occludes the vaginal entrance.

Labia majora (lā'-bē-ə mə-jōr'-ə). The outer, larger lips of the vagina, extending from the mound of Venus and tapering to below the vaginal opening. They protect the vagina and urethra and contain sebaceous and apocrine glands. Labia can be smooth or have many folds. One side can be smaller or larger than the other. They are often covered with pubic hair.

Labia minora (lā'-bē-ə mə-nōr'-ə). Hairless inner vaginal lips. When a woman is aroused, the labia minora swell, thicken, and darken. They secrete a sebum that helps lubricate the vagina.

Mound of Venus. Loosely translated from *mons veneris* (mänz' ve'-nə-rəs), and also referred to as *mons pubis* (mänz' pyü'-bəs). The fatty tissue mounded over the pubic bone, covered by skin and hair.

Ovaries (ō'-və-rēs). Two grape-sized organs that produce eggs and sex hormones such as estrogen, progesterone, and even small amounts of testosterone. A woman is born with all the eggs she will ever carry already in her ovaries; out of a possible 200,000 to 400,000 eggs, only about 400 ova will be released during a woman's childbearing years.

Prepuce (prē'-pyüs). See *clitoral hood.*

Urethra (yü-rē'-thrə). The narrow canal, located in the lower half of the front of the vaginal wall, that carries urine from the bladder and discharges it.

Uterus (yü'-tə-rəs). The womb; an organ for containing and nourishing an egg from fertilization through birth. An empty uterus weighs about four ounces; during menstruation, it can weigh eight ounces.

Vagina (və-ji'-nə). The word *vagina* is derived from Latin, meaning "sheath for a sword." A bit warlike, n'est-ce pas? The vagina is a three- to four-inch-long tube of muscles and fibers. When relaxed, its thick folded walls, known as *rugae,* touch, so that almost no opening exists. When stimulated, the vagina enlarges, becoming wider and longer. The first layer of the vaginal walls is a mucous membrane that is capable of secreting fluids. Under the mucosa are layers of muscles and connective tissue that are rich in blood and nerve endings. Bacteria keep the moist vaginal climate slightly acidic, helping prevent "unfriendly" bacteria from proliferating.

Vestibule (ves'-tə-byül). Entrance to the vagina.

Vulva (vəl'-və). A catch-all phrase that refers to the exterior of the female sexual organs: the vaginal opening, inner and outer labia, clitoral hood, clitoris, urethral opening, and everything else that is visible between the anus and the mound of Venus.

Yoni (yō'-nē). A term for *vagina* originating from Sanskrit terminology, meaning "origin" and "source."

MALE ANATOMY

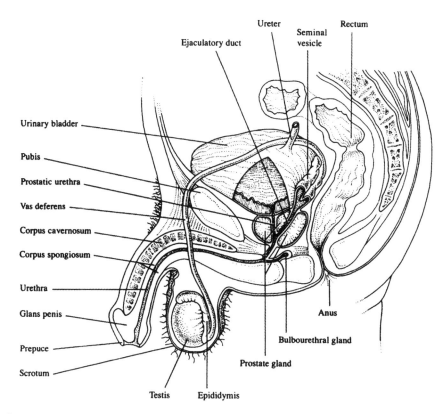

Reprinted with permission from James Green, author of *The Male Herbal.*

Cowper's glands (kaü'-pərz). Two small glands, comparable to the female Bartholin's glands, found at the base of the penile shaft, lying on either side of the urethra below the prostate gland. Before ejaculation, they produce a clear alkaline secretion that neutralizes any acid remaining in the urethra.

Epididymis (e-pə-di'-də-məs). A system of extensively coiled long ducts above each testicle. After sperm is produced, it is stored in the epididymis, where it becomes mature and motile.

Foreskin (f_r'-skin). A fold of skin that surrounds and protects the glans of the penis. It is also called the *prepuce* and is comparable to the clitoral hood.

Frenulum (fren'-yə-ləm). A connecting fold of membrane on the underside of the penis, where the shaft and glans meet. It is an extremely sensitive spot.

Glans (glanz). The cone-shaped head of the penis. It has very thin skin and is rich with nerves, which makes it very sensitive to touch.

Leydig's cells (lī'-digz). Epithelioid cells of the testes that produce androgens, namely testosterone.

Lingam (liŋ'-gəm). A term for *penis* originating in Sanskrit terminology.

Meatus (mē-ā'-təs). A natural body passage. The opening of the glans at the head of the penis is properly called a meatus.

Penis (pē'-nəs). The male organ of copulation, which also serves as the channel by which urine leaves the body. The penis contains spongy tissue, called *erectile tissue;* when a man is aroused, the tissue becomes engorged with blood and the surrounding muscles contract, causing the penis to become erect. When flaccid, the penis can range in size from 2.8 to 5.6 inches; when erect, the penis is usually five to seven inches long.

Prostate (präs'-tāt). A partly muscular, partly glandular, chestnut-shaped organ located below the neck of the bladder, where the seminal vesicles and urethra join. The prostate secretes a milky, alkaline fluid that is a major constituent of semen.

Scrotum (skrō'-təm). The pouch of skin that encloses the testicles.

Semen (sē'-mən). A milky fluid released during ejaculation consisting of sperm suspended in secretions of accessory glands.

Seminal vesicle (se'-mə-nəl ve'-si-kəl). A pair of glandular sacs located on either side of the reproductive tract. They produce most of the fluid in semen.

Testicles (tes'-ti-kəls). Reproductive glands that produce sperm. They also produce about 95 percent of a man's testosterone. The testicles are suspended in the scrotum below the penis; being held at a distance from the body allows sperm to stay slightly cooler than body temperature.

> *Testicle* comes from the Latin *testis,* which is also the root of *testament* and *testify.* Men used to swear an oath by placing their hands over their testicles.

Urethra (yu̇-rē'-thrə). The canal that carries urine from the bladder to the meatus of the penis. It also conducts spermatic fluids.

Vas deferens (vas' de'-fə-rənz). One of a pair of thick-walled ducts that carry sperm from the epididymis to the seminal vesicle ducts.

SEXUAL CHEMISTRY

Like the tides in the ocean, levels of hormones, neurotransmitters, and other physiological chemicals rise and fall in the body. The sexual impulse and reproductive ability are dependent on body chemistry, as are most physiological processes. Researchers are still in the early stages of learning about these compounds and their effects upon the body and the psyche. Those that we will apply to discussions later in this book are presented below.

Dehydroepiandrosterone

Dehydroepiandrosterone (DHEA) is the most abundant hormone in the body; it is sometimes called the "mother" sex hormone because many other sex hormones are derived from it. DHEA is produced mainly by the adrenal glands but also in small amounts by the ovaries, the testicles, and the brain.

High levels of DHEA can increase libido, support the health of the immune system, counteract depression, and lower cholesterol levels. Low levels of DHEA have the opposite effect, including contributing to weight gain. Most birth control pills decrease DHEA.

DHEA levels are highest from our teens through our twenties and during puberty and pregnancy. They slowly decrease as we age. Practices that increase DHEA include meditation, exercise, stress-reduction techniques, and orgasm.

Endorphins

Endorphins are neuropeptides that bind to opioid receptors in the brain and have potent analgesic properties. They are sometimes called "opiates of the mind." They can calm emotions, relieve pain, and reduce anxiety. Exercise, physical touch, orgasm, and sitting still all stimulate the brain to release endorphins.

Estrogens

Estrogens are substances (such as sex hormones) that regulate the menses and stimulate the development of female secondary sex characteristics. They are manufactured in the ovaries, testes, and adrenal glands. Estrogen improves cognition, performance, mood, vigilance, and reaction. It also improves the sense of smell and taste, prevents depression, reduces stress, and decreases appetite.

Alcoholism, liver disease, obesity, the first two weeks of the menstrual cycle, intercourse, and high levels of oxytocin can all contribute to elevated estrogen levels. Lack of sex, anorexia, hysterectomy, and menopause contribute to decreased levels of estrogen. Normal levels of estrogen help prevent osteoporosis and heart disease. Low estrogen levels can make a woman susceptible to these diseases and also diminish her ability to produce vaginal lubrication, which can interfere with sexual pleasure. Low estrogen levels may also cause vaginal atrophy, or thinning of the vaginal walls, which can lead to pain, bleeding, and increased risk of infection. For this reason, many health care providers recommend that a menopausal woman take estrogen supplements. However, not all women require hormone replacement therapy, as it's called.

Despite the marketing claims of the pharmaceutical industry, synthetic estrogen and other hormones are not the same as natural hormones. Physiological harmony, the standard-bearer of health, is disrupted when synthetic compounds are thrown into the sanctuary of a woman's body. In fact, they are often responsible for causing hormonal imbalance.

There are many natural substances that encourage the body to produce its own estrogen. For example, many herbs are phytoestrogenic, meaning that they simulate or stimulate the production of estrogen in the body. These include alfalfa herb, aniseed, black cohosh root, black haw bark, cramp bark, dong quai, false unicorn root, fennel seed, fenugreek seed, hops strobile, licorice root, motherwort herb, nettle leaf, parsley leaf, pomegranate seed, red raspberry leaf, red clover flower, rose hip, sage leaf, sarsaparilla root, saw palmetto berry, shepherd's purse herb, vitex berry, wild yam root, willow bark, and yarrow herb.

Foods that promote estrogen production include animal products (meat, eggs, and dairy products), apples, beans, buckwheat, cherries, dates, eggplant, flaxseeds, garlic, green, leafy vegetables, oats, olives, peaches, plums, sesame seeds, soy foods, strawberries, string beans, tomatoes, whole grains (brown rice, barley, oats, and whole wheat), and yams.

There are three main types of estrogenic compounds found in the body: estrone, estradiol, and estriol.

Estradiol

Estradiol is secreted by the ovaries and is considered the most potent of the three types of estrogen found in the body. Estradiol levels are highest before menopause. In postmenopausal women, the liver converts estradiol and estrone into estriol.

During a woman's childbearing years, estradiol stimulates buildup of the uterine lining in preparation for a baby, and after childbirth it promotes lactation. It promotes bone health, vaginal moisture and elasticity, and cardiovascular fitness.

Estriol

Estriol, like estradiol, promotes fitness for the vaginal lining and cardiovascular system, but it is specifically beneficial for the postmenopausal woman. Estriol is also important during pregnancy. During birth, estriol levels increase by a factor of one thousand; they return to normal two to three weeks after delivery. High levels of estriol are believed to contribute to a lower risk of breast cancer.

Estrone

Estrone stimulates the development of breast tissue and, along with estradiol, the buildup of the endometrial lining in the uterus. It is primarily a postmenopausal estrogen, meaning that it doesn't play much of a physiological role until menopause.

Follicle-Stimulating Hormone

Follicle-stimulating hormone (FSH) is produced in the pituitary gland and stimulates development of the follicles in the ovary in preparation for ovulation.

Luteinizing Hormone

Luteinizing hormone (LH) is produced in the pituitary gland and stimulates development of the corpus luteum. LH levels are highest during the first few weeks of pregnancy.

Oxytocin

Oxytocin is a peptide secreted by the pituitary gland and widely distributed throughout the body. It stimulates the uterine contractions that occur with orgasm and childbirth, increases sensitivity to touch, speeds ejaculation, decreases postpartum bleeding, may contribute to "forgetting" the pain of childbirth, and causes the let-down reflex in a nursing mother who hears her baby (and in some cases other babies) cry. The drug Pitocin, which is often used to stimulate labor, is a form of oxytocin.

Oxytocin stimulates the production of estrogen, testosterone, prolactin, and vasopressin. Oxytocin levels are increased by touch and especially inter-course; supplementing with choline may also increase oxytocin levels. Lack of estrogen, lack of touch, and the consumption of alcohol will decrease oxy-tocin levels.

Progesterone

The hormone progesterone, like estrogen, is instrumental in the ovulation and menstruation cycles. It is produced by the ovaries, corpus luteum, and adre-nal glands. It is also an end product of the body's metabolizing of cholesterol. It is primarily a female hormone; men have only minute quantities.

Progesterone is the dominant hormone in women during the last two weeks of the menstrual cycle and during pregnancy. When it drops sharply before menstruation, it stimulates menstrual bleeding and can cause depres-sion, edema, and irritability.

High levels of progesterone decrease sex drive. (It's sometimes given to sex offenders in the form of the drug Provera.) It can cause women to be sex-ually passive and irritable, as well as more nurturing toward their children. At high levels, it is mildly anesthetic; at low levels, it is sedative. It inhibits uterine contractions, oxytocin sensitivity, and LH production. It helps protect against premature labor in pregnancy and promotes lactation.

Progesterone levels increase during pregnancy, nursing, and the premen-strual phase and decrease after menopause. Phytoprogesteronic herbs include alfalfa, flaxseeds, lady's mantle, sarsaparilla, vitex, wild yam, and yarrow.

Prolactin

Prolactin is secreted by the pituitary gland. Men need prolactin for the pro-duction of sperm; however, elevated prolactin levels can decrease testos-terone production, contributing to erectile dysfunction. In women, prolactin levels peak midway through the menstrual cycle and stay high until the menses begin. If a woman becomes pregnant, prolactin levels remain high, stimulating mammary tissue growth and, eventually, lactation. When a baby nurses, the mother's prolactin levels increase by a factor of ten; they return to normal levels within two or three hours.

Prolactin can decrease libido in men and women. The more a mother nurses, the more likely her sex drive will be diminished. Prolactin also decreases alertness and sensitivity and can contribute to fatigue and depression.

Prolactin levels can be boosted by exercise, stress, nausea, jet lag, nipple stimulation, high-protein meals, opiates, and sleep. They are decreased by meditation.

Prostaglandins

Prostaglandins are fatty acids that perform hormonelike actions in the body. They are produced in the uterus and found in high concentrations in sperm.

In women, prostaglandins contribute to the contraction and relaxation of the uterus. Women who suffer from intense menstrual cramps often have elevated prostaglandin levels. Prostaglandins are also thought to trigger labor and orgasm.

Prostaglandin E (PGE) helps regulate uterine tone, protecting against cramps, and can ward off menstrual headache, edema, breast tenderness, and emotional distress. PGE also helps prevent blood platelets from clumping, thereby reducing the risk of heart attack and stroke.

Raw nuts, seeds, yogurt, and evening primrose, borage, hemp, and flaxseed oils provide the raw materials the body needs to make anti-inflammatory prostaglandins. A diet that is high in animal products (meat, eggs, and dairy products) can contribute to inflammatory prostaglandin production. Bromelain, an enzyme found in pineapple, can decrease prostaglandin production.

Testosterone

Testosterone is a steroid hormone produced in the adrenals, testicles, and ovaries. It is responsible for producing and maintaining male secondary sex characteristics. Women have twenty to forty times less testosterone than men. For both men and women, testosterone is a major factor in determining sex drive. Levels fluctuate daily and seasonally.

Aggression, assertiveness, competitiveness, self-confidence, and aloofness are byproducts of testosterone. When testosterone levels are elevated, men may become irritable and angry. High testosterone levels have been implicated in episodes of violence and psychotic behavior.

Exercise, competition, and a meat-based diet elevate testosterone levels; excess exercise, stress, vegetarianism, and progesterone decrease them. Testosterone inhibits the production of prolactin and improves the function of adrenaline and vasopressin.

Vasopressin

Vasopressin is a peptide hormone secreted by the pituitary gland and is widely distributed throughout the body. It is sometimes referred to as the "monogamy molecule," because it discourages extreme sexual and emotional patterns and modulates testosterone activity. Vasopressin has vasoconstrictor and antidiuretic properties.

THE ORIENTAL PERSPECTIVE

The traditional Oriental system of healing has been proven effective over thousands of years of practice. You will find references to this system of healing throughout this book. For those versed only in Western perspectives, however, the Oriental mechanism of diagnosis and treatment may be foreign—no pun intended—because the traditional Oriental understanding of anatomy, physiology, and epidemiology is quite different from that of Western medicine.

To help you understand and begin to implement Oriental diagnoses and therapies, a quick lesson in energetics and terminology is necessary.

The Five Elements

In Oriental tradition, human beings are a microcosm of the universe. Just as nature is ordered by five primordial powers—Wood, Fire, Earth, Metal, and Water—so, too, is the human body infused with these five elements. Each element corresponds to a particular organ or bodily system.

- Wood—Liver and Gallbladder
- Fire—Heart and Small Intestine
- Earth—Stomach and Spleen
- Metal—Lungs and Large Intestine
- Water—Kidneys and Bladder

These elements are the foundation of physiological harmony. An imbalance in one element can cause imbalance in others. (See illustration on page 21.)

When an organ system is referenced in the context of Oriental medicine, the initial letter of the organ's name is capitalized. This helps differentiate, for example, the Western understanding of the liver (the singular organ) from the Oriental understanding of the Liver (the organ, the system it is associated with, and its energy).

The Flow of Energy

The human body is infused with *chi*, which translates as "breath" and means "life force" or "vital energy." Chi flows throughout the body on meridians, or energy pathways, bringing life force to each of the organs and bodily systems that contribute to health. When chi is excessive, deficient, or blocked (stagnant), health is negatively impacted.

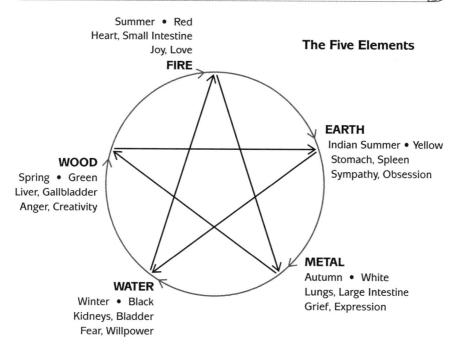

Summer • Red
Heart, Small Intestine
Joy, Love
FIRE

The Five Elements

WOOD
Spring • Green
Liver, Gallbladder
Anger, Creativity

EARTH
Indian Summer • Yellow
Stomach, Spleen
Sympathy, Obsession

WATER
Winter • Black
Kidneys, Bladder
Fear, Willpower

METAL
Autumn • White
Lungs, Large Intestine
Grief, Expression

Certain points along the body's meridians may be stimulated to affect the flow of chi. Acupuncture, acupressure, and massage make use of these vital points to keep chi flowing freely.

Yin versus Yang

Yin and yang are the vital polarities that permeate the universe, from the tiniest to grandest dimensions. They are not opposites but different sides of a continuum, merging into one another. They are yin and yang only in relation to each other; one does not exist without the other. Each contains elements of the other. The black-and-white yin-yang symbol shows a spot of white in the black, and a spot of black in the white. In the same manner, women (yin) have "male" hormones in their body, and men (yang) have "female" hormones in their body.

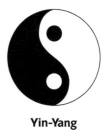

**Yin-Yang
Symbol**

In traditional Oriental medicine, ailments are often described in terms of a yin-yang imbalance. A yang deficiency (yin excess), for example, could result in a wet, cold condition, such as lower back pain, lethargy, edema, and a feeling of always being cold. A yin deficiency (yang excess) could result in a dry,

YIN	YANG	YIN	YANG
Agitation	Calm	Liver, heart, spleen, lungs, kidneys	Gallbladder, small intestine, stomach, large intestine, bladder
Alkaline	Acid		
Anabolism	Catabolism	Lower part of body	Upper part of body
Aromatic	Without aroma	Matter	Energy
Autumn	Spring	Midday	Midnight
Belowground	Aboveground	Moist skin	Dry skin
Black	Red	Moon	Sun
Blood, mucus, urine, sweat	Filtering processes of the body	Negative	Positive
Cave	Mountain	Night	Day
Centripetal	Centrifugal	Organs on the right side	Organs on the left side
Chaos	Order	Ovum	Sperm
Chronic illness	Acute illness	Pale	Ruddy
Cold	Hot	Particle	Wave
Complacent	Filled with desire	Passive	Active
Cool body and personality	Warm body and personality	Plants that grow quickly	Plants that grow slowly
Dark	Light	Receptive	Dynamic
Death	Life	Relaxation	Determination
Decomposes easily	Preserves well	Right brain	Left brain
Deep	Shallow	Salt	Sugar
Deficient	Excess	Salty, bitter, sour	Sweet, pungent
Descending	Ascending	Sense of touch	Sense of sight
Dreamy	Hyperactive mentality	Serene	Focused
Earth	Heaven and air	Shady side of slope	Sunny side of slope
Enjoyment	Accomplishments	Shakti	Shiva
Estrogen	Testosterone	Slow	Quick
Even numbers	Odd numbers	Soft	Hard
Feet	Head	Speaks softly	Speaks loudly
Feminine	Masculine	Solid organs	Hollow organs
Flaccid	Tense	Space	Time
Front of body	Back of body	Thoughts, feelings	Actions, expressions
Green, blue, purple	Yellow, orange, red	Timid	Aggressive
Heavy	Light	Vowels	Consonants
Hidden	Revealed	Water	Fire
Ice	Steam	Weak	Strong
Inhalation	Exhalation	West and north	East and south
Interior	Exterior	Wet	Dry
Introverted	Extroverted	Winter	Summer
Intuitive	Logical	Yoni	Lingam
Left side of body	Right side of body	Female	Male

warm condition, such as night sweats, insomnia, nervous exhaustion, and dizziness. Treatment is focused on restoring balance to the affected system or organ.

Heat increases metabolic activity, boosts circulation, and dilates blood vessels. Excess heat is associated with redness and inflammation. Sweet and pungent foods and herbs tend to increase heat.

Cold slows circulation and metabolic activity. Excess cold is associated with achy joints, chills, hypothyroid conditions, nighttime urination, and poor circulation. Cold, sour, bitter, and salty foods and herbs tend to be cooling.

Dampness is associated with the buildup of fluids. Excess dampness may contribute to mucus congestion and excess secretions. Dairy products and starchy foods can increase dampness.

Dryness is associated with lowering fluid levels. Excess dryness may cause dry skin and vaginal dryness. Spicy foods, diuretics, and antihistamines can aggravate dry conditions.

Nurturing the Kidneys

The Kidneys, representative of the Water element, govern sexual vitality and mental energy. Maintaining yin-yang balance and preventing chi blockage in the Kidneys is imperative to sexual health and libido.

To support Kidney vitality and, therefore, sexual vitality, avoid stress, over-work, and loud noises. Do not allow your lower back to become chilled, min-imize your intake of icy foods and beverages, and get adequate sleep every night. If the Kidney system is depleted, take a nap between 3 and 7 P.M. Even if the nap lasts only a few minutes, it will be a potent restorative.

Kidney Yin

Kidney yin deficiency may manifest as low libido, dry skin (including vaginal dryness), erectile dysfunction, low sperm count, premature ejaculation, semi-nal emissions (wet dreams), night sweats, constipation, hair loss, constant hunger, aggressive tendencies, loud behavior, insomnia, an aversion to heat, a desire for quick sex with minimal foreplay.

To cultivate Kidney yin, incorporate into your diet sea vegetables, fish, roots, greens, olive oil, plain yogurt, and small amounts of honey. Yin can also be built by swimming, taking baths, listening to the sound of water (fountains, waterfalls, or streams) gardening, being in nature, rest, and exposure to moonlight.

Kidney Yang

Kidney yang deficiency may manifest as erectile dysfunction, low libido, inability to orgasm, paleness, low energy, poor appetite, timid voice, fluid retention, lack of ambition, aversion to heat, and poor listening skills.

To cultivate Kidney yang, increase the amount of time you spend outdoors in the sun, take saunas, and stay warm, most beneficially from fire, such as a campfire, fireplace, or wood stove.

VOCABULARY OF THE MEDICINE CABINET

Natural medicines, such as herbs, homeopathic remedies, and flower essences, have a variety of physiological effects. Knowing the vocabulary that describes those effects can help you choose the medicine that best meets your needs.

Abortifacient: Capable of inducing abortion.

Adaptogen: Increases the body's resistance to stress, working through hormonal response.

Alterative: Alters one's condition. Restores body functions. Increases blood flow to tissues, detoxifies, aids assimilation, stimulates metabolism, and promotes waste and excretion.

Anabolic: Increases constructive metabolism.

Analgesic: Relieves pain.

Anaphrodisiac: Curbs sex drive.

Anesthetic: Deadens sensation.

Anodyne: Lessens pain by diminishing nerve excitability.

Anticoagulant: Prevents clotting of blood.

Antidepressant: Elevates mood and counteracts depression.

Antifungal: Inhibits growth of fungal organisms.

Anti-inflammatory: Soothes inflammation.

Antioxidant: Prevents free-radical damage, which is believed to contribute to cancerous growths.

Antipyretic: Lowers fever.

Antirheumatic: Eases pain, swelling, and stiffness in joints and muscles.

Antiseptic: Prevents bacterial growth, inhibits pathogens, counters sepsis.

Antispasmodic: Prevents or eases cramps or spasms.

Antitussive: Relieves coughing.

Antiviral: Inhibits viral replication.

Aphrodisiac: Increases sexual desire and potency.

Aromatic: Is fragrant or pungent; improves flavor of bitter herbs. Often stimulates digestive tract.

Astringent: Tightens, tones, and dries.

Bitter: Stimulates flow of digestive secretions, as well as those of the pituitary, liver, and duodenum.

Cholagogue: Promotes bile flow from the gall bladder.

Choleretic: Stimulates bile production in the liver.

Demulcent: Soothes irritated tissues, especially of the mucous membranes.

Deobstruent: Removes obstructions.

Depurative: Cleanses the systems, particularly the blood.

Diaphoretic: Promotes perspiration.

Discutient: Dissolves tumors and abnormal growths. Used internally in moderation and also topically.

Diuretic: Increases secretion and expulsion of urine by promoting activity of the kidneys and bladder.

Emmenagogue: Stimulates uterus. Normalizes female reproductive system.

Euphoric: Produces an uplifting effect, physically and mentally.

Febrifuge: Reduces or eliminates fevers.

Galactagogue: Increases the production of mother's milk.

Germicidal: Destroys germs, that is, microorganisms causing disease.

Hallucinogen: Induces hallucinations.

Hemostatic: Arrests bleeding.

Hepatic: Strengthens and tones the liver.

Hypotensive: Reduces blood pressure.

Mucilaginous: Lubricates, soothes, and heals.

Mucolytic: Reduces the viscosity of mucus.

Nervine: Calms and nourishes the nerves.

Nutritive: Supplies nutrients to build and tone the body.

Oxytocic: Stimulates uterine contractions. Can be used to assist or induce labor.

Parturient: Assists in labor and delivery.

Phytoandrogenic: Provides the raw materials to help the body make its own androgen hormones.

Phytoestrogenic: Provides the raw materials to help the body make its own estrogen.

Phytoprogesteronic: Provides the raw materials to help the body make its own progesterone.

Progesteronic: Aids the body in the production or activation of progesterone.

Refrigerant: Cools body temperature.

Regenerative: Aids in the repair of bones, flesh, tissue, and cartilage.

Soporific: Induces sleep.

Rejuvenative: Renews body, mind, and spirit. Can counteract stress and increase endurance.

Restorative: Helps rebuild a depleted condition and restores normal body functions.

Rubefacient: Increases blood flow to the surface of the skin; draws out deep impurities.

Sedative: Slows down body functions. Quiets the nerves.

Stimulant: Quickens various body functions and improves circulation.

Tonic: Promotes general health and well-being. Builds energy, blood, and chi.

Vasoconstrictor: Narrows blood vessels, thus elevating blood pressure.

Vasodilator: Expands blood vessels, thus reducing blood pressure.

Vulnerary: Encourages wound healing by promoting cellular growth and repair.

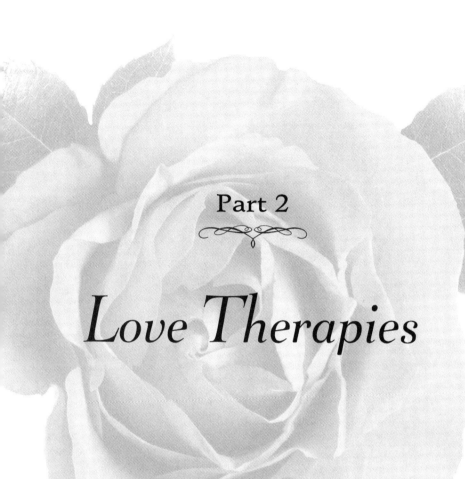

Part 2

Love Therapies

Sexercises: Strengthening the Love Muscles

e've all heard the lecture again and again. To stay healthy, we must exercise. To reduce stress, we must exercise. To lose weight, we must exercise. Somehow most of us still find ourselves unable to fit three twenty-minute exercise sessions into our schedule each week. But would it make a difference if I told you that you'd have the best sex of your life if you started exercising?

It's true. Regular exercise is one of the most efficient and inexpensive methods for promoting the "urge to merge." Psychologically, exercise relieves depression, reduces stress, relaxes the mind and body, and opens the heart of those who live behind emotional armor. Physically, it encourages strength, stamina, flexibility, and sensitivity. Chemically, it boosts the production of endorphins, adrenaline, and testosterone, all of which contribute to arousal. As a result, exercise also boosts libido and intensifies orgasms.

Exercising for twenty minutes three times a week can effect an astonishing change in your health, psyche, and sex life. The hardest part is just getting started. Once you do, you'll find that exercise is almost addictive—when you miss sessions, you'll feel restless and unsettled.

Making a commitment to exercise doesn't mean that you have to pay membership fees at a health club or start running marathons. Anything that increases your heart rate qualifies as exercise, and that includes cleaning the house, going for a walk, playing tag with your kids, dancing, gardening, and any other everyday activity that is undertaken with energy and enthusiasm. Making love itself is good exercise; it burns about 100 calories per session.

There are also many exercises designed specifically for boosting sexual vitality, either for an individual or between two people in a relationship. Some focus on the strength and flexibility of the muscles used in making love; others work to increase the flow of sexual energy through the body; still others harmonize the energies between two people in a relationship. You'll find that regular practice of these exercises increases your orgasmic ability, improves your stamina as a lover, enhances your sensitivity to your lover's needs, and endows you with strong sexual confidence.

Anything done to excess can drain energy and libido. Therefore, while it's important to get adequate exercise, it's also important not to overdo it.

KEGEL EXERCISES

The Kegel pelvic exercises have been known for thousands of years by practitioners of tantra as *mool bandha,* or "root locks." They are named after Dr. Arnold Kegel, who popularized them in North America in the 1950s as a treatment for stress-related incontinence. Kegels release tension, improve circulation, and strengthen muscles in the pelvic area. For women, they can be used to strengthen muscles weakened by childbirth and to increase the occurrence and intensity of orgasms. For men, they give greater staying power and also massage the prostate, contributing to prostate health. Kegels can also help men differentiate between orgasm and ejaculation.

To practice Kegels, you must tighten and then release the pubococcygeus muscles, which control the flow of urine and the anal sphincter. To find them, stop midstream the next time you are urinating. Can you feel the muscles in the pelvic area that allow you to halt the flow of urine? Then release. That tightening and then release amounts to one Kegel contraction.

When you practice Kegels, inhale while tightening and exhale while releasing. Hold each contraction for one to five seconds, and be sure to relax fully between contractions. Do the exercises three times daily, starting with twenty-one contractions at each session and working your way up to one hundred. Kegels are a very subtle exercise; if you practiced them in a room full of people, no one would ever notice. Kegels are, therefore, a great way to make good use of time when you're stuck in traffic, waiting in line, riding in a crowded elevator, and so on.

A variation of Kegels for men is to hang a damp washcloth over the erect penis while performing Kegels. With each Kegel, the washcloth will be carried up and down, serving as a weight of sorts. When the washcloth becomes easy to manage, start using a hand towel instead.

Once you've undertaken Kegel exercises seriously, you'll notice dramatic improvement in your orgasmic ability within a few weeks.

THE DEER

The Deer, also known as Stoking the Golden Stove, is one of the most important Taoist exercises for promoting long life and sexual vitality. The Deer moves blockages of energy, stimulates hormonal production, and relieves a wide range of reproductive disorders. This exercise can also help prevent prostate problems, hemorrhoids, and erectile dysfunction. There are male and female versions.

For women, sit up straight on a bed, chair, or the floor, and place a heel of a foot gently against the clitoris. Rub the hands together to warm them, and then massage around each breast (not nipples) in a slow, circular motion thirty-six times. Massage inward to make your breasts grow larger and outward to make them become smaller. If your breasts are overly large, tender, or prone to lumps, massage away from the heart. Then lower your hands to your sides and do thirty-six deep Kegels.

For men, The Deer is performed standing or while sitting on a chair or a bed. Rub the hands together to warm them. Hold the scrotum with one hand. With the palm of the other hand, massage right below the navel in a circular motion eighty-one times. Then switch hands and directions and massage again. Follow with thirty-six Kegels.

The Deer should be practiced twice daily, in the morning when you wake up and at night before you go to bed. It is essential to focus on the exercise, rather than thinking about what you're going to wear or have for lunch. Be mindfully present during your practice.

THE MOUNTED ARCHER

This Taoist exercise, also known as The Horseman, strengthens the kidneys, improves blood quality and circulation, calms the mind, and improves digestion.

Stand with your legs shoulder width apart and cross your arms in front of your chest. Keeping your heels on the floor, bend your knees, lower your upper body, and lean forward as if you were riding a horse. Pull one arm back as if you were drawing back a bowstring. Inhale, then resume the crossed-armed position. Repeat eight times, alternating arms. Practice daily.

MALE TONIFYING EXERCISE

In the Taoist tradition, the simple act of urinating can build sexual energy and strengthen kidney chi in men. But it's important to do it right. Stand on tiptoe, tighten the buttocks, keep the waist and back straight, hold in the stomach, and clench the teeth. Urinate forcibly, all the while exhaling slowly. This practice also helps treat erectile dysfunction and premature ejaculation.

THE WILD DUCK

The Wild Duck is a beneficial Taoist exercise for women. It can help in cases of menstrual concerns (such as painful or irregular periods), low libido, and leukorrhea. It tonifies the lower abdomen, including the kidneys, liver, spleen, and reproductive center.

Stand on the balls of the feet and stretch upward, simultaneously inhaling and raising the arms. Then drop your heels to the floor, and as you slowly lower your arms, bend at the waist until your head is between your knees, all the while gently exhaling. Stand and repeat.

When you've done the standing stretch five times, sit down on the floor or another firm surface. Extend your legs in front of you and place your hands on your thighs. Slowly exhaling, bend toward your legs and stretch your arms, attempting to touch your feet with your hands. When you've stretched as far as you can, begin to inhale and slowly return to your original position, keeping your arms extended.

Practice The Wild Duck daily for maximum benefit.

SQUATTING

Squatting as a general practice—to stretch, to rest, to watch—is a wonderful tonic for the reproductive system. It opens the pelvis, moving blockages, releasing tension, and improving the circulation of chi in the area. Just squat, breathe, and relax.

HIP CIRCLES

Like squatting, regularly doing hip circles will move blockages and improve chi circulation in the pelvic area. Hip circles also help you feel more grounded in your pelvic area, rather than in your head.

Stand with your feet shoulder width apart. Bend your knees as if you were about to sit, keeping your spine straight and your hands on your hips. Rotate to the right and then to the left, as if you were dancing. Repeat thirty-six times.

PELVIC LIFTS

Pelvic lifts strengthen the lower back and buttocks. They also increase circulation and energy in the pelvic region.

Lie on your back and bend your knees enough to place your feet flat on the floor about hip width apart. Place your arms at your sides. Tightly squeeze the muscles of the buttocks while contracting the abdominal muscles and pressing the small of the back to the floor. Exhaling, push the hips toward the ceiling, drawing the buttocks off the floor. Keep the abdominal and buttocks muscles held tightly. Hold for a few seconds at the high point. Lower slowly to the floor, rolling the spine down vertebra by vertebra from the middle back until your buttocks reach the floor. Rest for thirty seconds, then repeat. Start with five lifts and work up to twenty.

KIDNEY RUB

The kidney rub can be a fun exercise to perform with a partner. As explained on page 174, the kidneys govern sexual energy. A kidney massage, therefore, will strongly benefit libido and sexual vitality. The kidneys respond best to stimulation of the back. To perform the kidney massage, rub up and down over the bare lower back thirty-six times every morning and evening. The massage will warm and energize this vital area.

THE BUTTERFLY

This is an excellent exercise to open and relax the pelvis, which can make you more flexible and open to a wide variety of love positions.

Sit on the floor with your knees bent and the soles your feet touching each other. Gently bring your knees up and down, like the wings of a butterfly perched on a flower, and try to touch the floor several times.

CAT STRETCH

Cats take stretching to a new dimension, and we could learn a thing or two from them. This exercise helps relieve tension in the back, allowing chi to move more freely. Get down on your hands and knees with your arms and thighs vertical. While exhaling, slowly lower your head and arch up your back, making a convex curve. Then inhale, stretching your head up and arching your spine down, making a concave curve. Repeat seven times.

STRETCHING FOR PARTNERS

These stretching exercises also help to open the pelvis. Better still, they're a lovely way to play together!

Sit across from each other with your legs flat on the floor and spread wide, feet touching at the soles. Reach across and grasp hands. Swing back and forth so that one partner brings his or her head to the ground in front while the other leans back, and then vice versa. Use your arms to balance yourselves and create a smooth transition.

The second exercise has the partners sitting in the same position and grasping hands. Now swing back and forth in a circular fashion, first clockwise and then counterclockwise.

SHAKE, SHAKE, SHAKE!

Whenever you're feeling stressed or tight, turn on some groovy music and spend five minutes shaking every part of your body. Don't think about what you're doing; just do what feels good, letting your body take over. This wild and free movement releases tensions stored in the body. When you're done, sit cross-legged and quiet on the floor and feel the energy flow throughout your body.

DANCE, DANCE, DANCE!

Dancing loosens you up and makes you flexible for love. It aligns your vertebrae better than most chiropractic adjustments, improves circulation, and helps you let go of tight body patterns that keep you "uptight." Dancing with a partner can be its own kind of foreplay.

Dancing is like flying
It's really free.
Making love to music gets into me.
Tossing my head
Like a defiant child
Nothing lets me be so wild.
I feel I'm electric
I know I'm divine
Dancing takes me
Way beyond time.
I get lighter than light
And higher than air.
Being one with the music
It takes me all there.

YOGA

I highly recommend yoga, both for its overall health benefits and for its particular benefits for sexual vitality. Yoga harmonizes the nervous and glandular systems. Yoga postures that are especially beneficial for sexual energy and vitality include Cobra, Bow, Fish, Lotus, Tree, Curling Leaf, and Little Bird. Partners can benefit tremendously from taking a yoga class together. There are even newer forms of yoga, called Partner Yoga and Contact Yoga, that call for interactive yoga between partners.

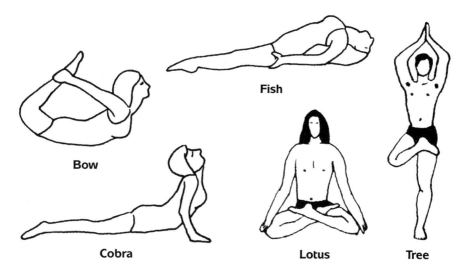

Fish

Bow

Cobra

Lotus

Tree

DEEP BREATHING

Breathing deeply increases our awareness of the present moment, promotes health, invites serenity, and massages the internal organs. During sex, deep breathing allows a man to make love longer without ejaculating and a woman to be more open to orgasm.

A deep breath is capable of containing seven pints of air; most people, however, inhale only a pint of air with each breath. That's unfortunate, because shallow breathing quickens the heart rate and increases stress levels.

Daily practice of deep-breathing exercises makes deep breathing a habit. Inhale slowly and deeply for a count of five, drawing breath all the way down into the belly and allowing the chest and belly to expand. As you inhale, do the contraction phase of Kegels (described on page 30). Hold for a count of five (unless you have high blood pressure, in which case you should begin to exhale immediately). Inhale an extra sniff of air, then exhale slowly to a count of five, relaxing the shoulders, pulling the belly inward, and releasing the Kegel contraction. Repeat seven times.

SYNCHRONIZED BREATHING

Breathing in harmony while making love can help lovers connect in a deep and powerful way. Partners can synchronize their breathing or alternate, so that one is breathing in while the other is breathing out, like a piston.

There are a couple of exercises that can help lovers learn to synchronize their breathing. In the first, the partners sit cross-legged with their backs touching and elbows interlaced. Though you may feel a gentle stretch in the shoulders while sitting like this, avoid pulling on your partner's arms. Breathe deeply together, feeling the breath of your partner fill his or her lungs.

In the second, the partners sit cross-legged on the floor facing each other. Press the palms of your hands together. Keep your wrists, elbows, and shoulders relaxed. Slow down your breathing and try to synchronize, always keeping eye contact. Allow the breath of life to dance between you!

4

Diet: Setting the Table for Passion

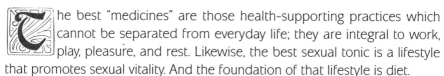he best "medicines" are those health-supporting practices which cannot be separated from everyday life; they are integral to work, play, pleasure, and rest. Likewise, the best sexual tonic is a lifestyle that promotes sexual vitality. And the foundation of that lifestyle is diet.

In the West, the abundance and variety of foods available at an average grocery store is astounding. Six different kinds of apples—in midwinter! A hundred kinds of breakfast cereal. Small frozen pizzas, large frozen pizzas, rising-crust frozen pizzas, frozen pizza dough, refrigerated pizza shells, organic whole-grain prebaked vacuum-packed pizza crusts. Not to mention candy, chips, and soft drinks galore! The sheer volume of choice available to the modern consumer can dull the mind.

With the plenitude available, it can be easy to slip into a "convenience" mindset. We buy what is least expensive and easiest to prepare. We allow our ancestrally inspired longing for high-fat, high-carbohydrate foods—which we needed in our hunter-gatherer days to resupply us with the huge amounts of energy we expended—to guide our modern-day fluorescent-lit shopping experience. The food we eat is far removed from its roots in the earth, and as a result, we suffer. We grow overweight, feel lethargic, have trouble sleeping, become prone to illness, endure headaches, develop allergies, and suffer from the mood swings and irritability associated with uncontrolled blood sugar. We even experience a decrease in libido and sexual vitality.

Unfortunately, much of Western civilization does not realize how closely the emotional, mental, and physical bodies are tied to diet. A growing number of movements—such as the vegetarian, organic, and raw foods movements—

are attempting to correct this situation. These movements combine the calls for ecological awareness and for better nutrition. Simply put, a healthy diet is better for us and better for the earth.

A simple change in diet, exchanging processed foods filled with preservatives for organic foods that are as close to their natural state as possible, can effect incredible changes in energy levels, emotional stability, mental acuity, and sexual vitality. Food is a tonic for human life. If we want to live better, feel better, and love better, we must eat better.

SEXUAL SUPERFOODS

Superfoods are unprocessed foods that pack a wide range of nutrients into a delicious healthful package. They provide a wide range of healing benefits to the human body. A superfood can be considered a sex tonic if it satisfies one or more of the following requirements.

1. It is highly nutritious and makes a significant contribution to overall health, thereby improving libido.

2. It nourishes the Liver System, which breaks down toxins and excess hormones in the body, helping maintain the immune system and hormonal balance. In traditional Oriental medicine, the Liver is responsible for sexual vigor.

3. It nourishes the Kidney System, which, according to Oriental tradition, governs sexual vitality.

4. It stimulates circulation, which moves blockages from, boosts sensitivity in, and improves the function of the sexual organs. Improved circulation also creates more warmth in the body, fueling the fires of passion.

5. It is an aphrodisiac, known to awaken feelings of sexual desire through physiological interaction or suggestive shape, color, or aroma.

The foods that follow satisfy one or more of these requirements. To reach and maintain peak sexual vigor, make them a regular part of your diet!

Fruits and Vegetables

Fruits and vegetables play a large role in the aphrodisiac pharmacopoeia. For the most part, the closer they are to their natural state, the more nutritive and aphrodisiac potency fruits and vegetables have. In fact, most fruits and vegetables are best eaten raw.

A few years ago I would have steered clients away from raw food, saying, "Cooked food is easier to digest, and raw foods will increase coldness and cool your passion." However, over the past few years, as I've gradually moved toward a vegan raw foods diet, I've found that raw foods have the opposite effect. They have improved my digestion and made me warmer, with improved circulation and heightened passion. They've filled me with incredible energy and happiness, not to mention helping me slim down and improve my body image.

The point is that raw foods have an incredible potential for supporting health and energy, generally but also specifically of a sexual nature. I now encourage clients to go raw—and you might want to try it, too.

Today, most fruits and vegetables are grown with the assistance of pesticides and herbicides, and livestock are injected with a wide range of hormones to force them to grow quickly, to achieve a larger size, and to increase their resistance to disease. Trace amounts of those pesticides, herbicides, and hormones make their way into the food on our tables, and they can cause the liver extreme stress as it works to remove these toxins from the body. Therefore, choose organic produce whenever it's available, and make sure that all meat, dairy products, and eggs you purchase derive from animals that were raised on organic feed and without the "assistance" of hormone treatments.

Apples

Apples belong to the Rose Family. As part of the Yuletide ritual, they were hung from Yule trees to symbolize the continuing fertility of the earth. They are alkaline in nature and contain high levels of fiber, vitamin A, vitamin B complex, vitamin C, phosphorus, potassium, silica, and iron. They can help lower cholesterol levels and blood pressure, stabilize blood sugar levels, promote weight loss, relieve the pain of arthritis, and counteract liver and gallbladder sluggishness. Eating apples stimulates the flow of saliva and cleans the teeth and gums, making your kisses sweet and delectable.

Other members of the Rose Family known for their sweetness, succulence, and aphrodisiac properties include apricots, cherries, peaches, and strawberries.

Artichokes

Artichokes contain cynarin, a compound that strengthens and helps regenerate the liver. They help detoxify the body and stimulate the production of bile. In the 1700s artichokes were peddled as aphrodisiacs by Parisian street vendors who would cry out, "Artichokes! Artichokes! Heats the body and the spirit. Heats the genitals!"

Asparagus

Cultivated by the ancient Arabs and Greeks as an aphrodisiac, asparagus not only has a suggestive shape but also is a genitourinary stimulant. The seventeenth-century English herbalist Nicholas Culpepper said that asparagus "stirreth up bodily lust in man and woman."

Avocados

The word *avocado* is an Anglicized version of *ahuacacuahatl,* an Aztec word meaning "testicle tree." Avocados are rich in protein, beta-carotene, vitamin B complex, vitamin E, fluorine, copper, and lecithin. An avocado has two to three times the amount of potassium found in a banana. And about 20 percent of an avocado is monounsaturated fat, which helps maintain high-density lipoprotein (HDL), or the "good" cholesterol. Avocado is a traditional remedy for erectile dysfunction and helps beautify the skin and hair.

Bananas

Bananas are rich in carbohydrates (mostly glucose and fructose), folic acid, vitamin B_6, vitamin C, potassium, and fiber. They also contain enzymes that aid in the production of sex hormones. They provide long-term energy and can improve stamina. In traditional Oriental medicine, they are considered cold and sweet, and they moisten the yin fluids of the body.

Beets

Beets have long been considered a food of beauty and energy. Aphrodite herself is said to have eaten beets to maintain her charms. Folk tradition says that two people who eat from the same beet are likely to fall in love. If only love were so simple! The French term for beets is *betterave,* which is also slang for "penis" or "man root."

Beets, being roots, are said to have a downward energy, affecting the lower organs and especially benefiting the colon, kidneys, bladder, spleen, and liver. Beets abound with beta-carotene, vitamin B complex, vitamin C, calcium, iron, phosphorus, sodium, and manganese.

Be aware that eating a lot of beets may cause your urine or stools to become red.

Berries

The sour flavor of berries is an indicator of their liver-activating potential. They encourage the metabolism of fats and thus improve circulation. Berries are also an excellent source of antioxidants.

Cabbage

Cabbage is a warming nutritive sexual tonic. It is rich in sulfur and iron and can improve circulation and, subsequently, passion.

Carrots

Carrots were highly regarded as an aphrodisiac by the ancient Greeks. Carrots help improve liver and kidney function, aid in the metabolism of calcium, lower cholesterol levels, and improve elimination.

Celery

Celery has a long history of use in aphrodisiac recipes. It contains androsterone, a hormone that is released from the human body in sweat and urine. Celery has a special affinity for the stomach, kidneys, and liver and can help neutralize acids in the body. It is rich in beta-carotene, folic acid, vitamin C, calcium, magnesium, potassium, silica, sodium, chlorophyll, and fiber. It can help counteract dry, damp conditions in the body, such as excess phlegm or yeast overgrowth. It can also be used to cool and detoxify the liver.

Cherries

Cherries have a warm, sweet energy. They are rich in beta-carotene, vitamin B_1, vitamin C, calcium, copper, iron, manganese, phosphorus, and potassium. The darker the cherry, the more rich in minerals it is.

On an esoteric level, cherries are ruled by Venus, the planet of love. In _The Magic of Food_ (Llewellyn Publications, 1995), author Scott Cunningham offers a cherry pie technique for bringing love into your life. Following his method, make the pie while visualizing love. Lightly trace a heart in the bottom of the crust before adding the cherries. Then eat one piece of pie every day while continuing to visualize love. If you have already found the one you love, you can strengthen that love by sharing a piece of pie every day.

Dark Green, Leafy Vegetables

Dark green, leafy vegetables are rich in beta-carotene, iron, protein, and chlorophyll. They help build the blood, strengthen mucous membranes, and improve energy and mood. Greens such as collards, kale, spinach, arugula, watercress—and their wild counterparts lamb's-quarter, malva, watercress, and dandelion—provide a wide range of minerals. For optimal health, eat a salad of dark greens every day.

Figs

Figs are warming and sweet in nature. They are restorative in function, improving energy levels in those who feel fatigued. They are rich in vitamin B_6, folic acid, calcium, copper, iron, magnesium, manganese, phosphorus, and potassium.

Flaxseeds

Flaxseeds are rich in omega-3 and omega-6 essential fatty acids, protein, and vitamin E. They have a high mucilage content that nourishes the body's sexual fluids. When consumed with plenty of fluids, they are also an excellent laxative. Three tablespoons of freshly ground flaxseeds eaten every day will support liver function, improve the metabolism of fats, and reduce inflammation.

In the eighth century, Charlemagne, King of the Franks, passed a law requiring his subjects to consume flaxseeds so that they would be healthier. In the twentieth century, Mahatma Ghandi said that when flaxseeds became a part of the regular diet of a people, greater health in the community would result.

Grapes

Grapes contain beta-carotene, B vitamins, vitamin C, boron, calcium, magnesium, potassium, fiber, malic acid, and citric acid. In the tradition of Oriental medicine, they are considered to be sweet, sour, neutral, and cooling.

Grapes have antibacterial, antiviral, and diuretic properties. They are considered therapeutic for the lungs, liver, kidneys, and spleen; they are also considered a tonic for the blood and for chi. They nourish the yin fluids of the body. Grape skins contain resveratrol, a compound that prevents blood platelet aggregation and elevates levels of high-density lipoprotein (HDL), which helps protect the arteries and encourages good circulation.

Mangoes

Mangoes are considered by many to be one of the planet's most delicious and fragrant fruits. As a yin tonic, they provide moistening fluids for the body and quench thirst. They are alterative and diuretic. They are rich in beta-carotene, niacin, vitamin C, flavonoids, vitamin E, iron, and potassium. They are also high in pectin, which can help lower blood cholesterol levels. Enjoy a mango in the bathtub with your beloved!

Okra

Okra is stiff and exudes a slimy fluid not unlike sexual fluids. It is a supreme nutritive vegetable for those who feel weak, exhausted, or depressed. It is rich in beta-carotene, vitamin B complex, vitamin C, calcium, iron, phosphorus, potassium, and sodium. It is also an excellent source of electrolytes, which help balance the body's fluids, and pectin, which can help lower blood cholesterol levels.

Peaches

Peaches belong to the Rose Family. In the Taoist tradition, peaches are considered to be a longevity tonic. They are rich in beta-carotene, vitamin C, calcium, boron, magnesium, phosphorus, potassium, and antioxidant flavonoids.

Persimmons

Suck the sweet orange flesh out of a perfectly ripe persimmon for a totally sensuous experience. Persimmons are sweet and cooling and help tonify the yin (moistening fluids) of the body. They are a good source of beta-carotene, vitamin C, calcium, magnesium, phosphorus, and potassium.

Plums

Like peaches and apples, plums belong to the Rose Family. In Chinese mythology, plums symbolize wisdom, longevity, and resurrection. They are rich in vitamin B_1, vitamin C, calcium, iron, phosphorus, and potassium. They are a good source of energy and are considered to be a tonic for the brain, nerves, and blood. In traditional Oriental medicine, plums are thought to help people open up emotionally.

Pomegranates

Pomegranate comes from the Latin term for "apple of many seeds." With its blood-red color, the pomegranate has long been a symbol of fertility, birth, and sexuality.

Pomegranates contain pelleterine, an alkaloid that is similar to the hallucinogen mescaline and is associated with spiritual states of consciousness. In traditional Oriental medicine, pomegranate is considered to be sweet and sour and is a yin tonic that builds the kidneys, liver, blood, and bladder. Pomegranate flesh is a rich source of vitamin C and potassium; the seeds contain phytoestrogenic compounds.

Shiitake Mushrooms

According to traditional Oriental medicine, shiitake mushrooms can make women more open to love. They are also being studied for their potential to prevent cancer.

Truffles

The underground fruiting body of a particular forest fungi, the truffle is a rare delicacy. Truffles also have a long history of use as an aphrodisiac and are especially high in minerals. Interestingly, they have been found to contain a particular phytosterol, or plant hormone, that is similar to a hormone found in boars' testicles and secreted in boars' saliva when they are in heat.

Watermelon

Watermelon is a rejuvenating blood tonic and is very alkalinizing. It is also a potent antioxidant and has anticoagulating and diuretic properties. It is a good source of beta-carotene, vitamin C, potassium, and silicon. Watermelon is a traditional remedy for strengthening the kidneys. It contains cucurbocitrin, a compound that dilates the capillaries and, thus, improves circulation. Eat the seeds as well as the flesh!

Whole Grains

Whole grains contain both the male and female energies of grasses and are universal symbols of fertility and abundance. When you plant a whole grain, it sprouts and grows into a grass plant. When you eat a whole grain, you take in that tremendous energy.

Whole grains help keep blood sugar levels stable, which, in turn, calms us. Grains that are especially beneficial for libido include barley, buckwheat, corn, millet, oats, rice (no wonder it's thrown at weddings), and wild rice.

It's been observed that, for many Americans, wheat and wheat-based products make up two-thirds of the diet. Yet wheat is one of the most common allergens. There's a large population of people with an undiagnosed wheat allergy, and eating wheat causes them to feel fatigued and congested. Rather than getting stuck in the toast, bagel, croissant, pancake, and pasta way of life, expand your horizons. There are many other wonderfully delicious grains out there.

Most people are familiar with grains as cooked food, but many can also be eaten as sprouts, used in cereals, or dehydrated into Essene breads. (Essene breads are made from sprouted grains and baked at a low temperature; see the recipe for Sprouted Herb Bread on page 53.) Grains that are sprouted are easier to digest. In addition, sprouting increases a grain's enzymatic activity and increases its vitamin C and vitamin E content.

Sugar and wheat are stressors for the liver. In excessive amounts, sugar impairs estrogen metabolism in the liver, promotes yeast overgrowth, weakens the immune system, and aggravates endometriosis. Wheat, in excessive amounts, irritates the liver and causes fluid retention. If you are working to improve the health of your liver, limit your intake of or avoid foods that contain sugar and wheat.

Beans

Beans are traditional symbols of fertility; the ancient Teutonic people considered them a symbol of sexual pleasure, perhaps because of the bean flower's striking resemblance to female genitalia. In the South, black-eyed peas and rice are eaten on New Year's Day to ensure a prosperous and fertile year.

Beans that are especially beneficial for libido include adzuki beans, garbanzo beans, and lentils. Black beans and black soybeans are potent kidney tonics.

Soybeans are an excellent food for sexual vitality, particularly for women. They are rich in phytosterols, including estrogenlike isoflavones, and can relieve many of the symptoms associated with premenstrual syndrome and menopause. They can also boost sex drive. Soy products like tofu, tempeh, and miso deliver all the benefits of soybeans.

Some individuals have trouble digesting beans. Fermentation seems to improve their digestibility and does not interfere with their nutritive potency. If you have trouble digesting beans, try fermented bean products, such as tempeh, unpasteurized miso, and unpasteurized tamari.

Sea Vegetables

Sea vegetables are rich in minerals, including calcium, iron, and iodine. They nourish the thyroid gland and the entire endocrine system, thereby supporting libido. They also help improve metabolism.

Seaweeds such as kelp, dulse, hiziki, and nori are usually available in dried form at natural food stores. These plants have been collected from the deep, mineral-rich waters of the salty seas and provide nutrients that are not often present in land vegetables.

Nuts and Seeds

Nuts and seeds contain the spark of life—the design and pattern for new life. For example, a pumpkin seed can replicate itself many times over; when planted, it sprouts and becomes an awesome vine bearing several pumpkins, each resplendent with nourishing seeds. When we eat nuts and seeds, we ingest all the nourishment and energy that is needed to sustain the new plant, as well as phytosterols, plant hormones that have a structure similar to that of human hormones.

Nuts and seeds are excellent sources of nutrients. They are rich in beta-carotene, vitamin B complex, vitamin D, vitamin E, calcium, protein, essential fatty acids, and trace minerals. They are high in fat, but fat that is beneficial. Nuts and seeds can, for example, actually help reduce levels of low-density lipoprotein (LDL), or the "bad" cholesterol. And raw nuts contain lipase, an enzyme that helps the body digest fats. Almonds, hazelnuts, hempseeds, pine nuts, pistachios, poppy seeds, walnuts, pumpkin seeds, sesame seeds, and sunflower seeds are particularly rich in zinc, which helps protect the prostate gland.

Nuts and seeds are infinitely more nutritive when raw than when roasted. Why? Returning to the pumpkin seed example above, a raw pumpkin seed contains the reproductive energy necessary to spark new life; a roasted, salted seed would not grow.

Soaking nuts and seeds overnight and rinsing them the following morning removes enzyme inhibitors, which can inhibit digestion, and softens them, enhancing their digestibility. It may also "bring them to life," as many will sprout.

Bee Products

Bees grant us wondrous superfoods for sexual vitality: honey and bee pollen.

Honey is energizing and rich in minerals. Honey mixed with ginger was recommended as an aphrodisiac by the ancient Arab physician Avicenna (980–1037). The Middle Eastern tradition also calls for honey mixed with powdered ginger and aniseed and applied to the genitals as a method for increasing virility.

Bee pollen, considered the sperm of flowers, contains 185 nutrients, including all the amino acids essential to human health. It is highly nourishing, boosts energy, enhances sexual vitality, and improves sperm production. Start by taking just a few grains, building up gradually to one teaspoon daily. However, if you have pollen allergies, take only a grain a day; taking too much can cause an allergic reaction.

Support local beekeeping companies whenever possible. They will, in general, take exceedingly great care with the health and safety of bees, which grant them income and perform vital pollinating services for our planet. We must respect bees, as we cannot live without them!

The Phenylethylamine Connection

When people are in love, their brains produce a chemical called phenylethy-lamine; this same chemical shows up during the warm glow of postcoital bliss. Strangely enough, phenylethylamine is also found in chocolate and rose water, making these two substances potent aphrodisiacs.

Chocolate was the love tonic of the Aztec emperor Montezuma (1466–1520), who reputedly drank some fifty cups daily before visiting his harem of six hundred women. During the 1800s, physicians recommended chocolate to boost libido, and to this day it is well known for its ability to inspire passion. For best effect, allow it to melt slowly and sensuously in your mouth.

When buying rose water, be sure that the packaging specifies that the rose water is distilled; otherwise, you may end up with a synthetic product. Add rose water to desserts such as fruit smoothies, rice pudding, and baklava.

Culinary Herbs

Many classic culinary herbs are considered aphrodisiacs. The herbs in the fol-lowing list have a warming, stimulating effect on the body and help improve circulation. Use lavish amounts of them in your cuisine.

- Aniseed
- Black pepper
- Cardamom
- Cayenne
- Cinnamon
- Coriander
- Cumin
- Curry (a blend of herbs)
- Fenugreek
- Garlic
- Ginger
- Nutmeg
- Paprika
- Parsley

- Rosemary

- Sage

- Turmeric

- Vanilla

Aphrodisiacs of the Sea

In general, all creatures of the sea are considered to be potent aphrodisiacs because they contain high levels of phosphorus, calcium, and iodine. Phosphorus is known to improve sex drive and responsiveness. Calcium is vital for skeletal health, calms the emotions, and promotes restful sleep. Iodine is found in high concentrations in the thyroid gland, which is important in regulating metabolism. A person with an iodine deficiency might feel listless and sluggish and have a diminished libido.

Fish

Oily fish such as anchovies, herring, mackerel, salmon, sardines, and tuna are rich in essential fatty acids, which build the body's lubrication systems. They support the health of the kidneys, which govern sexuality.

Oysters

Oysters, which resemble the female genitalia, are rich in zinc, protein, phosphorus, and selenium; they also contain high levels of mucopolysaccharides, which improve the elasticity of tissues and boost output of seminal fluids. Oysters were prized by Casanova for their seductive effect.

Eel

In traditional Japanese culture, eel is considered a supreme sexual tonic, in part because of the long, phallic shape of the fish.

Caviar

Caviar is a highly valued Russian remedy for restoring potency.

Nuoc-man

Nuoc-man is a spicy fish-based sauce served with dishes from a wide range of Asian cultures. It is rich in essential fatty acids and phosphorus. You can find it in most grocery stores.

Edible Flowers

Flowers are the sexual organs of plants; visually, aromatically, and energeti-

Factory-Farmed Fish or Wild Fish?

Factory-farmed fish are sometimes said to be good alternatives to wild fish, because we can eat them without depleting native fish populations. Many wild fish populations are now endangered due to overfishing. However, factory-farmed fish are subjected to antibiotics, fungicides, and other chemicals, and the farms where they are raised are often sources of tremendous pollution. For this reason, wild fish are considered to be more healthful than those that are factory farmed. However, many fish, whether wild or factory-farmed, are contaminated with heavy metals, and pregnant women are cautioned against eating fish in general to avoid possible heavy-metal toxins. It makes you wonder: If eating fish holds dangers for a developing fetus, what kind of danger does it hold for the rest of us? At one time fish was considered a healthy alternative to red meat, but that time is quickly passing.

cally, they are strong aphrodisiacs. To show your beloved that he or she is adored, decorate your food with organic edible flowers such as violets, rose petals (with the white heels removed), daylilies, and hibiscus. Make food a healthful, beautiful, and flavorful expression of your love.

Aphrodisiac Beverages

Most aphrodisiac beverages are alcoholic, and, while aphrodisiac in moderation, they become anaphrodisiac in excess. It's important, therefore, to remember that the purpose of an aphrodisiac beverage is to inspire passion and release inhibitions, not to cause loss of control.

Alcohol itself is an aphrodisiac. It relaxes the mind and body, releases inhibitions, and can call passion to mind. Honey wine, also known as mead, was given to ancient Teuton brides for a month after their wedding to help them feel more responsive to sexual overtures from their new husbands. (And from this practice the word *honeymoon* evolved.) Chartreuse, a yellow or green aphrodisiac liqueur, contains warming spices like allspice. Benedictine is another aphrodisiac liqueur. It's interesting to note that both Chartreuse and Benedictine were invented by monks and produced in monasteries. Liqueur de Damiana is a Mexican drink said to incite passion, and traditionally it is given to a bride on the morning of her wedding by her mother-in-law. Other traditional aphrodisiac alcohols include apricot brandy, champagne, cognac, palm wine, tequila, and vermouth.

Many imbibers would feel better if they avoided wines containing the preservative sulfite. Sulfite can cause allergic reactions, including breathing difficulty. It also increases the severity of hangovers.

Make your own love potion by tincturing (steeping in alcohol or an alcohol substitute, as described in the "Herbal Tinctures" section in Chapter 6) some of the passion-inspiring herbs given in Chapter 6. My favorites include cinnamon, cardamom, cloves, vanilla bean, nutmeg, aniseed, muira puama, damiana, rose petals, vitex berries, and ginseng root. You can tincture one herb singly or in combination with other herbs. Also try adding honey to the final tincture for a delicious, sweet liqueur.

Alcohol is not the only beverage you can use to make a toast to love. Try it with morning smoothies or fresh juice. My favorite love tonic drink these days is the juice from young coconuts. And remember, the best aphrodisiac of all is to be deeply in love. To good health and great love!

> The term *aphrodisiac* derives from the name of Aphrodite, the Greek goddess of love, fruitfulness, and beauty. An aphrodisiac is a substance that puts you in the mood for love, whether it be food, herbs, good conversation, moonlight, or even lingerie. Some aphrodisiacs have a direct stimulating effect on the erogenous zones. Some affect the mind, causing relaxation, releasing inhibitions, or inspiring passion. Others endow the user with stamina, allowing longer lovemaking sessions. Still others are simply reminiscent of sex in their shape, texture, or smell. (And according to the ancient Doctrine of Signatures, plants give us hints about their appropriate usage by the way they look, smell, taste, and grow.)
>
> Taken as a supplement, aphrodisiacs can be enjoyed thirty to sixty minutes before a lovemaking session. However, they are best put to use as an integral element of daily life, inspiring passion and sensuality throughout the day and offering the utmost of their tonifying properties.

ANAPHRODISIACS

Anaphrodisiacs are the opposite of aphrodisiacs. They decrease sexual vitality and passion. In this classification are lemonade, valerian, vinegar, tobacco, excessively refined sugars and carbohydrates, and cold showers. Icy foods, such as ice cream, cold sodas, and cold milk, can also cool your passions and cause congestion in the reproductive organs.

As Shakespeare warned in *Macbeth*, "Alcohol provoketh desire, but taketh away performance." Excessive drinking interferes with testosterone production and increases estrogen production; it decreases physical sensitivity, slows nerve functioning, and depresses the emotions. In men, prolonged excessive drinking has an adverse effect on erectile and ejaculatory functions and can even cause the male genitals to shrink. For women, it may lead to, menstrual irregularity, infertility, and the inability to orgasm.

RECIPES FOR PASSION

Food, not just mere filling for the belly, can also pleasure the soul, fuel the body, and promote good health. The ideal food for inciting passion is light, moist, sweet, easily digested, and raw. Moist foods lend their yin to sexual fluids. Naturally sweet foods, such as fruits and vegetables, provide energy and stamina. Raw foods contain enzymatic sparks of life.

Select unrefined foods that provide a wide range of colors and satisfy the senses. Make snacks an opportunity for health by eating nourishing foods. Let nuts, seeds, yogurt, fruit, and vegetables replace candy and ice cream.

RAW ASPARAGUS SOUP

It won't take long after mealtime before you'll feel the asparagus energy in this soup increasing circulation to your sex centers. These springtime shoots have long been considered potent aphrodisiacs.

½ cup raw macadamia nut,
soaked overnight, then rinsed

½ cup raw almonds,
soaked overnight, then rinsed

2 cups spring water

1 teaspoon Celtic salt

1 clove garlic, chopped

Juice of 1 lime

1 bunch asparagus (about 20 stalks),
with the tips removed and saved

6 stalks celery, chopped

4 scallions, chopped

Place the nuts, water, salt, garlic, lime juice, and stalks of asparagus in a blender and blend. Pour over the asparagus tips, celery, and scallions. Serve at room temperature.

MAKES TWO SERVINGS.

WILD THING SOUP

Want to feel more wild? Enjoy the organic harvest of freshly picked wild greens. They are far more nourishing than just about any greens you can find at the grocery store.

4 cups mixed wild greens, washed and chopped
(try dandelion, violet, nettle, malva, lamb's-quarter)

4 cups water

1 cup raw almonds,
soaked overnight, then rinsed

1 small onion, chopped

1 ripe avocado, peeled

1 clove garlic, chopped

1 teaspoon curry powder

$\frac{1}{2}$ teaspoon Celtic salt, pepper, or Nama Shoyu tamari

Combine all the ingredients in a blender or food processor and blend.

MAKES TWO GENEROUS SERVINGS.

CARROT GINGER SOUP

This bright orange, sweet, and spicy soup is incredibly easy to make.

3 cups spring water

1 cup chopped carrots

1 cup raw almonds,
soaked overnight, then rinsed

1 avocado, peeled

1 clove garlic

$\frac{1}{2}$ inch fresh ginger root

1 tablespoon Nama Shoyu tamari

A handful of cilantro, chopped

Combine all the ingredients except the cilantro in a blender and blend. Garnish with fresh chopped cilantro.

MAKES TWO SERVINGS.

SPROUTED HERB BREAD

Try this herb-inspired alternative to flour-based bread.
It is fiber rich and flavorful!

½ cup flaxseeds

2 cups sprouted whole wheat berries
(see *Sprouting Wheat* below)

3 tablespoons rosemary

3 tablespoons basil

⅛ cup chopped onion

3 cloves garlic, chopped

1 carrot, chopped

Soak the flaxseeds in water and cover for fifteen minutes. Place all ingredients in a food processor and purée. Form the dough into small, flat, round loaves. "Bake" the loaves in the hot sun or in a food dehydrator set to 100°F. When one side is dry, flip the loaves and bake the other side.

MAKES TWO LOAVES.

Sprouting Wheat

To sprout wheat, obtain a widemouthed glass jar with a sprouting lid (available in most natural food stores). Place 1 cup of wheat berries and 2 cups of water in the jar, and let steep overnight. In the morning, pour off the water (I usually give it to my houseplants). Rinse the berries and place them back in the jar. Rinse them again later that same day and twice more the next day (that's four rinsings total). By this time the berries should have "come to life," sprouting tails as long as the berries themselves.

FLAVORED HONEY

Use this herbal honey in salad dressings and to flavor tea. My favorite essential oils are rose, neroli, rose geranium, peppermint, and jasmine.

2 drops essential oil

¼ cup honey

Mix the essential oil into the honey.

MAKES ¼ CUP.

LOVE TONIC SMOOTHIE

Start your day with a toast to love. This smoothie is a real energy booster. It is rich in calcium and offers just a hint of rose to open your heart to love.

1 cup plain yogurt
(vegans can use almond
or sunflower yogurt)

1 peeled ripe mango

½ ripe banana

1 teaspoon honey

1 teaspoon rose water

½ teaspoon bee pollen

¼ teaspoon cardamom powder

Combine all the ingredients in a blender. Blend and enjoy.

MAKES TWO SERVINGS.

ALMOND MILK

Dairy products are a common allergen, and almond milk is a good substitute for cow's milk. The almond milk you find in stores has been pasteurized, destroying their vital nutrients. It takes only a few minutes to make your own.

1 cup raw almonds,
soaked overnight, then rinsed

4 cups water

2 dates

½ teaspoon vanilla extract

Combine all the ingredients in a blender and blend. Strain through a cheesecloth, squeezing out the "milk." This milk will keep for four days in the refrigerator.

MAKES 1 QUART.

DRIED FRUIT SOAK

This fruity mix can be enjoyed as a power breakfast.
It has the consistency of chunky porridge but is packed with colors,
flavors, and nutrients, particularly vitamin E and zinc.

1/8 cup raw almonds

1/8 cup dried unsulfured apricots

1/8 cup chopped figs

1/8 cup raw pumpkin seeds

1/8 cup black sesame seeds

1/8 cup sunflower seeds

1 cup spring water

Combine all the ingredients in a bowl and cover with water. Soak overnight. Enjoy the next morning.

MAKES ONE SERVING.

MARVELOUS MUESLI

Why start your day with a meal that makes you feel tired and polluted?
Muesli is a traditional European breakfast fare. It is satisfying
to the palate and packed with nutrients.

2 cups rolled oats

1 cup raw sunflower seeds

1/2 cup dried unsulfured apricots,
pitted and chopped

1/2 cup raw pumpkin seeds

1/2 cup unsulfured raisins

Combine the ingredients and store in a jar in the refrigerator. For a truly nutritious breakfast, mix 1/2 cup of muesli with 1/2 cup of yogurt, and add slices of half a banana or half an apple.

MAKES ABOUT 4 1/2 CUPS.

LOVER'S SALAD

*Get creative! There are plenty of alternatives to plain lettuce salad,
including this colorful and crunchy mixture.*

½ cup grated beets

½ cup chopped fennel leaves and bulb

¼ cup raw sunflower seeds

A handful of violet or pansy blossoms

A handful of organic rose petals,
with the white heels removed

Combine all the ingredients and serve.

MAKES TWO SERVINGS.

MISO TAHINI SALAD DRESSING

*Most bottled salad dressings contain hard-to-digest heated oils.
Enhance the dance of love with this dressing, which is filled
with "healthy" oils and can be enjoyed without guilt.*

½ cup spring water

3 tablespoons raw tahini

1 tablespoon unpasteurized miso

1 clove garlic, chopped

Juice of two limes or lemons

½ inch fresh ginger root

Combine all the ingredients in a blender. Blend, then place in a glass
jar, seal, and store in the refrigerator.

MAKES ¾ CUP.

CARROT SALAD

*Stimulate your sexual root chakras with raw roots.
Connect to orange energy and feel your passion rise!*

8 carrots, grated

6 tablespoons extra-virgin olive oil

4 tablespoons raw pumpkin seeds

2 tablespoons lemon juice

Combine all the ingredients. Let sit for thirty minutes before serving.

MAKES FOUR SERVINGS.

GUACAMOLE

Share a dip together, not in a pool but in a luscious bowl of spicy guacamole. Serve with raw vegetable slices, chips, or crackers, or use as a sandwich spread.

2 large ripe avocados, peeled

2 tablespoons lemon or lime juice

2 medium tomatoes, chopped fine

$\frac{1}{2}$ cup finely chopped onion

$\frac{1}{2}$ teaspoon salt

$\frac{1}{4}$ cup chopped pine nuts

$1\frac{1}{2}$ teaspoons fresh cilantro leaves

Mash the avocado with a fork. Add the lemon or lime juice, tomato, onion, salt, nuts, and cilantro.

MAKES ABOUT 2 CUPS.

PASSION PESTO

Pesto can be presto-quick. This delicious mix offers the health benefits of garlic, raw nuts, and herbs. Use it as a dip or a spread. I like to warm it and serve it over fresh zucchini that has been cut into spaghetti-like strips.

3 cups fresh basil leaves

1 cup extra-virgin olive oil

3/4 cup chopped fresh parsley

$\frac{1}{2}$ cup pine nuts

5 cloves garlic

1 teaspoon salt

Combine all the ingredients in a blender and purée.

MAKES FOUR TO SIX SERVINGS.

LOVE BALLS

End your meal with a dessert that tastes decadent
but is really heaven-sent.

1 cup tahini

½ cup honey

½ cup raw pumpkin seeds

2 tablespoons chocolate powder

1 teaspoon powdered ginseng

1 teaspoon vanilla extract

½ teaspoon cinnamon

½ teaspoon powdered cardamom

1 tablespoon chopped mint leaves

Sesame seeds or grated coconut

Combine all the ingredients except the sesame seeds or coconut and roll into small balls. Roll the balls in the sesame seeds or coconut until they are coated. Chill before serving.

MAKES ABOUT THIRTY BALLS.

FRUIT DESSERT

We know that eating more fruits and vegetables is the key
to better health and, yes, better sex. Why wait?

¼ cup each dried unsulfured figs,
Turkish apricots, and peaches
(soaked overnight in spring water)

1 teaspoon rose water

¼ teaspoon cinnamon powder

¼ teaspoon grated ginger

¼ teaspoon grated organic orange rind

Edible flowers, such as rose petals
(with the white heels removed) or tulip petals

Combine all the ingredients, using the flower petals as garnish.

MAKES TWO SERVINGS.

BANANA MANGO PUDDING

This creamy dish is sweet and sensuous. Enjoy a dessert
that makes you feel both beautiful and healthy.

4 ripe bananas

4 dates, pitted

2 ripe mangoes

½ cup pine nuts, soaked overnight, then rinsed

Sliced strawberries

Combine all the ingredients except the strawberries in a blender or food processor and blend. Garnish with slices of strawberries.

MAKES FOUR SERVINGS.

TANTALIZING TRAIL MIX

This mix is a good companion when you're hiking,
traveling, or even as an anytime snack.

1 cup raw pumpkin seeds

1 cup raw almonds

1 cup raw sunflower seeds

1 cup raisins

½ cup chopped unsulfured Turkish apricots

2 tablespoons bee pollen

Combine the ingredients.

MAKES 4½ CUPS.

STUFFED DATES

Simple and sweet, this treat has taken the place of chocolate in my life.

Dates

Raw almond butter

Raspberries

Cut the dates lengthwise and remove the seeds. Stuff with raw almond butter, and top with a raspberry.

5

Nutritional Supplements: Balancing and Rebuilding Sexual Health

he primary source of nutrition should always be a healthy diet. A balanced, varied range of organic, unprocessed, preferably raw food served up for breakfast, lunch, dinner, and all the snacks in between should supply adequate vitamins, minerals, and nutrients for a healthy body, a sound mind, and an ardent sexual appetite. If we all ate this way, we would have little use for supplements.

That said, there are situations in which diet is not adequate to supply the nutrients an individual needs, and supplements become necessary. For example, the high levels of progesterone in birth control pills can decrease a woman's clitoral sensitivity and increase her need for B vitamins, vitamin C, and zinc. A woman taking birth control pills might also want to take a daily multivitamin and mineral supplement and dine daily on one of the passion-inspiring recipes given in Chapter 4.

There are several nutrients that have a direct effect on sexual vitality and may be added as supplements to the diet when necessary. Food is always the first choice as a supplement, but these nutrients are also available in pill form. If you intend to take these supplements in pill form, look for ones that are free of artificial dyes and preservatives, and consult with your health care provider or a nutrition advisor before beginning the supplement regimen. Pills allow the user to pack in an incredible amount of a nutrient, and, as with just about everything, excess can be detrimental to your health. Your health care provider or a nutrition advisor will be able to give you guidelines for establishing a safe, healthy supplement program.

ARGININE

Action: Arginine, an amino acid, is a precursor to nitric oxide, a compound that is responsible for vasodilation and, thus, plays a role in blood flow to the genitals and increases arousal. Arginine appears to stimulate the release of growth hormone from the pituitary gland. It also relaxes smooth muscle contractions in the arteries of the penis, resulting in stronger erections.

Use: Arginine can improve libido in both sexes and strengthen erections in men. Applied topically in a cream, it can be used to intensify orgasms.

Recommended dosage: 1,000–2,000 mg twice daily, taken with food.

Caution: Those carrying the herpesvirus or suffering from diabetes should avoid taking arginine as a supplement, except under the supervision of a health care professional.

Natural sources: Chocolate, coconut, eggplants, nuts, oats, tomatoes, and wheat.

BETA-CAROTENE (VITAMIN A)

Action: Beta-carotene is a precursor to vitamin A The body converts beta-carotene to vitamin A, which is necessary for the production of sex hormones. It strengthens mucous membranes, prevents atrophy of the genitals, and can help increase sperm levels.

Use: Supplementation with beta-carotene can counteract vaginal dryness and thinning of the vaginal walls in postmenopausal women and improve sperm count in men.

Recommended dosage: 25,000–50,000 IU of beta-carotene daily.

Natural sources: Apricots, beet greens, broccoli, cabbage, cantaloupes, carrots, dandelion greens, grapefruit, green, leafy vegetables, green peppers, kale, lamb's-quarter, mangoes, mustard greens, nori, oranges, papaya, parsley, persimmons, peppers, pumpkin, romaine lettuce, spinach, sweet potatoes, Swiss chard, tomatoes, watermelon, winter squash, yam, and yellow squash.

B-COMPLEX VITAMINS

Action: Taken as a whole, the B-complex vitamins support the production of hormones in both men and women.

Use: Both men and women who suffer from inadequate hormone levels may benefit from supplementation with B-complex vitamins.

Recommended dosage: 50–300 mg daily.

Natural sources: Beans, brown rice, eggs, green, leafy vegetables, poultry, nutritional yeast, wheat germ, and whole grains.

CALCIUM

Action: Calcium is vital for the health of bones and teeth. It also calms the emotions and supports good sleep.

Use: Ingested in adequate amounts throughout adolescence and the menstrual years, calcium can prevent many of the concerns associated with menopause, most notably osteoporosis. It also may relieve cramping associated with dysmenorrhea and some symptoms of premenstrual syndrome.

Recommended dosage: 1,000–1,500 mg daily.

Natural sources: Almonds, beans (black, garbanzo, pinto, soy, and white), blackstrap molasses, Brazil nuts, broccoli, carob powder, clams, collards, dairy products, dandelion greens, egg, figs, flounder, green, leafy vegetables, hazelnuts, kombu, lentils, milk, miso, oats, oyster, peanuts, salmon, sardines, scallops, seaweeds, sesame seeds, shrimp, sunflower seeds, tofu, and turnip greens.

CHOLINE

Action: Choline, another B-complex vitamin, aids in the production of the neurotransmitter acetylcholine, which relays nerve messages between the brain and the sexual organs and can intensify orgasms. Choline can help improve mood and memory and enhance the brain's perception of pleasure.

Use: Those who have trouble achieving orgasm or who feel particularly tense or anxious about sex may benefit from supplementation of choline.

Recommended dosage: 25–500 mg daily.

Natural sources: Avocados, beans (especially garbanzo beans, lentils, split peas, and soybeans), beef liver, cabbage, cauliflower, corn, eggs, fish (particularly salmon), green beans, milk, nutritional yeast, oats, peanuts, potatoes, rice, soybeans, and wheat germ.

DIMETHYLGLYCINE

Action: Dimethylglycine (DMG) can boost energy, support endurance, improve libido, and benefit the entire urogenital system.

Use: Dimethylglycine can be used to treat vaginal dryness, cryptorchidism, and low libido.

Recommended dosage: 250 mg daily.

Natural sources: Nutritional yeast, pumpkin seeds, rice bran, sunflower seeds, and whole grains.

ESSENTIAL FATTY ACIDS

Action: Essential fatty acids (EFAs) are needed for proper hormone function; they also help promote soft skin and vaginal moisture. Low levels of EFAs can cause women to experience more cramping and men to lack sufficient ejaculate.

Use: Supplementation with EFAs may counteract vaginal dryness and cramping and improve ejaculate production.

Recommended dosage: If you're taking an EFA supplement, follow the dosage guidelines on the package label.

Natural sources: Cod liver oil, corn oil, fish (particularly eel, mackerel, and salmon), flaxseeds, hempseeds, peanut oil, purslane, safflower oil, sesame seeds, soybean oil, sunflower seeds, walnuts, and wheat germ.

GAMMA-LINOLENIC ACID

Action: Gamma-linolenic acid (GLA) is an essential fatty acid that invigorates the sexual organs and normalizes hormonal output.

Use: GLA has been found useful in treating low libido, erectile dysfunction, inability to orgasm, and premature ejaculation.

Recommended dosage: If you're taking a GLA supplement, follow the dosage guidelines on the package label.

Natural sources: Barley, black currant seed oil, borage seed oil, evening primrose oil, hempseeds, oats, and spirulina.

IRON

Action: Iron transports oxygen throughout the body; low levels can manifest as lack of energy and low libido. Iron is needed for production of hemoglobin. Vitamin C aids the absorption of iron; therefore, a vitamin C deficiency can lead to an iron deficiency.

Use: Supplementation with iron may benefit those with low energy or libido, as well as those who have been diagnosed as iron deficient.

Recommended dosage: 10–25 mg daily for men; 18–30 mg for women. Take only if needed.

Natural sources: Apricots, beans (particularly black beans, garbanzo beans, lentils, lima beans, navy beans, pinto beans, soybeans, and split peas), beef, beef liver, blackstrap molasses, bran, carrots, chicken (dark meat), chicken liver, dandelion greens, eggs, fish, green, leafy vegetables, green peppers, Jerusalem artichokes, kidneys, millet, miso, nori, oatmeal, oysters, parsley, persimmons, prunes, pumpkin seeds, raisins, seaweeds (dulse, hiziki, kelp, kombu), sesame seeds, shellfish, spinach, squash, sunflower seeds, turkey (dark meat), venison, watercress, and wheat bran.

Caution: Excessive levels of iron can cause constipation and may increase the risk of heart attack.

MAGNESIUM

Action: Magnesium helps prevent many of the health concerns associated with menopause. Magnesium is needed for the production of sex hormones and may be helpful in treating prostate problems. It is also a muscle relaxant and plays an important role in skeletal, muscle, and nerve function.

Use: Supplement with magnesium in cases of muscle spasms, cramps, and premenstrual syndrome, especially when PMS is accompanied by mood swings.

Recommended dosage: 500–750 mg daily.

Natural sources: Almonds, apricots, artichokes, avocados, bananas, barley, beans (especially black-eyed peas, kidney beans, lentils, lima beans, split peas, and soybeans), beef, beet greens, blackstrap molasses, bran, Brazil nuts, brown rice, buckwheat, carrots, cashews, celery, chard, cheese, chocolate, corn, crabs, dandelion greens, dates, dulse, figs, fish (particularly flounder, halibut, salmon, sole, and tuna), green, leafy vegetables, kelp, milk, millet, oatmeal, oranges, peas, peaches, peanuts, pecans, peppers, pine nuts, pork, potatoes, prunes, quinoa, rye, seaweeds, seeds (especially pumpkin, sesame, sunflower), shrimp, spinach, soybeans, squash, tofu, tomatoes, triticale, walnuts, watermelon, wheat, wheat germ, whole grains, and wild rice.

NIACIN (VITAMIN B$_3$)

Action: Niacin, also known as vitamin B$_3$, is one of the B-complex vitamins. It stimulates histamine release, which increases mucous membrane secretions, enables orgasm, and causes that "flush" or glow that occurs on the face, neck, and chest when arousal is high. Niacin also improves circulation and tactile sensations.

Use: Niacin can be used to correct erectile dysfunction and help women be more orgasmic.

Recommended dosage: 25–300 mg daily. For a "niacin rush," which can make a sexual encounter feel hot and intense, take 100 mg about fifteen minutes before getting started.

Natural sources: Avocados, barley, beans, bee pollen, beef, broccoli, chicken, clam, fish (particularly anchovies, haddock, halibut, mackerel, salmon, swordfish), kidneys, liver, mushrooms, nutritional yeast, oysters, peanuts, pork, potatoes, raspberries, rice, sesame and sunflower seeds, soybean, squash, strawberries, tempeh, tomatoes, tuna, turkey, watermelons, wheat, wheat germ, and whole grains.

Caution: Large doses of niacin can contribute to acid indigestion.

PANTOTHENIC ACID (VITAMIN B$_5$)

Action: Pantothenic acid, also known as vitamin B$_5$, is needed for hormonal function.

Use: People with hormonal deficiencies may benefit from supplementation with B$_5$, but note that it is part of the vitamin B complex.

Recommended dosage: 25–500 mg daily.

Natural sources: Anchovies, asparagus, avocados, beans (especially lentils and soybeans), bee pollen, beef, broccoli, buckwheat, cabbage, chicken, chicken liver, clams, corn, cottage cheese, crabs, eggs, fish (particularly flounder, haddock, herring, mackerel, salmon, sardines, and trout), flaxseeds, greens, liver, lobster, meat, milk, nutritional yeast, nuts (cashews, hazelnuts, peanuts, pecans), papaya, peas, pineapples, potatoes, royal jelly, sesame seeds, shiitake mushrooms, sunflower seeds, watermelons, wheat germ, whole grains, yams, and yogurt.

PYRIDOXINE (VITAMIN B$_6$)

Action: Pyridoxine, usually known as vitamin B$_6$, is another B-complex vitamin. It helps convert the amino acid histidine into histamine and plays a vital role in the production of ejaculate and testosterone. A B$_6$ deficiency is often associated with low libido.

Use: Supplementation with B$_6$ can facilitate orgasmic ability in women and boost libido.

Recommended dosage: 25–300 mg daily.

Natural sources: Apples, asparagus, avocados, bananas, barley, beans (particularly garbanzo beans, lentils, lima beans, navy beans, and soybeans), bee pollen, blueberries, brown rice, buckwheat, carrots, cheese, corn, crabs, eggs, fish (particularly cod, halibut, herring, mackerel, salmon, sardines, trout, tuna), flax, hazelnuts, kale, lettuce, mangoes, milk, molasses, nuts (particularly Brazil nuts, chestnuts, peanuts, and walnuts), nutritional yeast, onions, oranges, organ meats, peas, potatoes, poultry meat, prunes, sesame and sunflower seeds, spinach, squash, sweet potatoes, tomatoes, watermelons, wheat bran, and wheat germ.

SELENIUM

Action: The antioxidant selenium is concentrated in the testes and believed necessary for sperm production. It works synergistically with vitamin E. Selenium is best obtained from food or in the form of selenomethionine, a compound derived from selenium-rich sea vegetables.

Use: Selenium supplements may be helpful in cases of muscle weakness, lack of mental alertness, and depression.

Recommended dosage: 50–400 micrograms daily.

Natural sources: Barley, beef (particularly kidney and liver), beets, black-eyed peas, blackstrap molasses, Brazil nuts, broccoli, cabbage, carrots, cashews, celery, cheese, chicken liver, cod, eggs, fish, garlic, green, leafy vegetables, honey, kelp, lentils, lobster, meat, milk, mushrooms, nutritional yeast, onions, oysters, peanuts, poultry, rice (brown), salmon, scallops, seaweeds, shrimp, soybeans, spinach, sprouts, squash, sunflower seeds, tomatoes, tuna, wheat, whole grains, and yogurt.

SUPEROXIDE DISMUTASE

Action: Superoxide dismutase is an antioxidant enzyme that increases libido, supports sexual stamina, and prevents premature aging.

Use: Supplementation with superoxide dismutase can counteract low libido.

Recommended dosage: 100 IU daily.

Natural sources: Barley grass, broccoli, Brussels sprouts, green, leafy vegetables, nutritional yeast, and wheat grass.

VITAMIN C

Action: Vitamin C strengthens the body, clears heat, nourishes the adrenal glands, and supports collagen activity so that the skin remains elastic and supple. It is also an excellent antioxidant. Look for a vitamin C supplement that also includes bioflavonoids, which have a chemical activity similar to that of estrogen.

Use: Supplementation with vitamin C can reduce excessive bleeding during menstruation, normalize menstrual cycles, relieve hot flashes, increase vaginal lubrication, and counteract phimosis.

Recommended dosage: 1,000 mg of vitamin C with 500 mg of bioflavonoids daily.

Natural sources: Avocados, Brussels sprouts, cabbage, cauliflower, collard greens, cantaloupes, grapefruits, kale, mangoes, oranges, papaya, red peppers, rose hips, spinach, strawberries, and tomatoes.

VITAMIN E

Action: Vitamin E, a natural antioxidant, is sometimes referred to as "the sex vitamin." It stimulates vasodilation and improves blood flow to all parts of the body, including the sexual organs, thereby aiding in erection and orgasm. Vitamin E supports the production of sex hormones, increases stamina, boosts fertility, and nourishes the pituitary gland. It also eases the symptoms of hot flashes, limits or slows the thinning of vaginal walls, reverses or improves cases of vaginal dryness, helps improve sperm count, and counteracts loss of libido.

Use: Women who suffer from hot flashes, thin vaginal walls, vaginal dryness, and difficulty achieving orgasm may benefit from supplementation with vitamin E, as may men who suffer from erectile dysfunction and low sperm count. Vitamin E can also be helpful for both men and women with low libido, hormone deficiencies, and fertility problems.

Recommended dosage: 100–1,200 IU daily.

Natural sources: Almonds, asparagus, beet greens, blackberries, brown rice, dandelion greens, dark green, leafy vegetables, eggs, hazelnuts, kale, leeks, lettuce, liver, lobster, milk, nuts, oats, parsley, peanuts, purslane, quinoa, safflower oil, salmon, spinach, sprouted grains, sunflower seeds, sweet potatoes, tomatoes, tuna, vegetable oils, walnut oil, wheat germ, and whole grains.

ZINC

Action: Zinc stimulates the thymus gland to manufacture thymosin, which aids in the production of sex hormones and neurotransmitters. Zinc is needed for normal genital development, vaginal lubrication, and sperm count and motility. Be aware that zinc levels decline with age, and that coffee, alcohol, and smoking deplete the body of zinc.

Use: Supplement with zinc to counteract low libido, prostatitis, erectile dysfunction, vaginal dryness, and low sperm count.

Recommended dosage: 22.5–50 mg daily.

Natural sources: Adzuki beans, almonds, beans, bee pollen, Brazil nuts, brown rice, buckwheat, cashews, cheese (particularly Swiss), corn, crabs, eggs, garlic, green, leafy vegetables, herring, kelp, lobster, maple syrup, milk, mushrooms, mussels, nutritional yeast, oatmeal, oysters, peanuts, peas, potatoes, poultry, pumpkin seeds, rice bran, rye, sesame seeds, sunflower seeds, tuna, walnuts, wheat bran, wheat germ, and whole grains.

Herbs: Natural Sexual Vitality

erbs offer a safe, natural way to nourish the body and boost sexual vitality. They are multifaceted, multidirectional, and multidimensional. A single herb can have many beneficial effects, some immediate, some long-range, some physical, some emotional. Herbs can be directly heal- ing, while they can also support the body's own healing mechanisms. For thousands of years, millions of people have used herbs to improve health. That, in part, includes building sexual vigor, treating sexual dysfunction, and nourishing reproductive health.

Herbs aren't like aspirin. They aren't always packaged up in neat little standardized pills. They have wide-ranging effects, and they affect different people differently. They also tend to have a progressive effect; they work best when taken at an appropriate dosage over an appropriate length of time. So before using any herb as a health supplement, it's a good idea to educate yourself about it. Look it up in at least three herbal health books, and compare the descriptions. Consider consulting with an herbalist. Most important, if you are taking any medications—prescription or over-the-counter—consult with your health care provider before beginning a program of herbal supplements. Herbs and drugs can interact strangely, possibly leading to a serious health risk.

Herbs can be prepared as teas, tinctures, and capsules. These prepara- tions are easy to make at home. You can also find many premixed formula- tions at natural food stores and herb shops. Whether you make your own formulations or purchase commercial mixes, these time-tested botanicals are sure to spice up your love life!

HERBAL TEAS

Teas are soothing and warming. They can stimulate your senses, nourish your body, refresh your mind, and revitalize your energy. Having a cup of tea makes you take time out of a busy day to sip, savor, and reflect.

To make a tea from leaves and flowers, you must prepare an *infusion*. Bring 1 cup of water to a boil in a nonaluminum pot. Remove from heat and add 1 heaping teaspoon of dried herb or 2 heaping teaspoons of fresh herb. Cover and let steep at least ten minutes. Strain.

To make a tea from roots and barks, you must prepare a *decoction*. (One caveat: A root that is particularly high in volatile oils, such as ginger, is best infused rather than decocted.) Combine 1 heaping teaspoon of dried herb or 2 heaping teaspoons of fresh herb with 1 cup of water. Bring to a boil, reduce heat, and simmer, covered, for twenty minutes. Strain.

If you want to make a tea from a combination of herbs that must be infused and herbs that must be decocted, prepare the herbs that must be decocted first. When they have simmered for twenty minutes, remove the pot from the stovetop and strain. Then pour the hot water over the herbs that must be infused. Cover and let steep for at least ten minutes, then strain.

Return the spent herbs to the earth by adding them to your compost pile.

HERBAL TINCTURES

Tinctures are alcohol-based herbal extracts. Tinctures are made by steeping herbs in alcohol, which extracts the water-soluble and alcohol-soluble elements from them. As a result, the alcohol is imbued with the healing properties of the herbs. The alcohol must be at least 50 proof to activate the extraction process and to serve as a preservative. Most herbalists use vodka or brandy; vodka is the purest grain alcohol, and brandy has a sweetness that balances the flavor of some of the lesser-palatable herbs. The substance used to extract the herbs is known as the *menstruum*. The herbs being tinctured are known as the *mark*.

Tinctures are easy to use; just put a dropperful in a bit of warm water and drink. You can buy herbal tinctures at any herb shop or natural food store; however, they're also easy to make at home, using the following method.

Chop or grind the herbs. Place them in a glass jar, then fill the jar with brandy or vodka so that the alcohol rises to an inch above the herbs. Screw the cover on tightly, and place in a cool, dark location. Shake daily. After a month, strain the herbs from the menstruum, first through a strainer and then through a clean, undyed cloth. Squeeze the cloth tightly to force out the last few drops of precious liquid. Put the tincture in glass bottles—dark glass is preferable, as it protects the tincture from the deactivating effects of light. Label and date the bottles, and store away from heat and light. Stored properly, these alcohol-based tinctures will keep for many years.

Tinctures can also be made using vegetable glycerin rather than alcohol. Glycerin-based tinctures, known as glycerites, are excellent for those who are alcohol intolerant as well as for children, pregnant women, and nursing mothers. Glycerin is both a solvent and a preservative, with an effectiveness somewhere between that of water and alcohol. It is naturally sweet, slightly antiseptic, demulcent, and healing. Glycerites are prepared just like tinctures, but instead of alcohol, use a menstruum of one part water to two parts glycerin. A glycerite's shelf life is one to three years.

Apple cider vinegar—preferably organic—is another alternative menstruum for tincturing. It is also a digestive tonic and can be used to season food. For maximum potency, warm the vinegar before pouring it over the herbs. Do not use a metal lid to seal the container; contact with vinegar causes metal to rust, which will contaminate the tincture. A vinegar-based tincture will have a shelf life of six months to two years. Look for a vinegar that is 5.7 percent acetic acid (or thereabouts) for a longer shelf life. Discard a tincture if it smells strange or contains mold.

> The day of the new moon is traditionally considered the best time to start a new batch of tincture. The energy of the moon is thought to draw out the properties of the herbs.

HERB CAPSULES

To make herb capsules, simply grind small amounts of dried herbs to a powder in a grinder. (Some dried herbs, such as saw palmetto berries, are very hard and will likely destroy a grinder. If that seems like it would be the case with an herb you're considering, forget about making your own capsules and purchase ready-made ones.)

You can purchase empty capsules at natural food stores and herb shops. Look for the size "00" capsules. Pull apart each capsule, scoop herbs into it, and press the two capsule halves together again. Store in a sealed glass jar away from heat and light. And don't forget to label the jar, so that you'll remember what's in it.

AN HERBAL COMPENDIUM

Every culture has a set of herbal favorites that nourish sexuality. Here's a compilation of herbs from around the world that have served humanity pleasurably in both ancient and modern love potions.

Anise

Pimpinella anisum

Family: Apiaceae.

Part used: Seed.

Also known as: Huei-hsiang, saunf.

Properties: Aphrodisiac, aromatic, tonic.

Use: In Oriental tradition, anise warms the kidneys. Historically, the seed was baked into wedding cakes to stimulate wedding night vigor.

Energetics: Sweet, pungent, warm.

Dosage: 1 cup of tea or 40–60 drops of tincture three times daily.

Concerns: Avoid therapeutic doses during pregnancy except under the supervision of a health care professional.

Ashwagandha

Withania somnifera

Family: Solanaceae.

Part used: Root.

Also known as: Indian ginseng, winter cherry.

Properties: Anabolic, aphrodisiac, hormonal regulator, nutritive, rejuvenative, restorative.

Use: Ashwagandha relaxes blood vessels and promotes an overall feeling of well-being. It enhances libido, boosts fertility, and strengthens the adrenal glands. It is often used to treat nervous exhaustion, debility, involuntary semen emission without orgasm, and sexual dysfunctions associated with stress. It also counteracts diseases associated with aging.

Energetics: Bitter, sweet, warm.

Dosage: 1 cup of tea or 30–40 drops of tincture three times daily.

Concerns: Avoid during pregnancy. It may increase the potency of barbiturates; if you are taking barbiturates, consult with your health care provider before taking ashwagandha.

Asparagus

Asparagus officinalis, A. cochinchinensis

Family: Liliaceae.

Part used: Root.

Also known as: Tian men dong, shatavari.

Properties: Aphrodisiac, cardiotonic, kidney tonic, rejuvenative, reproductive tonic.

Use: Asparagus increases orgasmic ability, boosts sperm count, and nourishes the ovum. It is often used to treat erectile dysfunction, and it is excellent for women who have had hysterectomies. On the emotional side, asparagus fosters deep feelings of love and compassion.

Energetics: Cool, bitter, sweet, moist.

Dosage: 1 cup of tea or 30–40 drops of tincture three times daily.

Concerns: Safe when used appropriately.

Asafoetida

Ferula foetida, F. assa-foetida, F. rubricaulis

Family: Apiaceae.

Part used: Resin.

Also known as: Hing.

Properties: Antiseptic, hypotensive, sedative.

Use: In Tibetan medicine, asafoetida is considered one of the best aphrodisiacs. It releases and moves stagnation in the body's chi pathways.

Energetics: Pungent, bitter, hot, dry.

Dosage: 1 cup of tea or 1 to 2 "00" capsules three times daily.

Concerns: Do not give to children under the age of two. In rare cases, it may cause diarrhea. Avoid therapeutic doses during pregnancy and in cases of ulcers.

Atractylodes

Atractylodes lancea, A. macrocephala

Family: Asteraceae.

Part used: Rhizome.

Also known as: Bai zhu.

Properties: Chi tonic, restorative.

Use: This traditionally Oriental herb boosts energy levels. It is warming in nature, helping to dry damp conditions in the body.

Energetics: Bitter, sweet, warm.

Dosage: ½ cup of tea or 20 drops of tincture three times daily.

Concerns: Avoid in cases of bleeding ulcers or dehydration.

Basil

Ocimum basilicum

Family: Lamiaceae.

Part used: Herb.

Also known as: Sweet basil, lui le, tulsi.

Properties: Antidepressant, circulatory stimulant.

Use: Basil was once used by Italian women as an aphrodisiac and love charm. It is energizing and improves circulation.

Energetics: Pungent, warm, dry.

Dosage: 1 cup of tea or 10–30 drops of tincture three times daily.

Concerns: Do not take therapeutic doses for extended periods. Pregnant women and young children should not ingest therapeutic doses.

Black Pepper

Piper nigrum

Family: Piperaceae.

Parts used: Peppercorn, unripe fruit.

Also known as: Hu jiao, marich.

Properties: Aromatic, circulatory stimulant, rubefacient, stimulant.

Use: Black pepper warms the genitourinary tract and stimulates sexual impulses.

Energetics: Pungent, hot.

Dosage: ½ cup of tea or 20 drops of tincture three times daily.

Concerns: Safe when used appropriately. Men who experience premature ejaculation should avoid black pepper.

Burdock

Arctium lappa

Family: Asteraceae.

Parts used: Root, seed.

Also known as: Wu shih (root), ni ban zi (seed).

Properties: Adrenal tonic, aphrodisiac, nutritive, rejuvenative.

Use: In Chinese and Hawaiian cultures, burdock is considered an aphrodisiac. It helps one feel grounded in the body.

Energetics: Bitter, cool, dry.

Dosage: 1 cup of tea or 10–30 drops of tincture three times daily.

Concerns: Safe when used appropriately. Avoid the seeds during the first trimester of pregnancy.

Caraway

Carum carvi

Family: Apiaceae.

Part used: Seed.

Also known as: Yuan-sui.

Properties: Aromatic, mild stimulant.

Use: Caraway is often recommended in Oriental sex manuals. It sweetens the breath and relaxes the uterus. According to tradition, if chewed and added to a lover's food, it will keep the lover faithful.

Energetics: Pungent, warm.

Dosage: ½ cup of tea or 20–50 drops of tincture three times daily.

Concerns: Safe when used appropriately.

Cardamom

Elettaria cardamomum

Family: Zingiberaceae.

Part used: Seed.

Also known as: Grains of paradise, bai dou kou, ela.

Properties: Aphrodisiac, aromatic, cerebral stimulant, tonic.

Use: Cardamom relieves chi deficiency, depression, and spermatorrhea (the involuntary emission of sperm, without orgasm). It can be used to promote erotic vigor.

Energetics: Pungent, bitter, sweet, warm, dry.

Dosage: 1 cup of tea or 10–20 drops of tincture three times daily.

Concerns: Safe when used appropriately. Men who experience premature ejaculation should avoid cardamom.

Catuaba

Erythroxylum catuaba

Family: Erythroxylaceae.

Part used: Bark.

Also known as: Chuchuhuasha, tatuaba, pau de reposta.

Properties: Antiseptic, antiviral, aphrodisiac, brain tonic, central nervous system stimulant, tonic.

Use: The Minas people of South America have a saying that reveals the nature of catuaba: "Until a father reaches sixty, the son is his; after that, the son is catuaba's." This South American herb enhances sexual desire, generally by decreasing stress. It is used to treat erectile dysfunction and low libido.

Dosage: 1 cup of tea or 10–20 drops of tincture three times daily.

Concerns: Safe when used appropriately. Though it is in the same family as coca (from which cocaine is derived), catuaba does not contain cocaine alkaloids.

Cinnamon

Cinnamomum cassia, C. verum

Family: Lauraceae.

Part used: Inner bark.

Also known as: Cassia, rou gui, tvak.

Properties: Aphrodisiac, mild stimulant.

Use: Cinnamon is a sexual tonic that has been used in love potions since medieval times. It improves circulation. In Oriental tradition, it also warms and tonifies the kidneys.

Energetics: Sweet, pungent, hot, dry.

Dosage: 1 cup of tea or 30–50 drops of tincture three times daily.

Concerns: Avoid in cases of hemorrhoids, dry stools, bloody urine, or excess heat, such as fever and inflammation. It may exacerbate premature ejaculation. Avoid therapeutic dosages during pregnancy.

Cistanches

Cistanche salsa

Family: Orobanchaceae.

Part used: Root.

Also known as: Broomrape, rou cong rong.

Properties: Aphrodisiac, phytoandrogenic, phytoestrogenic, reproductive restorative.

Use: Cistanches is a traditional remedy for erectile dysfunction. It helps restore muscle tone after illness.

Energetics: Sweet, salty, sour, warm, moist.

Dosage: 1 cup of tea or 20–40 drops of tincture three times daily.

Concerns: Safe when used appropriately.

Clary Sage

Salvia sclarea

Family: Lamiaceae.

Part used: Herb.

Also known as: Muscatel sage.

Properties: Aphrodisiac, euphoric, nerve and muscle relaxant.

Use: Clary sage is energizing and uplifting. It contains phytosterols, or plant hormones that provide the body with raw material for the production of human hormones.

Energetics: Pungent, warm.

Dosage: ½ cup of tea or 10–20 drops of tincture three times daily.

Concerns: Safe when used appropriately.

Clove

Syzygium aromaticum

Family: Myrtaceae.

Part used: Bud.

Also known as: Ding xiang, lavanga.

Properties: Anesthetic, aphrodisiac, aromatic, rubefacient.

Use: Clove is a traditional ingredient in love potions for attracting the opposite sex. In Oriental tradition, it warms the kidneys. One can chew cloves to freshen the breath. When a small amount of clove-infused massage oil is applied to the genitals, it creates a pleasant numbing effect that can allow for prolonged lovemaking. Never apply undiluted clove oil.

Energetics: Pungent, warm.

Dosage: ¼ cup of tea or 10–20 drops of tincture three times daily.

Concerns: Safe when used appropriately.

Cordyceps

Cordyceps sinensis

Family: Clavicipitaceae.

Part used: Cordyceps fungus and entire larval carcass it grows upon.

Also known as: Winter bug summer herb, vegetable caterpillar, dong chóng xìa cao.

Properties: Kidney tonic, restorative, sedative.

Use: Sixteenth-century Chinese herbalist Li Chih Shen, who is said to have lived to be 256 years old, noted that cordyceps was equal to ginseng as a tonic. It relieves fatigue and can be used to treat erectile dysfunction and spermatorrhea. It also builds bone marrow, skeletal muscles, and chi.

Energetics: sweet, neutral, dry.

Dosage: 1 cup of tea or 20–60 drops of tincture three times daily.

Concerns: Safe when used appropriately.

Coriander

Coriandrum sativum

Family: Apiaceae.

Part used: Seed.

Also known as: Dhanyaka.

Properties: Aphrodisiac, mild stimulant.

Use: Coriander is said to promote harmony in relationships and to improve a bad mood. It is a traditional ingredient in love potions; in fact, it's mentioned in the tales of *The Arabian Nights* as an aphrodisiac, and during medieval times it was thought to encourage women to part with their virtue. The first-century Greek physician Dioscorides recommended adding coriander seeds to wine to increase semen output.

Energetics: Pungent, cool.

Dosage: 1 cup of tea or 30–40 drops of tincture three times daily.

Concerns: Safe when used appropriately. Excessive use can have a narcotic effect.

Cotton Root

Gossypium hirsutum, G. herbaceum

Family: Malvaceae.

Part used: Bark.

Also known as: Upland cotton, mian hua gen.

Properties: Aphrodisiac, nutritive, uterine tonic, yang tonic.

Use: By constricting blood vessels, cotton root improves circulation to the reproductive area and enhances orgasmic capability. It is being investigated as a male contraceptive agent. In Ayurvedic medicine, cotton root is used as a tonic and aphrodisiac.

Energetics: Sweet, sour, warm, dry.

Dosage: ½ cup of tea or 20 drops of tincture three times daily.

Concerns: Avoid during pregnancy. Large doses may cause nausea and vomiting and may lead to sterility in men if used over an extended period of time. Avoid in cases of urogenital irritation.

Cubeb

Piper cubeba

Family: Piperaceae.

Part used: Unripe fruit.

Also known as: Tailed pepper, kankola.

Properties: Antiseptic, stimulant, yang tonic.

Use: Applied topically to the genitals as an ointment, cubeb will help remedy premature ejaculation. The application gives a tingling feeling, which has led to its use in Arab culture as an aphrodisiac. Cubeb can be taken internally to treat spermatorrhea, leukorrhea, bladder inflammation, and abscess of the prostate. In the past it was used to treat gonorrhea.

Energetics: Pungent, warm.

Dosage: ¼ cup of tea or 20 drops of tincture three times daily; topical applications as needed.

Concerns: Avoid in cases of acute digestive and kidney irritation.

Cyperus

Cyperus rotundus

Family: Cyperaceae.

Part used: Rhizome.

Also known as: Sedgeroot, chufa, nutgrass, xiang fu, musta.

Properties: Stimulant, tonic, vasodilator.

Use: Cyperus relieves congested chi, depression, and moodiness.

Energetics: Pungent, bitter, warm, dry.

Dosage: 1 cup of tea or 20–40 drops of tincture three times daily.

Concerns: Safe when used appropriately.

Damiana

Turnera aphrodisiaca, T. diffusa

Family: Turneraceae.

Part used: Herb.

Properties: Antidepressant, aphrodisiac, stimulant, urinary antiseptic, yang tonic.

Use: Damiana is high in phosphorus, which may contribute to its energizing ability. It improves orgasmic ability, boosts nerve sensitivity, and strengthens the reproductive system. It's used in Central America to treat erectile dysfunction and premature ejaculation. Damiana counteracts testicular atrophy and remedies sexual problems related to anxiety. There are some reports of people having unusually erotic dreams while taking damiana. The herb has been used by livestock breeders to encourage mating.

Energetics: Pungent, bitter, warm, dry.

Dosage: 1 cup of tea daily or 15 drops of tincture three times daily.

Concerns: Avoid in cases of high blood pressure, urinary tract infections, kidney disease, or liver disease. Damiana is not recommended for use by pregnant women or nursing mothers. Otherwise safe when used appropriately.

> Some lovers enjoy sharing a ritual smoke of damiana before making love. Combine a pinch of peppermint leaf with a pinch of skullcap leaf and two pinches of damiana leaf. Add a few shredded rose petals, then roll up in smoking paper and smoke.

Deer Antler

Cervus nippon

Family: Cervidae.

Also known as: Velvet antler, cornu cervi, lou rong.

Properties: Aphrodisiac, energy tonic, gland tonic, kidney yang tonic, rejuvenative, restorative.

Use: That's right, the antlers of a deer are a potent sexual supplement, especially for men. It's not an herb, technically, but it is a very powerful remedy. The deer used for this remedy are raised on farms, and their antlers are sawed off (by a veterinarian or a trained specialist, using an anesthetic). The antlers regrow every spring. You can find deer antler in Chinese pharmacies in capsules, in tinctures, and as sliced rounds. Deer antler stimulates sperm production and testosterone secretion. It increases energy, builds the blood, and eases lower back pain. It is an excellent source of vitamins, minerals, amino acids (including arginine), and phytosterols. It can be used to treat erectile dysfunction and nocturnal emissions.

Energetics: Salty, sweet, warm, dry.

Dosage: 1 cup of tea two times daily or 15–20 drops of tincture three times daily.

Concerns: Deer antler is not recommended for people with yin deficiency. Those who are concerned about animal rights can find plenty of alternatives to this remedy.

Dendrobium

Dendrobium nobile

Family: Orchidaceae.

Part used: Herb.

Also known as: Shi hu.

Properties: Demulcent, kidney tonic.

Use: Dendrobium is superb for building sexual vigor. It tonifies kidney yin, increases sexual fluids, and prevents fatigue.

Energetics: Sweet, salty, cool, moist.

Dosage: 1 cup of tea or 20–40 drops of tincture three times daily.

Concerns: Safe when used appropriately. Dendrobium is an endangered herb; use only cultivated—never wildcrafted—supplies.

Dill

Anethum graveolens

Family: Apiaceae.

Part used: Seed.

Also known as: Mishreya.

Properties: Aphrodisiac, aromatic, mild stimulant.

Use: Dill is a wonderful aphrodisiac. It was a classic ingredient in medieval love potions.

Energetics: Pungent, warm.

Dosage: 1 cup of tea or 20–40 drops of tincture three times daily.

Concerns: Safe when used appropriately.

Dodder

Cuscuta chinensis, C. japonica, C. europaea

Family: Cuscutaceae.

Part used: Seed.

Also known as: Tu si zi.

Properties: Aphrodisiac, yang tonic, yin tonic.

Use: Dodder is used in traditional Chinese medicine to treat erectile dysfunction. It builds sperm and can be used as a treatment for involuntary seminal emission. It also strengthens the nerves.

Energetics: Sweet, neutral.

Dosage: 1 cup of tea or 20–40 drops of tincture three times daily.

Concerns: Safe when used appropriately.

Dong Quai

Angelica sinensis

Family: Apiaceae.

Part used: Root.

Also known as: Dang gui, tang kuei.

Properties: Aromatic, blood tonic, uterine tonic, yin tonic.

Use: Dong quai is a classic women's herb, but it also holds benefits for men. It increases a woman's sex drive, which can be particularly helpful for menopausal women. It can improve circulation and act as an energy tonic for both sexes. On the emotional side, dong quai supports calmness and fosters compassion. In Oriental tradition, it is used to disperse congestion in the pelvic region.

Energetics: Sweet, pungent, bitter, warm, moist.

Dosage: 1 cup of tea or 20–40 drops of tincture three times daily.

Concerns: Avoid during pregnancy, except under the guidance of your health care provider. It may increase menstrual flow. Do not use in cases of diarrhea, poor digestion, or bloating, or in conjunction with blood-thinning medications such as ibuprofen.

Epimedium

Epimedium aceranthus, E. grandiflorum

Family: Berberidaceae.

Part used: Leaf.

Also known as: Horny goat weed, yin yang huo.

Properties: Aphrodisiac, hormonal regulator, kidney tonic, nervous system tonic, vasodilator.

Use: Epimedium stimulates the sensory nerves, thereby increasing sexual desire and strength. It also strengthens the adrenal system, dilates capillaries, and improves circulation. It is a traditional remedy for erectile dysfunction. It's also a restorative for the reproductive system and increases sperm and testosterone production.

Energetics: Pungent, sweet, warm.

Dosage: ½ cup of tea or 15–30 drops of tincture three times daily.

Concerns: Those who have overactive sex drives and wet dreams should avoid epimedium. Large doses may cause vertigo, vomiting, dry mouth, and nosebleed. Use only for short periods of time.

Eucommia

Eucommia ulmoides

Family: Eucommiaceae.

Part used: Bark.

Also known as: Du zhong.

Properties: Aphrodisiac, kidney tonic, liver tonic, reproductive system tonic, sedative.

Use: Eucommia nourishes chi, builds deep vitality, and strengthens bones and muscles. It is often used to treat erectile dysfunction.

Energetics: Sweet, pungent, warm.

Dosage: ½ cup of tea or 20–30 drops of tincture three times daily.

Concerns: Avoid in cases of fever, infection, and yin deficiency. Large doses are sedative but not dangerous. Otherwise safe when used appropriately.

Evening Primrose

Oenothera biennis

Family: Onagraceae.

Part used: Oil from the seeds.

Properties: Demulcent, sedative, yin tonic.

Use: Evening primrose is often recommended for a variety of women's health problems. It's also helpful for men who produce insufficient ejaculate. It is an excellent source of gamma linolenic acid, an important essential fatty acid that helps the body produce energy. It heightens sexual response, can reduce menstrual cramps, and, as a side benefit, makes the skin softer and smoother.

Energetics: Sweet, cool.

Dosage: 1 or 2 capsules three times daily.

Concerns: Evening primrose may be contraindicated for people with epilepsy. Keep refrigerated as oils can go rancid.

False Unicorn

Chamaelirium luteum

Family: Liliaceae.

Part used: Rhizome.

Also known as: Helonias, blazing star, fairywand, studflower.

Properties: Diuretic, reproductive tonic, restorative.

Use: False unicorn can be used to treat endometriosis, hormonal imbalance, erectile dysfunction, ovarian cysts, and uterine prolapse. It boosts fertility and works well as a restorative after a woman discontinues using birth control pills. It's a wonderful complement to psychotherapy in helping one heal from sexual abuse.

Energetics: Bitter, warm, dry.

Dosage: 1 cup of tea or 15–30 drops of tincture three times daily.

Concerns: The bitter taste of this herb can cause vomiting. Excessive amounts may cause kidney and stomach irritation, blurred vision, and hot flashes. Do not use without employing birth control during sex unless pregnancy is desired. Discontinue use during pregnancy. False unicorn is at risk of becoming endangered in the wild; use only cultivated—never wildcrafted—supplies.

Fennel

Foeniculum vulgare

Family: Apiaceae.

Part used: Seed.

Also known as: Xiao hue xiang, shatapushpa.

Properties: Aphrodisiac, aromatic, diuretic.

Use: In Hindu culture, fennel is said to increase sexual vigor, and in Mediterranean culture, it is said to increase libido. It is a strong aphrodisiac and boosts energy levels. It also contains phytoestrogens.

Energetics: Pungent, sweet, warm, dry.

Dosage: 1 cup of tea or 10–30 drops of tincture three times daily.

Concerns: Large doses can stimulate the nervous system. Safe when used appropriately.

Fenugreek

Trigonella foenum-graecum

Family: Fabaceae.

Part used: Seed.

Also known as: Hu lu ba, methi.

Properties: Aphrodisiac, aromatic, diuretic, rejuvenative, restorative, stimulant, yang tonic.

Use: Fenugreek seeds were eaten by harem women to enhance their sexual allure. The seeds sweeten the breath and increase libido. In Oriental tradition, they are used to warm and nourish the kidneys.

Energetics: Bitter, warm.

Dosage: 1 cup of tea or 20–60 drops of tincture three times daily.

Concerns: Avoid during pregnancy. If you have diabetes, consult with your health care provider before use.

Galangal

Alpinia galanga, A. officinarum

Family: Zingiberaceae.

Part used: Rhizome.

Also known as: Siamese ginger, gao ling jiang, rasna.

Properties: Aphrodisiac, aromatic, stimulant.

Use: "It stimulates bodily lusts," wrote sixteenth-century physician Mattioli. The Indonesians agree; galangal is considered an important aphrodisiac in that region.

Energetics: Pungent, hot.

Dosage: ½ cup of tea or 20–40 drops of tincture three times daily.

Concerns: Daily use for longer than a month can irritate the digestive tract.

Garlic

Allium sativum

Family: Liliaceae.

Part used: Bulb.

Also known as: Da suan, lashuna.

Properties: Aphrodisiac, diuretic, vasodilator, yang tonic.

Use: In ancient Rome, garlic was a favorite herb of Ceres, the goddess of fertility. It is a tonic for the cardiovascular system and increases sexual desire.

Energetics: Pungent, hot, dry.

Dosage: 1 clove, 5–25 drops of tincture, or 1–2 capsules three time daily.

Concerns: Some people are allergic to garlic. Excessive use can cause emotional irritability and irritation of the stomach and kidneys. Avoid therapeutic doses during pregnancy, and avoid during the first three months of nursing, as it can cause breast milk to become unpalatable for infants. Avoid use the week before having surgery.

Ginger

Zingiber officinale

Family: Zingiberaceae.

Part used: Root.

Also known as: Gan jiang, ardra (fresh root), shunthi (dried root).

Properties: Aphrodisiac, stimulant.

Use: The great herbalist and mystic Hildegard of Bingen extolled the merits of ginger for its aphrodisiac properties for older men married to young, energetic women. It is considered an aphrodisiac in Chinese, Arab, Turkish, and Indian cultures. Ginger improves circulation to all parts of the body, relieves pelvic congestion, and helps restore yang energy.

Energetics: Pungent, sweet, hot, dry.

Dosage: ½ cup of tea four times daily, or 15 drops of tincture three times daily.

Preparation note: Ginger root is high in volatile oils, so it is best infused rather than decocted when prepared as a tea.

Concerns: Avoid large doses in cases of acne and eczema. Discontinue use if heartburn results. It may exacerbate premature ejaculation. Safe when used appropriately.

Ginkgo

Ginkgo biloba

Family: Ginkgoaceae.

Part used: Leaf.

Also known as: Maidenhair tree, bai gou.

Properties: Antioxidant, blood vessel dilator, cerebral tonic, circulatory stimulant, kidney tonic, rejuvenative.

Use: Ginkgo relaxes blood vessels. The resulting improved blood flow allows nutrients to be better distributed throughout the body and creates greater sensitivity in the sexual organs of men and women. It also helps reverse erectile dysfunction without altering blood pressure, unlike some pharmaceuticals that are used to treat this condition. Ginkgo prevents blood platelet aggregation, may boost sperm production, and increases the production of dopamine and adrenaline.

Energetics: Sweet, bitter, neutral, dry.

Dosage: 1 cup of tea or 20–40 drops of tincture three times daily.

Concerns: Side effects are rare, though headache and gastrointestinal complaints have been reported. Those with hemorrhaging tendencies should avoid ginkgo. Do not combine ginkgo with aspirin, as they both decrease blood platelet aggregation. Avoid use the week before having surgery.

Ginseng

Panax ginseng, P. quinquefolius

Family: Araliaceae.

Part used: Root.

Also known as: P. ginseng—Chinese ginseng, Korean ginseng, ren shen, lakshmana; *P. quinquefolius*—American ginseng, xi yang shen.

Properties: Aphrodisiac, chi tonic, rejuvenative, restorative, stimulant, tonic.

Use: In the sacred Hindu Vedas, ginseng is described as capable of bestowing "the power of the bull." In case you're wondering what that means, read on. This potent herb helps the body make better use of oxygen, thus enhancing physical endurance and mental alertness. It relieves fatigue and calms anxiety. It also strengthens adrenal glands, improves blood flow, supports endocrine function, increases testosterone levels in both men and women, boosts sperm counts, endows virility, and supports testicle and ovarian growth in young men and women, respectively. It even improves muscle tone.

Energetics: P. *ginseng*—Sweet, bitter, warm. P. *quinquefolius*—Sweet, bitter, neutral.

Dosage: 1 cup of tea or 20–60 drops of tincture three times daily.

Concerns: Avoid in cases of excess heat, such as inflammation, fever, and high blood pressure. Since ginseng can be energizing, avoid taking it within four hours of bedtime. Avoid during pregnancy. Avoid prolonged use for children. American ginseng is at risk of becoming endangered in the wild; use only cultivated—never wildcrafted—supplies.

Hops

Humulus lupulus

Family: Cannabaceae.

Part used: Strobile.

Also known as: Ch-ku-tsao.

Properties: Phytoestrogenic, anaphrodisiac, muscle relaxant, sedative.

Use: Hops is a strong sedative, and it can ease tension and anxiety. It can be used to subdue excessive sexual desire and to treat premature ejaculation due to sexual neurosis.

Energetics: Bitter, cold, dry.

Dosage: ½ cup of tea or 15–30 drops of tincture three times daily.

Concerns: Avoid during pregnancy and in cases of depression. The fresh plant may cause dermatitis in some individuals.

Ho Shou Wu

Polygonum multiflorum

Family: Polygonaceae.

Part used: Root.

Also known as: Fo-ti, Chinese knotweed.

Properties: Aphrodisiac, cardiotonic, chi tonic, diuretic, rejuvenative, yin tonic.

Use: This classic Chinese herb improves circulation, boosts libido, and relieves anxiety. In Oriental tradition, it helps in cases of liver or kidney deficiency. It can be used to minimize premature ejaculation.

Energetics: Bitter, sweet, warm.

Dosage: ¼ cup of tea four times daily, or 15–30 drops of tincture three times daily

Concerns: Avoid in cases of diarrhea.

Kava Kava

Piper methysticum

Family: Piperaceae.

Parts used: Root, upper rhizome.

Properties: Euphoric, muscle relaxant, sedative.

Use: Kava kava helps one feel more relaxed, peaceful, and sociable. It warms the emotions, calms anxiety, and enhances communication. It is said to stimulate clitoral size and make women feel sexually excited. An oil infused with kava kava can be applied to a man's erect lingam to give him more relaxed control.

Energetics: Pungent, bitter, hot.

Dosage: ¼ cup of tea or 15–30 drops of tincture three times daily; add some milk or coconut milk to the tea, because the active compounds in kava kava are fat soluble and will be assimilated better by the body when delivered with a small amount of fat.

Concerns: Excessive use can temporarily alter perception, so use it only when you intend to stay put for a while. It can cause temporary numbness in the mouth and tongue and a rubbery feeling in the limbs. Pregnant women and nursing mothers should avoid use. There have been recent reports implicating kava kava in cases of liver toxicity; until this controversial issue is cleared, I would recommend that people with liver dysfunctions avoid kava kava. This herb is at risk of becoming endangered in the wild; use only cultivated—never wildcrafted—supplies.

Licorice

Glycyrrhiza glabra, G. uralensis

Family: Fabaceae.

Part used: Root.

Also known as: Gan cao, yashtimadhu.

Properties: Adrenal tonic, chi tonic, demulcent, endocrine system tonic, nutritive, rejuvenative.

Use: Licorice nourishes the adrenal glands; it boosts energy levels, strength, and vigor. It also encourages feelings of peace and harmony. It contains phytosterols and can be used to balance hormones.

Energetics: Sweet, bitter, neutral, moist.

Dosage: ½ cup of tea or 30–60 drops of tincture three times daily.

Concerns: Avoid during pregnancy and in cases of edema, high blood pressure, or diabetes. Do not use in combination with digoxin drugs. Excessive use can cause sodium retention and potassium depletion.

Longan

Euphoria longan

Family: Sapindaceae.

Part used: Berry.

Also known as: Long yan rou.

Properties: Blood tonic, energy tonic, nervous system restorative, nutritive, sexual tonic.

Use: Longan berry is a good overall sexual tonic; it tonifies sexual fluids and female reproductive organs. It also calms anxiety. You can take it as a tea or tincture or incorporate it as an ingredient in your regular diet.

Energetics: Sweet, hot, moist.

Dosage: 1 cup of tea or 20–40 drops of tincture three times daily.

Concerns: Avoid in cases of diarrhea.

Lycii

Lycium chinense, L. barbarum

Family: Solanaceae.

Part used: Berry.

Also known as: Wolfberry, boxthorn, gou qi zi.

Properties: Aphrodisiac, blood tonic, energy tonic, nutritive, rejuvenative, yin tonic.

Use: Lycii berry strengthens the kidneys and liver, enhances libido, and promotes cheerfulness.

Energetics: Sweet, neutral, warm, moist.

Dosage: 1 cup of tea or 20–40 drops of tincture three times daily.

Concerns: Avoid during pregnancy and in cases of diarrhea, bloating, or excess heat, such as fever or inflammation.

Maca

Lepidium meyenii, L. peruvianum

Family: Brassicaceae.

Part used: Root.

Also known as: Ayak, ayuk willku, chichira, maca-maca, maka, Peruvian ginseng, quechua.

Properties: Adaptogen, aphrodisiac, immunostimulant, nutritive, rejuvenative, tonic.

Use: Maca root enhances sexual desire and improves fertility in both men and women. It can be used to treat erectile dysfunction and vaginal dryness. It increases strength and stamina and helps the body deal with stress. On the hormonal front, maca stimulates the hypothalamus and the pituitary gland, elevating estrogen and progesterone levels, and balances the adrenal glands, the thyroid, and the pancreas. Maca contains important essential fatty acids, including omega-3 and omega-5.

Energetics: Sweet, warm.

Dosage: 5 to 20 grams of the dried root daily or 30–40 drops of tincture three times daily.

Concerns: Safe when used appropriately.

Marjoram

Origanum majorana

Family: Lamiaceae.

Part used: Herb.

Properties: Aromatic, tonic.

Use: The sweet breath of Aphrodite is said to have created the fragrance of marjoram. Ancient Romans considered marjoram to be an aphrodisiac. It helps calm nerves and allay fear.

Energetics: Pungent, warm.

Dosage: 1 cup of tea or 20–40 drops of tincture three times daily.

Concerns: Avoid therapeutic doses during pregnancy.

Muira Puama

Ptychopetalum olacoides, P. unicatum

Family: Oleaceae.

Part used: Inner bark, root.

Also known as: Potency wood.

Properties: Aphrodisiac, central nervous system stimulant, tonic.

Use: Muira puama is famous in Brazil as a remedy for erectile dysfunction and for its ability to improve orgasmic ability. It can be used to enhance both the physical and psychological enjoyment of sex. It improves fertility, prolongs virility, lessens inhibitions, and relieves the emotions induced by sexual trauma. In a French study undertaken with 262 male test subjects, all of whom suffered from low libido and inability to achieve erection, 51 percent of those with erectile dysfunction reported improvement when taking muira puama, and 62 percent reported enhanced libido. The bark is chewed, made into a tea, and sometimes smoked.

Energetics: Pungent, warm.

Dosage: ½ cup of tea or 10–30 drops of tincture three times daily.

Concerns: Safe when used appropriately.

Mustard

Brassica nigra

Family: Brassicaceae.

Part used: Seed.

Also known as: Svetasarisha.

Properties: Circulatory stimulant, rubefacient.

Use: Mustard has a long history as an aphrodisiac. This hot seed warms the libido for both sexes.

Energetics: Pungent, hot.

Dosage: ½ cup of tea or 10–20 drops of tincture three times daily.

Concerns: Do not apply directly to the skin as it can cause blistering. Those with gastrointestinal and cardiovascular problems should avoid excessive use. Men who experience premature ejaculation should avoid mustard.

Nettle

Urtica dioica, U. urens

Family: Urticaceae.

Part used: Leaf, root, seed.

Also known as: Stinging nettle, bichu.

Properties: Adrenal tonic, circulatory stimulant, diuretic, kidney tonic, metabolic stimulant, nutritive, rubefacient, thyroid tonic, uterine tonic.

Use: Nettle, especially its seeds, have been used as a remedy for impotence for thousands of years. Second-century herbalist Galen (131–200 A.D.) wrote that nettle seeds "taken in a draught of mulled wine arouse desire"; nettle seeds soaked in honey is a traditional Arab cure for impotence. And since ancient times, fresh nettles have been used for the practice of flagellation, or, more properly termed, urtication: The genitals are whipped with fresh stinging nettles to increase blood flow to the area—a painful sort of herbal Viagra that is not for the unadventurous!

In a recent study undertaken at Budapest University, researchers found that men who ingested a formula of nettles and oatstraw experienced increased stamina, strength, sexual vitality, and testosterone levels. At the Advanced Study of Human Sexuality in San Francisco, the same combination was given to a group of forty men and women, and both genders experienced an increase in sexual desire. Nettle seeds have also been shown to have a positive effect on benign prostatic hyperplasia.

Energetics: Bitter, salty, cool, dry; the seed is warm.

Dosage: 1 cup of tea or 20–40 drops of tincture three times daily.

Concerns: Contact with the fresh plant will irritate the skin. Use only dried herb. Wear gloves when collecting. Safe when used appropriately.

Night-blooming Cereus

Selenicereus grandiflorus

Family: Cactaceae.

Parts used: Flower, stem.

Also known as: Cactus flower.

Properties: Aphrodisiac, cardiac stimulant, tonic.

Use: Night-blooming cereus helps restore muscle tone, and it is often used to treat erectile dysfunction.

Energetics: Bitter, warm.

Dosage: ½ cup of tea or 10–25 drops of tincture three times daily.

Concerns: Safe when used appropriately. Do not exceed the recommended dosage.

Nutmeg

Myristica fragrans

Family: Myristicaceae.

Part used: Kernel.

Also known as: Rou dou kou, jatiphala.

Properties: Aphrodisiac, circulatory stimulant, sedative.

Use: Nutmeg improves libido and can be used to treat erectile dysfunction and premature ejaculation. Myristicine, a compound derived from nutmeg, was part of the original formula for MDMA, or Ecstasy.

Energetics: Pungent, warm.

Dosage: ½ cup of tea or 20 drops of tincture three times daily.

Concerns: Avoid therapeutic doses during pregnancy. Do not exceed the recommended dosage.

Oat

Avena sativa, A. fatua

Family: Poaceae.

Part used: Spikelet (oatstraw).

Also known as: Yen-mai.

Properties: Antidepressant, aphrodisiac, cerebral tonic, endocrine tonic, nerve tonic, nutritive, rejuvenative, uterine tonic.

Use: The spikelets of oat, called oatstraw, have a relaxing effect; they nourish the nervous system and help the body handle stress. Oatstraw is rich in magnesium and polysaccharides that promote energy. It is an excellent herb to use during a convalescence. It also benefits the libido, makes tactile sensations more pleasurable, promotes vaginal lubrication, and makes it possible for women to experience multiple orgasms. It can be used to treat cases of erectile dysfunction and premature ejaculation.

Energetics: Sweet, cool, moist.

Dosage: 1 cup of tea or 20–40 drops of tincture three times daily.

Concerns: Safe when used appropriately. Those with gluten allergies may need to begin with small dosages and increase cautiously.

Parsley

Petroselinum crispum

Family: Apiaceae.

Parts used: Leaf, root.

Properties: Antiseptic, aphrodisiac, nutritive, sedative.

Use: Parsley is rich in zinc and freshens breath.

Energetics: Sweet, neutral.

Dosage: 1 cup of tea or 30–60 drops of tincture three times daily. Of course, fresh parsley can also be used as a garnish for the dinner plate.

Concerns: Avoid therapeutic doses during pregnancy and in cases of kidney inflammation.

Polygala

Polygala siberica, P. tenuifolia

Family: Polygalaceae.

Part used: Root.

Also known as: Milkwort, Siberian milkwort, yuan zhi.

Properties: Antiseptic, nervine, restorative, uterine stimulant.

Use: Traditionally, polygala is used to build strength of character and willpower and to promote vivid dreams. It promotes positive feelings, clears consciousness, calms the spirit, and quiets the heart.

Energetics: Sweet, sour, pungent, salty, neutral, dry.

Dosage: $\frac{1}{2}$ cup of tea or 10–30 drops of tincture three times daily.

Concerns: Avoid during pregnancy and in cases of gastritis or ulcers. Large doses may be emetic.

Poria

Poria cocos

Family: Polyporaceae.

Part used: Fungus.

Also known as: Indian bread, tuckahoe, hoelen, fu ling.

Properties: Cardiotonic, chi tonic, diuretic, nutritive, restorative.

Use: In Oriental tradition, poria is used to strengthen the kidneys and dispel excessive dampness. It is a good remedy for nervousness.

Energetics: Sweet, neutral, dry.

Dosage: 1 cup of tea or 40 drops of tincture three times daily.

Concerns: Safe when used appropriately.

Red Raspberry

Rubus idaeus

Family: Rosaceae.

Part used: Leaf.

Also known as: Fu-pen-tzu, gauriphal.

Properties: Astringent, hormonal regulator, kidney tonic, nutritive, prostate tonic, uterine tonic, yin tonic.

Use: Red raspberry leaf is a wonderful complement to therapy for victims of sexual abuse. It also nourishes the reproductive system and strengthens the entire genitourinary system.

Energetics: Bitter, cool.

Dosage: 1 cup of tea or 20–40 drops of tincture three times daily.

Concerns: Safe when used appropriately.

Rehmannia

Rehmannia glutinosa

Family: Gesneriaceae.

Part used: Root.

Also known as: Chinese foxglove, shen di huang (raw), shu di huang (cooked).

Properties: Cardiotonic, demulcent, diuretic, rejuvenative.

Use: Rehmannia is a tonic for the kidneys and the adrenal glands. It nourishes yin, improves vaginal lubrication, and boosts energy levels.

Energetics: Raw root: Bitter, sweet, cool. Prepared root: Bitter, sweet, warm.

Dosage: 1 cup of tea or 20–40 drops of tincture three times daily.

Concerns: Avoid in cases of loose stools, poor appetite, bloating, or a coated tongue.

Reishi

Ganoderma lucidum

Family: Polyporaceae.

Part used: Fruiting body.

Also known as: Lucky fungus, ling zhi.

Properties: Adaptogen, antiseptic, rejuvenative.

Use: In the Taoist tradition, reishi is said to enhance spiritual receptivity. It was used by monks to calm the spirit and mind. It is considered a symbol of feminine sexuality. Reishi helps normalize blood pressure and blood sugar levels. It also inhibits blood platelet aggregation.

Energetics: Bland, sweet, bitter, neutral.

Dosage: 1 cup of tea or 20–40 drops of tincture three times daily.

Concerns: Safe when used appropriately. There have been reports of dry mouth, digestive distress, nosebleed, and bloody stools when reishi is used for extended periods of time (at least 3 to 6 months).

Rose

Rosa spp.

Family: Rosaceae.

Parts used: Bud, flower.

Also known as: Mei gui hua, shatapatra.

Properties: Antidepressant, aphrodisiac, aromatic, blood tonic, diuretic, kidney tonic, sedative.

Use: The open rose is a symbol for the opening of the heart and vulva. Rose calms anger and relieves exhaustion. In Oriental tradition, it is used in cases of deficient kidney chi.

Energetics: Sweet, bitter, sour, neutral, cool.

Dosage: ½ cup of tea or 10–20 drops of tincture three times daily.

Concerns: Safe when used appropriately.

Saffron

Crocus sativus

Family: Iridaceae.

Part used: Stigma.

Also known as: Zang hong hua, kumkum.

Properties: Aphrodisiac, rejuvenative.

Use: Saffron stimulates circulation to the genitals. It relieves depression and can be used to treat impotence. In ancient Greek and Arab culture, saffron was thought to stimulate sensuality in women.

Energetics: Pungent, sweet, bitter, cool.

Dosage: ½ cup of tea two times daily, or 20 drops of tincture three times daily.

Concerns: Do not exceed recommended dosage; excessive use can lead to serious health risks. Avoid therapeutic doses during pregnancy.

Sarsaparilla

Smilax spp.

Family: Smilaceae.

Part used: Root.

Also known as: Tu fu ling, chopchini.

Properties: Aphrodisiac, rejuvenative, tonic.

Use: Sarsaparilla is rich in phytosterols, including smilasaponin, sarsaponin, and sarsaparilloside, which provide the raw material for the body to produce hormones. It also contains the trace minerals selenium and zinc. It strengthens the adrenal system and sexual organs. It makes men more virile and women more passionate. It is a traditional Mexican remedy for low libido and erectile dysfunction.

Energetics: Sweet, neutral.

Dosage: ½ cup of tea four times daily, or 30–60 drops of tincture three times daily.

Concerns: Safe when used appropriately.

Savory

Satureja hortensis (summer savory), *Satureja montana* (winter savory)

Family: Lamiaceae.

Part used: Leaf.

Properties: Aphrodisiac.

Use: In European tradition savory is used to promote marital bliss. Its genus name, *satureja,* derives from the same root as *satyr;* the satyrs were well known for their penchant for seducing maidens and fairy folk.

Energetics: Pungent, bitter, warm.

Dosage: 1 cup of tea or 20–40 drops of tincture three times daily.

Concerns: Safe when used appropriately.

Saw Palmetto

Serenoa repens

Family: Palmaceae.

Part used: Berry.

Also known as: Sabal.

Properties: Aphrodisiac, diuretic, nutritive, rejuvenative, reproductive tonic, urinary antiseptic, yang and yin tonic.

Use: Saw palmetto is best known for its ability to inhibit the conversion of testosterone to dihydrotestosterone (DHT), a substance that can contribute to swelling of the prostate. It also helps rebuild atrophying genitals, including thinning of the vaginal walls in women. It reduces the occurrence of nocturnal urination and can be used to treat erectile dysfunction, premature ejaculation, and "honeymoon cystitis" (irritation occurring from excessive sex). It improves orgasmic ability and boosts libido.

Energetics: Pungent, sweet, warm.

Dosage: ½ cup of tea or 10–60 drops of tincture three times daily.

Concerns: Safe when used appropriately. There have been rare reports of saw palmetto causing stomach distress.

Schizandra

Schisandra chinensis

Family: Schisandraceae.

Part used: Fruit.

Also known as: Fruit of the five flavors, wu wei zi.

Properties: Aphrodisiac, cerebral tonic, kidney tonic, rejuvenative, restorative.

Use: Schizandra increases staying power in men. It can be used to remedy general weakness, to relieve anxiety and depression, to reduce the occurrence of nocturnal emissions, and to treat sexual debility. It also helps one overcome trauma associated with sexual abuse.

Energetics: Sour, sweet, salty, pungent, bitter, warm.

Dosage: ½ cup of tea or 20–30 drops of tincture three times daily.

Concerns: Avoid in cases of excess heat, such as fever or infection. May be contraindicated for those with epilepsy, intracranial pressure, or high stomach acid levels.

Siberian Ginseng

Eleutherococcus senticosus

Family: Araliaceae.

Parts used: Root, root bark.

Also known as: Eleuthero, ci wu jia.

Properties: Adaptogen, aphrodisiac, cardiotonic, chi tonic.

Use: Siberian ginseng is an excellent treatment for a weakened nervous system or adrenal gland insufficiency. It relieves fatigue, improves stamina, and helps remedy erectile dysfunction.

Energetics: Sweet, bitter, neutral.

Dosage: 1 cup of tea or 20–40 drops of tincture three times daily.

Concerns: Safe when used appropriately.

Suma

Pfaffia paniculata

Family: Amaranthaceae.

Part used: Root.

Also known as: Brazilian ginseng, para todo.

Properties: Adaptogen, aphrodisiac, chi tonic, demulcent, hormonal regulator, nutritive, rejuvenative.

Use: Suma increases sexual stamina and helps the body make better use of oxygen. Its potential to increase male hormone production is under investigation.

Energetics: Pungent, sweet, neutral.

Dosage: 1 cup of tea or 40–60 drops of tincture three times daily.

Concerns: For the moment, safe when used appropriately. Suma is relatively new to the Western pharmacopoeia and its effects—and contraindications—are still being researched.

Tienchi Ginseng

Panax pseudoginseng

Family: Araliaceae.

Part used: Root.

Also known as: San qi ginseng.

Properties: Adrenal tonic, blood tonic, cardiotonic, chi tonic, circulatory stimulant, yin tonic.

Use: Tienchi ginseng improves coronary blood flow and, thus, circulation to the genitals. It can be used to treat erectile dysfunction.

Energetics: Bitter, neutral.

Dosage: ¼ cup of tea or 20 drops of tincture three times daily.

Concerns: Avoid during pregnancy and in cases of blood deficiency.

Tribulus

Tribulus terrestris

Family: Zygophyllaceae.

Part used: Fruit.

Also known as: Caltrop, puncture vine, goat's head, ci ji li, gokshura.

Properties: Aphrodisiac, kidney tonic, rejuvenative, tonic.

Use: Tribulus has been used since ancient times in India as a remedy for low libido in men and women. It can boost sperm count and remedy erectile dysfunction. It increases testosterone production by activating luteinizing hormone secretions from the pituitary gland. In women it increases levels of follicle stimulating hormone. It also improves the metabolism of fats, thus improving the circulation of chi and blood throughout the body.

Energetics: Sweet, bitter, cool.

Dosage: 1 cup of tea or 20–40 drops of tincture three times daily.

Concerns: Avoid during pregnancy except under the supervision of a health care professional. Avoid in cases of dehydration.

Vanilla

Vanilla planifolia, V. tahitensis

Family: Orchidaceae.

Part used: Cured seed pod.

Properties: Aphrodisiac, aromatic, stimulant.

Use: The word *vanilla* is derived from Latin and means "little vagina"; if you've ever seen a vanilla orchid, you'll know why. Vanilla is a mild urethral irritant and sexual stimulant.

Energetics: Sweet, warm.

Dosage: Add 1/4 to 1/2 teaspoon of vanilla extract to tea, juice, wine, or even your bath.

Concerns: Safe when used appropriately.

Vitex

Vitex agnus-castus

Family: Verbenaceae.

Part used: Fruit (berry).

Also known as: Chaste-tree berry, monk's pepper, man jing zi.

Properties: Phytoprogesteronic, anaphrodisiac, reproductive tonic.

Use: Vitex is a hormonal system normalizer. It also helps normalize the menses, shortening a long cycle or lengthening a short one. It is especially helpful for regulating the menstrual cycle of women who are discontinuing birth control pills.

Energetics: Sweet, bitter, neutral.

Dosage: 1 cup of tea or 20–40 drops of tincture three times daily.

Concerns: Avoid during pregnancy except under the supervision of a health care professional. Vitex can decrease the effectiveness of birth control pills. Rare individuals may experience contact dermatitis. Vitex has the reputation of decreasing sex drive in some people.

Yohimbe

Pausinystalia yohimbe, Corynanthe yohimbe

Family: Rubiaceae.

Part used: Bark.

Also known as: Johimbe.

Properties: Aphrodisiac, cardiac stimulant, cerebral stimulant, nerve stimulant, vasodilator.

Use: As a vasodilator, yohimbe increases the dilation of blood vessels, thus increasing blood flow to genitals. It also stimulates the ganglion nerves, which affect erection, and the "sex center" of the human brain in the hypothalamus. It increases levels of norepinephrine, which causes a temporary boost in energy. Yohimbe is used by vets to encourage lazy bulls and stallions to mate.

Energetics: Pungent, warm.

Dosage: 1 cup of tea or 40 drops of tincture; take only as needed.

Concerns: Do not use for more than three days in a row. Avoid in cases of high blood pressure, anxiety, prostate inflammation, peripheral vascular disease, bipolar conditions, liver disorders, or kidney disorders. Pregnant women, the elderly, and children should not ingest yohimbe. Adverse reactions may include nausea, vomiting, hypertension, excessive perspiration, salivation, tremors, dizziness, lack of coordination, headache, and skin flushing. Do not combine with alcohol, sedatives, antihistamines, diet pills, narcotics, blood pressure medications, monoamine oxidase (MAO) inhibitors, or tyramine-rich foods (including bananas, cheese, chocolate, sauerkraut, and red wine). Symptoms of overdose include pupil dilation, excess salivation, diarrhea, heart palpitations, and low blood pressure. Taking 1,000 mg of buffered vitamin C with yohimbe can minimize side effects.

Zallouh

Ferulas harmonis

Family: Orchidaceae.

Part used: Root.

Also known as: Shirsh zallouh.

Properties: Antioxidant, aphrodisiac, circulatory stimulant, rejuvenative.

Use: Zallouh has been used since ancient times to treat erectile dysfunction and to increase libido in both men and women. It contains ferulic acid, which dilates blood vessels and enhances circulation.

Energetics: Sweet, warm.

Dosage: 1 cup of tea or 20–40 drops of tincture three times daily.

Concerns: Avoid in cases of heart disease or diabetic neuropathy except under the supervision of a health care professional. There have been rare reports of zallouh causing headache.

HERBALIST LOVE POTIONS

The following recipes and potions were devised and graciously donated by several of my herbalist friends.

Sex is most enjoyable when the juices are flowing, but sometimes, due to a variety of issues, dryness prevails. Even when intercourse is juicy, some people are very sensitive to tissue friction, which can cause "honeymoon cystitis" or encourage an outbreak of herpes or another obnoxious syndrome. Fortunately, good-quality herbal oils and salves, used liberally on both partners, offer a safe, natural solution to petroleum-based lubrication.

No-Cook Herbal Salve

Salves save the day! When you or your beloved needs a little tenderness on an "ouchie," this herbal salve brings comfort.

Infused Herbal Oil (recipe on page 106)
Beeswax, cocoa butter, or shea butter
(2 ounces for every 2 cups of oil)

1. Heat the oil in a heavy pan over low heat until it's warm enough to liquefy the beeswax.

2. Add the beeswax. Stir until it is completely melted.

3. While the oil is warm, pour it carefully into salve containers.

4. When the salve has hardened, secure the lid and seal tightly.

5. Store in a cool, dark location and use within one year.

Infused Herbal Oil

Use this oil for massage or to soothe sore muscles.

Dried, chopped blossoms of chamomile, calendula, or Saint John's wort

Good-quality vegetable oil (such as olive, almond, sesame, avocado, or peanut)

1. Place the herbs in a clean glass jar with a tight-fitting lid. There should be enough blossoms to fill the jar about three-quarters of the way to the top.

2. Cover the herbs with the vegetable oil so that they are completely submerged. Leave two inches of headroom in the jar. Secure the lid and seal tightly.

3. Let the jar sit in a warm, sunny location for ten to twenty days. Shake often.

4. Line a clean container with cheesecloth or muslin, and pour the oil and flowers onto it. Let the oil drip from the flowers through cheesecloth or muslin to filter. When the flowers have stopped dripping oil, bottle the infused oil in a clean glass container.

5. Store in a cool, dark location and use within one year.

If you are using Saint John's wort, add this very important step to the infusion process. If it is not done, it can ruin all your effort. As the oil sits, moisture from the fresh herbs will evaporate and become trapped in the headroom and on the lid of the jar. Wipe out this moisture with a clean cloth daily or as needed. Do not shake the bottle until all the moisture is removed.

Healing a Broken Heart

Sometimes in life, love doesn't work out.
Here is a healing formula to bring comfort.

1 part hawthorn berry and/or flower

1 part organic rose petals

Prepare as a tea or a tincture, following the instructions on page 72.

David Winston, author of *Saw Palmetto for Men and Women* (Storey Books, 1999) and dean of the Herbal Therapeutics School of Botanic Medicine.

APHRODISIAC FORMULA FOR WOMEN

This recipe combines some of nature's best.

2 parts damiana herb

2 parts schizandra berry

1½ parts rosemary leaves

1½ parts organic rose flower

1 part clove bud

3 cups water

1. Combine all the herbs.

2. Place 3 tablespoons of the herb mixture into a Mason jar. Add 3 cups of boiling water. Cover and let sit overnight.

3. Strain the infused water from the spent herbs. Drink 1 cup of the tea before each meal during the day.

4. Continue this daily program for one to two months.

APHRODISIAC FORMULA FOR MEN

A potent herbal blend for men!

3 parts Syrian rue seed

3 parts muira puama inner bark

2 parts nettle seed

2 parts milky oat seed

1½ parts polygala root

1. Combine all the herbs in a Mason jar. Cover with vodka, so that the vodka rises one inch over the top of the herbs.

2. Let steep for one month, shaking every day.

3. Strain the infused vodka from the spent herbs through fine cheesecloth. Bottle in amber glass dropper bottles. Take 1½ dropperfuls in a bit of warm water three or four times daily on an empty stomach; continue for one to two months.

Matthew Becker, clinical herbalist and faculty member at the Rocky Mountain Center for Botanical Studies, where he teaches Herbal Therapeutics.

MAGIC ZOOM BALLS

A delicious herbal bonbon!

1 cup tahini (drain excess oil from the top)

1 cup cashew or almond butter

1 to 1½ cups honey (more or less to taste)

½ ounce damiana leaf powder

1 ounce Siberian ginseng powder

1 ounce *Panax ginseng* powder

1 ounce guarana powder (contains caffeine)

1 tablespoon cardamom powder

1 teaspoon mace

2 vials royal jelly and/or 2 tablespoons of Chambord
(or any thick sweet raspberry liqueur)

2 vials ginseng (available at natural food stores
and Oriental markets)

8 ounces unsweetened shredded coconut, toasted

1 cup finely chopped almonds

1 package bittersweet chocolate chips

Unsweetened cocoa powder

2 pounds bittersweet dark
dipping chocolate (optional)

1. Stir together the tahini, nut butter, and honey, until you have achieved a smooth mixture.

2. Combine the herbal powders and stir into the nut butter mixture.

3. Add the royal jelly, Chambord, ginseng vials, toasted coconut, almonds, and chocolate chips. Mix well. This usually requires mixing with your hands.

4. Add unsweetened cocoa powder to the mix until you have reached the desired thickness.

5. Roll the mixture into small balls. Place in the refrigerator until they are cool.

6. Melt the dipping chocolate in a double boiler. When the chocolate is completely melted, use a fork to dip the balls into it one at a time. Tap each ball against the side of the pot to get rid of excess chocolate. Set the balls on waxed paper to cool.

7. Store the balls in baking tins in a cool location. They will keep for a few weeks.

Rosemary Gladstar, author of *Herbal Healing for Women* (Fireside, 1993) and *Rosemary Gladstar's Family Herbal: A Guide to Living Life with Energy, Health, and Vitality* (Storey Books, 2001). She is the director of Sage Mountain Retreat Center and Botanical Sanctuary in Vermont.

COOKED HERBAL SALVE

A "must have" in every home medicine chest.
Can be used on sore muscles, cuts, and bruises.

2 cups good-quality vegetable oil
(such as olive, almond, coconut,
sesame, avocado, or peanut)

8 ounces fresh or dried, chopped blossoms
of chamomile, calendula, or Saint John's wort

2 ounces beeswax, cocoa butter, or shea butter
(if you're using coconut oil, skip this ingredient)

1. Add the oil to a heavy-bottomed, nonaluminum pot.

2. Stir in fresh or dried herbs.

3. Warm over low heat for thirty to sixty minutes. If you're using fresh herbs, keep uncovered so that moisture can evaporate. If you're using dried herbs, cover.

4. Line a clean container with cheesecloth or muslin, and pour the oil and flowers onto it. Let the oil drip from the flowers through cheesecloth or muslin to filter. When the flowers have stopped dripping, measure the amount of oil.

5. Reheat the filtered oil in a clean pot until it is warm enough to melt the beeswax, cocoa butter, or shea butter. Then add the beeswax, cocoa butter, or shea butter. (If you're using coconut oil as your base, you do not need to add beeswax, cocoa butter, or shea butter.) Stir until the ingredients are thoroughly combined.

6. While the oil is warm, pour it carefully into salve containers.

7. When the salve has hardened, secure the lid and seal tightly.

8. Store in a cool, dark location and use within one year.

Cascade Anderson Geller. As a voice for the green world, Cascade shares her experiences with plants and discusses the interconnection of plants and people—in the clinical herbal setting, the home, and, most importantly, outdoors in forest, field, and garden.

DAMIANA ROSE CORDIAL

This formula is a tonic for the nervous and reproductive systems.
Try drizzling it over fruit pieces or baked pears, adding it to orange juice,
tea, or carbonated water, or sipping it from little cordial glasses.
A little bit goes a long way. Try your belly button as a cordial cup!

1 ounce damiana leaf

2 cups brandy

1 ½ cups spring water

1 cup honey

1 tablespoon rose water

1 tablespoon vanilla

1. Place the damiana in a clean glass jar and pour the brandy over it. Stir well, then cover. Let soak for five days.

2. Strain the liquid from the leaves. Reserve the leaves, and store the liquid in a clean bottle.

3. Place the alcohol-drenched leaves in a clean glass jar. Pour the spring water over them. Stir well, then cover. Let soak for three days.

4. Strain the liquid from the leaves and reserve it. Compost the leaves.

5. Place the water in a saucepan. Warm it over low heat, then add the honey. Stir and heat just until the honey is melted and mixed into the water. Remove from heat.

6. When the honey water has cooled, combine it with the brandy extract. Add the rose water and vanilla. Pour into a glass jar, cover, and shake well. Let sit for one to four weeks before using.

Diana De Luca, author of *Botanica Erotica: Arousing Body, Mind and Spirit* (Healing Arts Press, 1998).

SENSUALITY PERFUME

Awaken your passion through the sense of scent.

200 drops spikenard essential oil

100 drops rose otto essential oil

50 drops lavender essential oil

1 drop blue chamomile essential oil

Combine all the oils. Apply this perfume to all your favorite body parts.

THE LOVE SHAKE

This is way beyond your average smoothie!

2 tablespoons organic chocolate powder

2 cups almond milk

4 dried figs (preferably organic Turkish), soaked

1 frozen banana

A touch of vanilla extract

2 tablespoons maca powder

Frozen organic raspberries (optional)

2 dropperfuls fresh damiana tincture
(optional)

2 dropperfuls ginger tincture (optional)

½ to 1 teaspoon red ginseng
powdered extract

Combine all ingredients in a blender and blend.

Christopher Hobbs, L.Ac., A.H.G., coauthor of the Peterson Field Guide *Western Medicinal Plants and Herbs* (Houghton Mifflin, 2002) and author of *Natural Therapy for Your Liver* (Avery, 2002).

APHRODISIAC DATE PARFAIT

After this, you may become the final dessert.

2-pound package of pitted dates

Brandy (I prefer apricot brandy.)

Vanilla ice cream

Whipped cream

Jasmine essential oil

Nuts (optional)

1. Chop up the dates.

2. Stir the brandy into the chopped dates until they are gooey. Refrigerate until chilled.

3. In a parfait glass, layer the date mixture with vanilla ice cream. Top with whipped cream to which 1 drop of jasmine essential oil per 8 servings has been added. Sprinkle with nuts, if desired. Chill again until ready to serve.

GOD-US "UNDRESSING" OIL

This recipe is medicine for the heart, our body's most erogenous organ, as well as a lovely massage oil. The directions for making it can be followed or not, as you will. It's dedicated to Rico, my best lover. As the God-Us undresses, apply sparingly to revealed body parts. Give thanks for embodiment. Apply oil liberally with Holy Wonder to genitals before the sacred connection.

Oil—The Carrier of Bliss:
1 pint organic virgin olive oil

4 ounces organic almond oil

1 ounce organic calendula oil

1 teaspoon organic jojoba oil

8 drops organic lavender essential oil

3 drops organic rose essential oil

The Herbs—Lovers of the Earth:
2 sprigs sweet basil, crushed, with stem removed

1 sprig rosemary, crushed, with stem removed

Petals from three fresh calendula flowers

1. On the new moon in Gemini (in cooler climates) or the new moon in Scorpio (in temperate climates), and with passionate care, combine the oil and herbs in a sturdy jar just big enough that the combined oil and herbs come almost to the top. Seal the jar.

2. Dig a hole and place the jar upright in it. Bury the jar in sand (or warm earth) as you give gratitude for your sexual vitality.

3. At the quarter moon, dig up the jar and shake it as you sing your most cherished love song. Bury it again. Give thanks for the earth's vitality.

4. Repeat the digging up, shaking, singing, and reburying of the jar with gratitude at the next full moon, third-quarter moon, new moon, and first-quarter moon.

5. On the second full moon after you first buried the jar, dig up the jar for the last time.

6. Strain the herbs from the oil into a cheesecloth. Twist and wring all of the remaining oil out of the cloth into a bowl. Discard the herbs into the compost. Siphon this herbed oil into a clean container.

7. Write the date and moon sign on the label, and call it "Parvati's God-Us UnDressing Oil."

Jeannine Parvati Baker, author of *Prenatal Yoga and Natural Childbirth* (Freestone Publishing, 2001) and *Hygieia: A Woman's Herbal* (Freestone Publishing, 1978) and coauthor of *Conscious Conception* (Freestone Publishing, 1986).

EASY MASSAGE OIL

This massage oil encourages passion.
It can also be dripped moderately over desserts to add flavor.

1 drop jasmine absolute

1 drop neroli essential oil

1 drop sandalwood essential oil

1 drop spikenard essential oil

1 drop ylang ylang essential oil

1 ounce vegetable oil (I prefer hazelnut, sunflower, or olive.)

Combine the essential oils in a small container and shake vigorously. Then add the vegetable oil and shake again until it is truly blended.

Jeanne Rose, founder of New Age Creations, the first body-care company in the United States to use aromatherapy, author of *Herbal Body Book* (Frog, Ltd., 2000) and *Herbs and Aromatherapy for the Reproductive System* (Frog, Ltd., 1994), and director of the home-study courses Herbal Studies Course and Aromatherapy Studies Course.

MALE SEXUAL VITALITY TONIC

This formula is an adaptogenic sexual tonic. It can enhance sexual health and performance in the healthy man, while it is also useful in cases of sexual weakness or exhaustion. It is especially indicated for male sexual impotence.

5 parts *Panax ginseng* root tincture

5 parts Jamaican sarsaparilla root tincture

4 parts saw palmetto berry tincture

4 parts oat "milky" seed tincture

2 parts cardamom seed tincture

Combine all ingredients. Take 40 drops in a bit of water or juice two or three times a day.

HERBAL ED'S SEXY SMOOTHIE

*After drinking this smoothie, I feel completely energized,
and sexual vitality and stamina are definitely enhanced.
All ingredients are approximate, so feel free to experiment.*

2½ cups soy milk

1 cup blueberries, strawberries,
other berries

2 tablespoons maca root powder

2 tablespoons wheat germ

1 tablespoon raw flaxseeds

1 tablespoon raw pumpkin seeds

Combine the ingredients in a blender and blend.

"Herbal Ed" Smith, founder of Herb Pharm (www.herb-pharm.com).

HEART AND SOUL TONIC

*To maintain good love, more is involved than mere engagement
on the sexual level. It is equally important for the heart and the soul
to be involved. In this tonic, the hawthorn is for the heart, the damiana
is for the sexual excitement, and the sacred basil is for the soul.
Chambord is added because it tastes so good!*

2 ounces hawthorn brandy
(berries steeped in brandy for six weeks)

2 ounces damiana brandy (damiana leaf and flower
steeped in brandy for six weeks)

8 ounces sacred basil infusion (sacred basil leaf
steeped in boiling water for four hours)

A splash of Chambord

Combine all ingredients. Store in the refrigerator, where it will keep
for several weeks.

Pam Montgomery, author of *Partner Earth: A Spiritual Ecology* (Destiny Books, 1997) and
director of Partner Earth Education Center and Green Nations Gatherings.

ASPARAGUS-EPIMEDIUM TEA

Epimedium is also known as horny goat weed. Meditate on that name while sharing this tea with your beloved over a large shrimp cocktail.

1 quart water

1 heaping teaspoon Chinese asparagus root

3 heaping teaspoons epimedium leaf

1. Drop the asparagus root into the water. Bring to a boil, cover, and simmer for twenty minutes.

2. Remove from heat. Add the epimedium leaf. Cover and let steep for twenty minutes.

3. Strain and share.

Lesley Tierra, author of *The Herbs of Life* (Crossing Press, 1992), *Healing with Chinese Herbs* (Crossing Press, 1997), and *A Kid's Herb Book* (Robert D. Reed Publishers, 2000) and coauthor of *Chinese Traditional Herbal Medicine* (Lotus Press, 1998).

A ROMANTIC LOVE POTION

An herbal beverage to enjoy by the glass.

1 quart red wine (or red raspberry
or pomegranate juice)

2 tablespoons rose water

1 teaspoon vanilla extract

1 teaspoon ginseng tincture

1 tablespoon damiana tincture

3 drops cardamom essential oil

½ teaspoon nutmeg powder

2 tablespoons honey (optional)

Combine all the ingredients. Let sit for a couple of days to allow the flavors to blend and mellow.

Kathi Keville, author of *Herbs for Health and Healing* (Rodale Press, 1996), coauthor of *Aromatherapy: A Complete Guide to the Healing Art* (Crossing Press, 1995), and director of the American Herb Association.

SUSUN WEED'S LOVE FEST MENU

Angel Hair Pasta: Whole wheat tastes best, and its B vitamins build sexual appetite.

Gar-Lick Bread: Whole wheat sourdough, doused with olive oil, covered with minced garlic, and baked at 350°F until hot and crisp (six to fifteen minutes). Make at least two pieces per person.

Sweet Potatties: Rub olive oil on one large sweet potato per person and bake, covered, for one hour at 350°F.

Wickedly Wild Salad: Prepare a mix of greens (chickweed, garlic mustard, lamb's-quarter, sheep sorrel, wild mints of all kinds, wild madder, dandelion leaves, plantain leaves, violet leaves) and flowers (dame's rocket, roses, nasturtiums, pansies, daylilies, tulips, lilacs, lavender flowers, chive blossoms). Toss with a dressing prepared from extra-virgin olive oil, tamari, and lavender vinegar.

Kava Kava Brew: At least twenty-four hours before your love fest, prepare your brew, using $1/2$ to 1 ounce of dried kava kava root per person. Chop up the roots and place in a glass jar or enamel pan. Pour 2 cups of boiling water per person over the cut roots. Cover and let steep, away from heat, until you're ready to drink it. Serve chilled or warmed, with honey and milk and a little cinnamon or nutmeg if you like. Hint: When your nose starts to tingle, drink another half glass of kava kava, no more. Then concentrate on love.

Susun S. Weed (www.susunweed.com), author of *Wise Woman Herbal for the Childbearing Year* (Ash Tree Publishing, 1985), *New Menopausal Years the Wise Woman Way* (Ash Tree Publishing, 2001), and *Breast Cancer? Breast Health!* (Ash Tree Publishing, 1997). She is the director of Wise Woman Center in Woodstock, New York.

CHINESE PATENT HERB FORMULAS

There are several Chinese patent formulas, some which are ancient, that can do wonders for sexual vigor. Patent medicines are ready-made herbal formulas, which are usually found in pill form. They are often used in combination with other therapies, such as acupuncture. For more information about these formulas, contact a practitioner of traditional Oriental medicine.

Cong Rong Bu Shen Wan

This formula tonifies kidney yin and yang and nourishes *jing,* or life essence. It is often recommended in cases of weak lower back, erectile dysfunction, and premature ejaculation.

Nan Xing Bu Shen Wan

This formula warms and tonifies the kidneys. It can be used to remedy coldness in the extremities, lower back pain, urinary incontinence, and sexual weakness.

Rehmannia Six Pills

Rehmannia Six Pills is recommended in cases of kidney yin deficiency. It calms the heart, builds the blood, and remedies low libido and/or erectile dysfunction resulting from illness.

Tian Wang Bu Xin Wan

This formula is recommended in cases of emotional instability, premature ejaculation, and sexual anxiety.

Tzepau Sanpien Pills

Tzepau Sanpien Pills strengthen the kidneys and thus improve sexual function. The formula remedies erectile dysfunction, weakness, and dizziness.

Yao Jian Shen Pian

This formula is often recommended in cases of kidney yang depletion, weak lower back, and fatigue, especially when due to sexual excess.

You Gui Wan

Also known as Yudai Wan, You Gui Wan can be used to treat incontinence, weakness following illness, and kidney depletion (especially the right kidney). It is often recommended in cases of erectile dysfunction, leukorrhea, premature ejaculation, and lower back pain.

Zan Yi Dan

This formula nourishes kidney yang and is recommended in cases of apathy, weak lower back, erectile dysfunction, and infertility.

Aromatherapy:
Essential Oils for Love

romatherapy is the practice of using the essential oils of plants for physical and emotional healing. Essential oils are aromatic, volatile, chemically rich substances that plants produce to support all of their life processes, including growth and reproduction. They attract pollinators, repel predators, and protect plants from disease. A single plant contains just a tiny amount of essential oil, but that small dose is potent and has wide-ranging effects. Doesn't it make sense that these precious oils could also benefit humanity?

Scientific research has shown that fragrance directly affects our consciousness. Scent can lift or depress the spirits, calm or excite the mind, inspire passion or promote good sleep, and much more. Essential oils are sharply aromatic; more importantly, they have a direct chemical effect on the olfactory system and the brain. When the molecules that make up essential oils are inhaled through the nose, they travel up the olfactory passages to the brain. These molecules are so small that they bypass the blood-brain barrier (a wall of tissue that prevents substances in the blood from crossing over into brain tissue) and enter the brain itself. Once in the brain, essential oils have a direct impact on the limbic system, the part of the brain associated with emotion, memory, and learning, and so evoke a powerful emotional response. They can also stimulate the production of neurotransmitters.

Essential oils can also be applied externally, where the small size of the molecules again contributes to the healing effect. The molecules penetrate the skin and enter the bloodstream, which carries them throughout the body.

Many essential oils have antiviral and immunostimulating properties.

Some are antibacterial, and unlike many of the synthetic antibacterial agents in use today, bacteria do not seem to develop a resistance to them.

ESSENTIAL OILS TO INSPIRE PASSION

The sense of smell is greatly underused in the realm of romance. Pleasantly fragranced oils, lotions, and other potions can encourage us to engage in healing touch therapy, such as massage, acupressure, or even foreplay. Equally important are the direct healing, soothing, energizing, stimulating, and aphrodisiac effects that aromatic essential oils can have on the human mind. Whether mixed with oil in preparation for a massage, warmed over a diffuser to scent the air, dabbed on the neck and navel as a delicate perfume, or spritzed onto the sheets and mattress to refresh the bed, essential oils have the power to turn our thoughts to passion.

The essential oils described here are handpicked from a vast array of choices and chosen for their powerful effects on human sexuality. Some are potent aphrodisiacs, others are wonderful tonics for the reproductive system, and still others promote emotional openness. When you want to encourage passion in the bedroom, these are the essential oils to turn to.

Cardamom

Elettaria cardamomum

Family: Zingiberaceae (Ginger).

Energetics: Sweet, pungent, warming.

Use: Cardamom fosters joy and clarity, and in Ayurvedic medicine it is considered to be an aphrodisiac. It is also a stimulant and a breath freshener.

Caution: Do not use undiluted.

Champa

Michelia champaca

Family: Magnoliaceae (Magnolia).

Energetics: Sweet, bitter, warm.

Use: Champa has a floral, sensuous scent. It aids in the release of anger and can help bring couples closer together. It alleviates frigidity and is considered to be an aphrodisiac.

Cinnamon

Cinnamomum cassia, c. verum

Family: Lauraceae (Laurel).

Energetics: Sweet, warm.

Use: Cinnamon essential oil invigorates the senses, calms the nerves, and improves circulation. It also increases desire and creativity. It is often used to treat erectile dysfunction and frigidity. One study found that the smell of cinnamon buns increased blood flow to the penis. Pumpkin pie spice also had this effect.

Caution: Do not use undiluted.

Clary sage

Salvia sclarea

Family: Lamiaceae (Mint).

Energetics: Sweet, bitter, pungent, warm.

Use: Clary sage arouses the emotions and helps one feel more grounded in the body. It is an antidepressant, an aphrodisiac, and a mild euphoric. It is often used in the treatment of amenorrhea, premenstrual tension, menopause, and postnatal depression.

Clove

Syzygium aromaticum

Family: Myrtaceae (Myrtle).

Energetics: Sweet, pungent, warm.

Use: Clove combats exhaustion and nervousness and is considered to be an aphrodisiac. It also has anesthetic properties and can be used to prevent premature ejaculation.

Caution: Do not use undiluted.

Coriander

Coriandrum sativum

Family: Apiaceae (Parsley).

Energetics: Pungent, warm.

Use: Coriander is a gentle stimulant and helps relieve depression and stress. It has a long history as an aphrodisiac and a love potion.

Dhavana

Artemesia pallens

Family: Asteraceae (Daisy).

Energetics: Sweet, warm.

Use: Dhavana essential oil is often used to calm anger. It has a special affinity for the reproductive system, improving circulation there and helping reduce both the size and occurrence of ovarian cysts.

Fennel

Foeniculum vulgare

Family: Apiaceae (Parsley).

Energetics: Sweet, warm.

Use: Folklore recommends fennel essential oil for promoting courage, self-esteem, and strength. Because it has phytoestrogenic activity, it is considered a tonic for the female reproductive system; it can be used to treat cramps and amenorrhea and to improve the flow of breast milk in nursing mothers. In Mediterranean tradition, fennel is used to curb the appetite and promote slenderness.

Geranium

Pelargonium graveolens, P. odorantissimum

Family: Geraniaceae (Geranium).

Energetics: Sweet, penetrating, cool.

Use: Geranium essential oil calms anxiety, reduces stress, alleviates fatigue, and stimulates sensuality. It helps one feel at ease, improves relationships, and aids in resolving passive-aggressive issues. Geranium essential oil has phytoestrogenic properties and can be used to treat PMS, excessive menses, menopause, and fertility and as a tonic for the reproductive system. It is a thyroid stimulant, antidepressant, antiseptic, aphrodisiac, cell regenerator, and hormonal balancer for both men and women.

Ginger

Zingiber officinale

Family: Zingiberaceae (Ginger).

Energetics: Pungent, sweet, warm.

Use: Ginger's stimulating fragrance helps open the heart and has aphrodisiac properties. It improves circulation, alleviates depression, and can be used to treat erectile dysfunction.

Caution: Do not use undiluted.

Jasmine

Jasminum officinale

Family: Oleaceae (Olive).

Energetics: Sweet, warm, stimulating.

Use: Essence of jasmine is available as an absolute, not an essential oil, but it still has potent healing powers. The fragrance of the absolute is rich and sensual. It relieves stress, helps move emotional blocks, calms fears and anxiety, and is mildly euphoric. Jasmine is sacred to Kama, the Hindu god of love (the Eastern version of Cupid), who uses it to anoint the tips of his arrows.

> An absolute is not a pure essential oil; it is extracted with a solvent. Absolutes should never be taken internally.

Keawa

Pandanus odoratissimus

Family: Pandanaceae (Screw Pine).

Energetics: Sweet, bitter, cool.

Use: Keawa essential oil has long been used in religious ceremonies in India and is said to attune the senses toward spirituality. It improves self-esteem, helps with issues of attachment, and assists one in letting go of resentment, anger, and grief. It is also considered a nerve tonic. It can be particularly helpful during life transitions.

Neroli

Citrus bigaradia, C. aurantium

Family: Rutaceae (Rue).

Energetics: Sweet, cool.

Use: Neroli essential oil, which is extracted from orange blossoms, has antidepressant properties and eases anxiety, stress, and grief. Neroli helps relieve first-encounter apprehensions when one is spending time with a new partner. It is used to calm premenstrual tension and cramps.

Nutmeg

Myristica fragrans

Family: Myristicaceae (Nutmeg).

Energetics: Stimulating, pungent, warm.

Use: The scent of nutmeg essential oil invigorates the brain and calms and strengthens the nerves. It has long been considered an aphrodisiac and is helpful for resolving erectile dysfunction and irregular menses.

Caution: Do not use undiluted.

Patchouli

Pogostemon cablin

Family: Lamiaceae (Mint).

Energetics: Sweet, warm.

Use: Patchouli calms anxiety, lifts spirits, stimulates the nervous system, overcomes frigidity, improves clarity, and attracts sexual love. It has antifungal, antidepressant, antiseptic, aphrodisiac, and regenerative properties. It is often used to treat yeast and other vaginal infections and to balance libido levels.

Rose

Rosa spp.

Family: Rosaceae (Rose).

Energetics: Sweet, cool.

Use: Rose is considered sacred to Aphrodite, the goddess of love. Its rich fragrance is deeply floral. Essence of rose is available as both an absolute and an essential oil; the oil is much more expensive. (Before you balk at the price, consider that it takes 180 pounds of rose blossoms to make just 1 ounce of the essential oil.) Rose is both sensual and romantic; it is the supreme heart opener. It is helpful for those who feel distanced from their emotional center. Rose promotes a sense of happiness, relieves anger and jealousy, deflates relationship conflicts, and helps heal grief caused by emotional trauma. To rekindle the spark of love, apply rose oil to the body while making love. In addition to being an aphrodisiac, rose is antidepressant, antiseptic, and rejuvenative. It strengthens the uterus, regulates menses, and relieves cramps. It can be used to treat uterine disorders, menorrhagia, menopause, erectile dysfunction, frigidity, and low sperm count.

> To have dreams of love, prepare a dilution of rose oil, using the proportions given for massage oil on page 129. Place a drop of the rose-scented oil on your forehead before sleep.

Sandalwood

Santalum album

Family: Santalaceae (Sandalwood).

Energetics: Sweet, bitter, warm.

Use: Sandalwood has a chemistry similar to that of the male hormone andros-terone. Its scent is earthy and reminiscent of the odors of the reproductive organs. It is regarded as spiritually uplifting, ecstatic, and erotic. It helps build sexual confidence and has been used to treat anxiety that can contribute to erectile dysfunction and frigidity. In tantra, sandalwood is used to awaken the kundalini energy. It has antifungal, antidepressant, antiseptic, aphrodisiac, and relaxing properties, and it is often recommended as a treatment for genito-urinary infections, such as cystitis.

Caution: Sandalwood is at risk of becoming endangered in the wild; use essential oil that was extracted from cultivated—never wildcrafted—supplies.

Tuberose

Polianthes tuberosa

Family: Amaryllidaceae (Amaryllis).

Energetics: Sweet, cool.

Use: Tuberose is often used in perfumes for its sweet, floral scent. It is avail-able only as an absolute. Tuberose is both an antidepressant and an aphro-disiac. It strengthens and evokes the emotions.

Vanilla

Vanilla planifolia, v. tahitensis

Family: Orchidaceae (Orchid).

Energetics: Sweet, warm.

Use: Vanilla calms the mind, appeases anger, and soothes irritability. It is be-lieved that the smell of vanilla may stimulate the release of the neurotrans-mitter serotonin, causing feelings of arousal and satisfaction. It is an aphrodisiac and a mild menstrual stimulant. Vanilla is available as an absolute or oleoresin.

Vetivert

Vetiveria zizanioides

Family: Poaceae (Grass).

Energetics: Sweet, bitter, warm.

Use: The essential oil of vetivert calms, comforts, grounds, uplifts, and sedates. Vetivert has antiseptic, aphrodisiac, and rejuvenative properties. It stimulates circulation and can also help women through postpartum depression and menopause.

Ylang ylang

Cananga odorata

Family: Annonaceae (Custard Apple).

Energetics: Sweet, bitter, cool.

Use: In the Malayan language *ylang ylang* means "flower of flowers." The flower of the ylang ylang tree, from which the essential oil is extracted, is a euphoric and is used to calm anger, anxiety, and fear. It can also be used to relax a nervous partner prior to sex. Ylang ylang is antidepressant, antiseptic, and aphrodisiac. It stimulates the senses, improves self-esteem, fosters a sense of peacefulness, and helps overcome frigidity. It is often recommended for treating PMS, hormonal imbalance, and erectile dysfunction, and is known to stimulate orgasmic ability. In Indonesia ylang ylang flowers are scattered on the beds of newlyweds to promote desire and bless the union with children.

AROMATHERAPY LOVE POTIONS

There are hundreds of ways to incorporate aromatherapy into your life, especially your love life. Aromatherapy doesn't have to be complicated. For an aphrodisiac effect, aromatherapy can be as simple as keeping fresh flowers in the home. You might also simply dab a drop of essential oil on the nape of your neck as perfume or anoint your bed with a few drops of a passion-inspiring essential oil. If you're interested in pursuing the therapeutic effects of essential oil to resolve a physical or emotional dysfunction, consult with a qualified aromatherapist.

When you're working with essential oils, keep in mind that quality is imperative. Be sure to use pure essential oils and not synthetic fragrances. Be suspicious of companies whose essential oils are all the same price; some essential oils are harder to extract than others, or are unusual or rare. These differences should be reflected in the price. Essential oils should be packaged in dark-colored glass bottles. The label on the bottle should give both the common name and the botanical name of the plant whose essential oil is contained in the bottle.

Store essential oils away from light, heat, plastic, and metal and beyond the reach of children. Be careful when using them, as some oils can stain clothing and damage the finish on furniture. Keep essential oils away from broken skin and mucous membranes such as those of the eyes, mouth, and genitals. Some essential oils can induce uterine contractions, so pregnant women should avoid them unless they are under the supervision of a qualified aromatherapist or health care professional.

Most essential oils are very potent and should be diluted in a carrier oil. I like to use almond, grapeseed, and apricot kernel oils because they are light and don't have a strong odor. When I want to create a more warming blend, I use a heavier oil, such as hazelnut or sesame.

The scent of an essential oil application should be subtle, not overpowering. Dizziness, nausea, and rashes can all be signs that you are overdoing it or that you are sensitive to a particular oil. If an essential oil mixture begins to irritate your skin, wash it off and apply vegetable oil directly to the irritation.

Following are a few of my favorite ways to inspire "scentual" delight with essential oils. For more information on aromatherapy uses, safety, and preparations, read *Aromatherapy: A Complete Guide to the Healing Art* by Kathi Keville and Mindy Green (Crossing Press, 1995).

Bath

Stir 2–8 drops of an essential oil into your bathwater. Mix in the oil before you get in the tub, so that it is well diluted.

Bath Salts

Combine ⅛ teaspoon (about 12 drops) of essential oil with ½ cup of sea salt, Epsom salt, baking soda, or borax (or a combination thereof). Add mixture to the bathwater before you get in the tub. You can mix up big batches of bath salts ahead of time, using just ½ cup at a time in the tub. A scalloped seashell is delightful as a bath salt scoop.

Bedding

When changing the sheets, anoint the mattress with a few drops of a clear-colored essential oil such as cardamom or coriander.

Body Powder

Combine ½ to 1 teaspoon (50–100 drops) of essential oil with 1 ounce of orris-root powder. Add ½ pound of dried, powdered herbs. (I like to use lavender.)

Chakra Anointment

According to Mindy Green, author of *Natural Perfumes* (Interweave Press, 1999) and *Calendula* (Keats Publishing, 1998) and coauthor of *Aromatherapy: A Complete Guide to the Healing Art,* a classic tantric ritual involves anointing a woman's chakras. Before intercourse, the woman is worshipped as shakti, the embodiment of the creative force. She is anointed with five different fragrances on different areas of her body, arousing her five senses and lifting her spirits so that she can manifest as a goddess.

The sites of anointment are:

- Jasmine—hands
- Patchouli—neck and cheeks
- Amber or ambrette seed—breasts and genitals
- Spikenard—hair
- Sandalwood—thighs

Each oil should be diluted (5 drops of essential oil in $\frac{1}{2}$ ounce of body lotion or oil) before application to the body.

Diffusers

There are aromatherapy diffusers of all sorts that can fill your home with the beautiful fragrance of essential oils. Some are powered by candles, others by electricity. They range in price depending on the materials they are made from.

Facial Spray

Combine 1 teaspoon of vodka, $\frac{1}{4}$ teaspoon (25 drops) of essential oil, and 4 ounces of distilled water or aloe vera juice. (If you use aloe vera juice, keep this spray refrigerated.) Spritz onto the face after washing and before bed. The spray may also be applied throughout the day for moisture and a pleasant cooling effect.

Foot Bath

Add 10 drops of essential oil to 2 gallons of very warm water. Drop in those tired feet and enjoy!

Foot Powder

Add 8 drops of essential oil to $\frac{1}{2}$ cup of arrowroot powder, baking soda, white clay powder, or cornstarch (or a combination thereof).

Hair Rinse

Add 2 drops of essential oil and 2 tablespoons of apple cider vinegar to a cup of herbal tea of your choice. Apply after shampooing for sensuously fragrant hair.

Inhalations

Essential oils can be used like smelling salts. Hold a bottle of essential oil an inch or two from your nose and take ten deep, slow breaths, inhaling through your nostrils and exhaling through your mouth.

Steam inhalations can be especially helpful for breaking up congestion and clearing sinus passages; they're also a wonderful facial treatment. To prepare a steam inhalation, bring 2 cups of water to boil in a large pot. Stir in 4 drops of essential oil. Tent a towel over both your head and the aromatic pot. Breathe in the steam for at least ten minutes, coming up for air when it becomes too hot.

Massage Oil

Mix 25 drops of essential oil with 2 ounces of a carrier oil. To allow the skin to benefit from the therapeutic effects of the oils, don't bathe for at least an hour after the massage.

EDIBLE MASSAGE OIL

¼ cup almond oil

2 tablespoons chopped beeswax

2 tablespoons cocoa butter

2 vitamin E capsules

½ teaspoon nonalcoholic glycerin flavoring, such as strawberry

¼ teaspoon (25 drops) rose, jasmine, or neroli essential oil

Combine almond oil, beeswax, and cocoa butter and warm over low heat until they are melted together. Let cool, then add the vitamin E, glycerin, and essential oil. This massage oil can be used as a moisturizer or a lubricant, but it should not be used with latex.

Perfume

Apply a single drop of your favorite essential oil to your temples, the nape of your neck, your throat, behind your ears, your pubis, and the insides of your wrists. To perfume the hair, every time you wash your hairbrush, dab 1 or 2 drops of essential oil of jasmine or rose onto the brush.

Sauna

Add 10–15 drops of essential oil to 16 ounces of water. Throw a bit at a time onto the hot rocks in the sauna. (Caution: Never use the oils undiluted in the sauna; the heat in combination with the oils can cause an explosion.)

Scented Shampoo and Conditioner

Add 20 drops of essential oil to 4 ounces of good-quality unscented shampoo or conditioner.

Spritzer

Combine 20 drops of essential oil, 1 tablespoon of vodka, and 8 ounces of water. Pour into a mister bottle. Spritz into the air, onto the sheets, or onto each other should you get overheated!

ANOINTING BALM

¼ cup almond oil

2 teaspoons honey

1 tablespoon grated beeswax

2 tablespoons grated cocoa butter

2 vitamin E gel capsules

¼ teaspoon jasmine, neroli, rose, or ylang ylang essential oil

½ teaspoon vanilla glycerite (optional)

A few drops of peppermint essential oil (optional)

Combine the almond oil, honey, beeswax, and cocoa butter in the top of a double boiler and heat. When all ingredients have liquefied, blend. Remove from heat and allow to cool, then add the contents of the vitamin E capsules and the essential oil. If desired, add the vanilla glycerite (for sweetness) and the peppermint essential oil (to produce a pleasant tingle on the body).

Homeopathy: A Dose for What Ails You

omeopathy is based on the law of similars, or the philosophy that "like cures like." It was developed from the work of Dr. Samuel Hahnemann (1755–1843), who sought an alternative to the barbaric medicinal practices of his time and wanted to offer a safer, more effective form of treatment.

A homeopathic remedy is a tremendously diluted solution of a substance that would, in the body of a healthy person, produce symptoms similar to those of a particular illness. The solution contains an infinitesimal amount of the substance; you might say it contains just a ghost or pattern replica of the substance. Exposure to the pattern replica, however, triggers a powerful healing response from the body. In other words, by stimulating the body's own healing response, a homeopathic remedy encourages the body to heal itself.

Homeopathic remedies can effect amazingly fast-acting and profound cures. The degree of success, however, depends on selecting the right remedy for a person's constitution. Some basic guidelines for choosing and using homeopathic remedies follow, but you may also benefit from consultation with a professional homeopath to gain insight into the best remedies for your constitution. Note that homeopathy often calls for very small doses of substances that in large doses could be toxic. Do not confuse homeopathic remedies with herbal remedies.

USING HOMEOPATHIC REMEDIES

Homeopathic remedies come in the form of small pellets, alcohol solutions, and water solutions. The usual dosage is four pellets, or as many liquid drops as the package label recommends, taken under the tongue four times daily. Rather than swallowing the pellets whole, allow them to dissolve slowly.

For best results, do not eat or drink for ten minutes before and after taking a homeopathic remedy.

HOMEOPATHY FOR SEXUAL VITALITY

Homeopathy offers useful methods for balancing body, mind, and spirit and, therefore, can be a powerful ally in healing sexual dysfunctions that have both physical and mental roots. Homeopathy helps the natural healing energy of the body realign itself and, in so doing, improves health issues of all kinds, including those that affect sexual vitality.

Note that homeopathic remedies have different effects on different people, depending on the temperament of the individual. The effects described here, then, are of a general nature and may not encapsulate your experience with a particular remedy.

Agnus Castus

Source: Chaste tree (*Vitex agnus-castus*).

Use: Agnus Castus alleviates depression that is accompanied by a sense of foreboding. It improves orgasmic ability and is recommended for use when sexual organs have "cooled their fire"—for example, erectile dysfunction, especially in older people, and a distaste for intercourse in women. *Agnus Castus* is also recommended for women who have light menses or who are sterile.

Berberis

Source: Root of barberry (*Berberis vulgaris*).

Use: Berberis is recommended for those who have a suppressed sex drive. It is particularly helpful for those who appear pale and have sunken cheeks, dry mucous membranes, a feeling of constriction in the genitals, and rapidly changing symptoms.

Caladium Seguinum

Source: American arum.

Use: This remedy is recommended in cases where leakage of sexual fluids occurs without any excitement. It also helps those who suffer from cold sweating around the genitals.

Calcarea Carbonica

Source: Carbonate of lime.

Use: Calcarea Carbonica is recommended for those who experience an excessive sex drive, premature ejaculation, or sharp menstrual cramps.

Cantharis

Source: Spanish fly (*Lytta vesicatoria, Cantharis vesicatoria*).

Use: Cantharis is recommended in cases of weak ejaculation, loss of normal erection, temporary erectile dysfunction, and frigidity. It is also helpful for those who have excessive sex drive, especially in cases where excess has led to irritation of the genitals. It is sometimes indicated for those with violent tendencies.

Carbo Vegetabilis

Source: Vegetable charcoal.

Use: Carbo Vegetabilis suppresses libido and can be used to prevent premature ejaculation. It is often recommended for those who feel exhausted and have low vitality, as well as those who have not "felt like themselves" since an accident or illness.

Cinchona Officinalis

Source: Peruvian bark.

Use: Cinchona is a remedy for intense, hypersensitive individuals who have a hard time sharing their feelings. It helps individuals with lascivious fantasies balance their sexual desire.

Conium

Source: Poison hemlock (*Conium maculatum*).

Use: Conium can be used to treat erectile dysfunction as well as painful premature ejaculation. It is particularly helpful for those who feel emotionally paralyzed due to excess or lack of sex.

Gelsemium

Source: Root of yellow jasmine (*Gelsemium semperivens*).

Use: Gelsemium can help curb the frequency of wet dreams and the leakage of semen when passing a stool. It is indicated for those who have facial pallor, with dark circles around the eyes, and a feeble mind. It can also help relieve fears, phobias, and overexcitement that impair a person's ability to function and enjoy life.

Graphites

Source: Black lead.

Use: Graphites is indicated for those who experience extreme sexual excitement. It can help women who have scanty menses, sore nipples, and a distaste for intercourse, as well as men who have high levels of sexual desire but are debilitated, having premature or no ejaculation. *Graphites* can prevent or limit flatulence for those who tend to become gassy when they are sexually excited.

Ignatia

Source: Saint Ignatius bean (*Ignatia amara*).

Use: Ignatia opens emotional doors and aids recovery from grief. It is recommended for those who are irritable and cry easily, and it can aid the recovery or normalization of libido after grief or trauma. Use if grief causes menses to cease.

Lycopodium

Source: Club moss (*Lycopodium clavatum*).

Use: Lycopodium is recommended for the person who fears solitude, responsibility, and intimacy and who is prone to oversensitivity and angry outbursts. It can be used to treat cases of enlarged prostate, urination difficulties, cold penis, incomplete ejaculation, tenderness in the ovaries, painful intercourse, and liver and digestive problems. It might be recommended for a person who tends to fall asleep during intercourse. It is especially helpful for resolving erectile dysfunction, especially when the dysfunction is psychological in nature.

Natrum Muriaticum

Source: Salt, chloride of sodium.

Use: Natrum Muriaticum is recommended for those who are irritable, feel like crying, and lack desire and energy for sex. It can be used to prevent or limit loss of pubic hair, vaginal dryness, and genital odor (when it is atypically strong or unpleasant).

Phosphorus

Source: Phosphorus.

Use: Phosphorus is best suited for those with a fiery personality, who are full of light and life. It calms nervous tension and anxiety, and can help those who are easily confused, lack perspective, and burn out easily. It also helps regulate excessive sexual desire and can prevent or limit premature ejaculation.

Sabal Serrulata

Source: Saw palmetto (*Serenoa repens*).

Use: This remedy improves tissue strength in the genitals, builds sexual vitality, and decreases fear of sexual intimacy.

Selenium

Source: Selenium.

Use: Selenium is helpful for men who have great sexual desire but suffer from exhaustion, erectile dysfunction, insomnia, memory loss, or melancholy. It is the most effective remedy for premature ejaculation that is accompanied by weakness in the back.

Sepia

Source: Inky juice of cuttlefish (*Sepia officinalis*).

Use: Sepia is recommended particularly for dark-haired, dark-eyed women who are unhappy and overburdened and for men who have low sex drive, mental fatigue, and frequent erections. It can help those of both sexes who feel exhausted after intercourse. It also can ease symptoms of burning in the urethra. It is indicated for those with hormonal imbalances, such as premenstrual syndrome, cramps, heavy menses, and hot flashes, as well as prolapsed uterus and pain during intercourse.

Staphysagria

Source: Stavesacre, also known as palmated larkspur (*Delphinium staphysagria*).

Use: Staphysagria is recommended for those who are oversensitive, easily excited, and prone to sudden outbursts of passion and violence. It helps individuals come to terms with repressed feelings of shame and anger and can be of great help in cases where incest issues impair healthy sexual enjoyment. It also can help relieve cross-dressers from feelings of shame. It is indicated for women who experience physical pain with a new sex partner.

Yohimbe

Source: Bark of yohimbe (*Pausinystalia yohimbe*).

Use: Yohimbe helps increase sensation in the sexual organs. It can help improve and prolong erections that are otherwise impaired by atherosclerosis and diabetes.

Zincum Metallicum

Source: Zinc.

Use: Zincum Metallicum is recommended for those who fidget and touch their genitals excessively, have excessive sex drive, and experience chronic wet dreams. It also can prevent or limit hair loss and is used to treat depression.

9

Flower Essences: The Blossoming of Sexual Harmony

lower essences are potentiated plant preparations that carry the vibrational energy patterns of specific flowers. As an energy medicine, they strengthen the relationship between body, mind, and spirit. They do not have a strong aroma or flavor but, rather, just a hint of the flower that was used in preparing them.

Flower essences can help release some of the emotional barriers that keep us from sexual bliss. They are strong allies in healing emotional patterns that block true joy and intimacy.

OBTAINING AND USING FLOWER ESSENCES

Flower essences are made by soaking flowers in spring water for several hours in the sun. The water is then collected and bottled.

Flower essences are available at most health food stores and herb shops. You can also make your own. Just fill a clear glass bowl with about 12 ounces of spring water. Collect organically grown flower blossoms at their ripest in the early hours of the morning. Use a leaf as a "napkin" to pinch them off so that you don't touch them directly. Gently drop the flowers into the water and let them soak for three to four hours in direct sunlight. Then remove the flowers, again using a leaf so that you don't touch them. Add an equal amount of brandy to the water. Now you have made a "mother tincture."

To make a stock bottle, from which you'll obtain doses of the flower essence, place 2–4 drops of mother tincture in a clean, glass 1-ounce eyedropper bottle, using a nonmetallic (preferably glass) funnel. Then fill the bottle almost to the top with spring water. Add 1 teaspoon of brandy as a preservative. Store away from extreme heat, extreme cold, and electromagnetic devices.

Before measuring out a dosage of flower essence, shake the bottle. The usual dosage is 7 drops under the tongue or taken with a glass of water three or four times daily. You can also add flower essences to bathwater, massage oils, and body lotions. Try applying them to the sensitive skin on the insides of the wrists and to the "third eye" at the center of the forehead.

CHOOSING THE RIGHT FLOWER ESSENCE

Flower essences work well individually and in combination, using up to six different essences. You'll find that the healing effects range from subtle to dramatic. Most people find that flower essences, used over time, bring clarity, a sense of well-being, and an improved self-image.

Aspen

Aspen eases anxiety, apprehension, and phobias pertaining to sex.

Banana

This tropical essence helps you find balance between the left and right sides of the brain. It can help resolve sexual insecurity in men and decrease machismo.

Basil

Basil lends strength to those who tend to seek sexual relationships outside of their main partnership and aids couples who want to get to the root of a conflict. It encourages a sense of completeness and can help resolve conflicts about sexual abuse.

Black-eyed Susan

This flower essence helps "shine the light" on buried sexual issues, such as rape or incest, and encourages the transformation of pain.

Clematis

Clematis helps those who feel unconnected to the physical body regain that connection.

Crab Apple

Crab Apple helps overcome feelings of "dirtiness" or shame about sexuality.

Easter Lily

Easter Lily helps integrate spirituality and sexuality. It can bring perspective to those who repeatedly choose unsuitable partners and help those who have experienced sexual abuse overcome feelings of uncleanliness about sex.

Elm

This essence eases anxiety about sexual performance and helps resolve feelings of inadequacy.

Fuchsia

Use Fuchsia when you want to let go of sexual and emotional repressions.

Hibiscus

Hibiscus fosters responsiveness and warmth. It is especially helpful for women who have been sexually traumatized.

Holly

Holly opens the emotional heart and helps overcome chronic suspicion. It eases feelings of jealousy, insecurity, and neediness.

Mariposa Lily

Mariposa Lily alleviates lingering trauma resulting from sexual abuse during childhood. It can help overcome feelings of not being loved and not having been adequately mothered. It can move you closer to the feminine aspect of creation.

Mimulus

Mimulus helps overcome shyness. It eases general fear and anxiety.

Rescue Remedy

Rescue Remedy is a combination of five flower essences. It is also sold under the name *Five-Flower Essence.* It helps relieve shock after physical and emotional trauma, including arguments and heartbreak. Take 2 drops under the tongue as often as needed.

Nasturtium

This essence is indicated for those who are "too into their heads" to have an interest in sex; it helps them come out of their shells. It also can be used to increase vitality.

Scarlet Monkeyflower

When you're going through therapy, Scarlet Monkeyflower can help give you the courage to express your emotions. It also helps restore sexual harmony after anger.

Sticky Monkeyflower

Sticky Monkeyflower helps balance feelings about sexual issues. It can help dispel fears of intimacy and release emotional pain resulting from past relationships.

Walnut

Walnut helps its user feel protected from outside influences, shoring up those who are oversensitive.

10

Feng Shui: Creating a Love Palace

eng shui, translated from the Chinese as "wind and water," is the Oriental art of placement. Feng shui has been used for more than five thousand years to harmonize the chi that flows around and through our environment. Just as chi flows through the body (see page 20), so chi flows through the home. Feng shui teaches us how to make that natural energy work for us.

THE BAGUA

The *bagua* is a grid that divides a space into nine sectors, each associated with a particular aspect of life: career, relationship, family, prosperity, health, helpful people/travel, children and creativity, new knowledge, and reputation. (See illustration.) The career sector is at the entrance to the space, and determines where the other sectors fall. The bagua can be applied to an entire house or to a single room. Proper arrangement of living quarters in a particular sector strengthens the energy you derive from it; when the energy in all nine sectors is strong and balanced, the people who live in the home have strong and balanced chi.

Feng shui also prescribes the auspicious arrangements of elements within a particular room. With proper feng shui, the bedroom becomes the bedrock of passion and marital harmony; the kitchen, a realm of healing nourishment; the living room, an oasis of relaxation; and the bathroom, a temple in which to purify the body.

In our continuing quest for great sex, love, and health, we will focus on

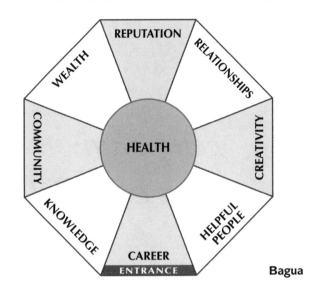

Bagua

the bedroom and the relationship sector. No matter how small or simple your space, you can create positive feng shui to encourage greater joy in life. The guidelines and tips offered here will carry you a long way toward positive feng shui, but if your interest is not satiated, consider having a professional feng shui master come to your home for a consultation.

ACTIVATING THE RELATIONSHIP SECTOR

To attract a new love relationship into your life, consider energizing the relationship sector. Paint that sector bright red or hang a red tapestry on the wall, and install red lanterns or red lights. Place a bird feeder, or a statue of Venus or a loving couple, in the yard in that sector. Once a week or during the new moon, light red or pink candles in the relationship sector as a love charm.

After you have found your beloved, it's time to change the feng shui energy in the relationship sector from attraction to simple vibrancy. Repaint the area its original color or take down the tapestry. Take down the red lights and install strong, warm indoor lighting. Keep the area clean, uncluttered, and fresh to allow these qualities to imbue the relationship. Do not keep trash or dirty laundry in the relationship sector.

Keeping plants in the relationship sector can attract all kinds of potent sexual energies. Flowers to consider include:

- Hibiscus: to encourage sexual fulfillment

- Gardenias: to attract love and happiness

- Peace lily: for harmony
- Roses: to open the emotional heart
- Orchids: to inspire sexual energy

Flowers should be fresh or made of silk (which should then be kept dusted); dried flowers are not recommended. When fresh flowers begin to wilt, dispose of them immediately, because decomposing flowers represent dying energy.

Do not keep prickly cacti in the home, as they create "cutting chi," or negative energy. (Kept outdoors, cacti represent protection.) Avoid bonsai, as well, because they represent stunted growth.

Invite magic and passion into your love life by creating a love altar in the relationship sector. For good love medicine, include a vase with two fresh or silk flowers and two red or pink candles. Write a love poem, or copy down one of your favorites, and prop it up against a wall or screen behind the altar. Over the altar, scatter pieces of rose quartz (signifying love and equanimity), seashells (representing depth and the feminine aspect), pearls (signifying lasting love), and/or garnets (signifying passion and constancy). You might even consider including two fresh red peppers to signify the spice of life. Set a photo of you and your beloved, which was taken in a time of happiness, in a prominent location in the altar. If you are still in search of a beloved, place an item that symbolizes a loving couple on the altar.

> When you have a gift for your lover, activate it by placing the gift on the love altar a couple of days before presenting it to your mate.

BEDROOM FENG SHUI

Improving the feng shui of the bedroom is a powerful mechanism for improving or attracting a romantic relationship. With proper arrangement and décor, the bedroom becomes a sanctuary of comfort, serenity, and sensuality. We spend one-third of our lives in the bedroom, so it behooves us to make it a wonderful, inspiring palace of pleasure. May you wake and sleep in beauty!

The Entryway

Entering the bedroom must be easy; blockages or obstacles at the bedroom door can cause blockages or obstacles in your love life. To minimize disharmony, there should be just one entry to the bedroom, and the door should open inward rather than outward.

Place a plant, wind chimes, or a mobile at the entrance to encourage movement, rather than stagnation, in your love life. A bell will encourage the flow of positive chi.

The Bed

When you're starting a new relationship, a secondhand bed or a bed that has been used for a previous partner can carry negative energy. It is best to purchase a new bed. If you can't do that, sprinkle the bare mattress with 1 cup of baking soda mixed with 30 drops of lavender essential oil and let it sit for a day, with the bedroom windows open. Then vacuum up the baking soda. You can also smudge the bed by burning over it aromatic herbs such as sage, artemisia, or cedar; use a shell or ashtray to catch the ash. At the very least, get new sheets.

> After you've had an argument with your lover, refresh your relationship by washing the bedsheets with 1 cup of salt added to the wash water.

Your bed should be rectangular and comprised of a standard mattress and box spring, or a futon mattress and base. Circular beds lead to disorientation; water beds encourage "wishy-washy" support in a relationship. Beds that are made by pushing two smaller mattresses together can cause a subconscious split in the relationship; in this case, the cure is to place a red sheet that spreads across the breadth of the bed between the mattresses and the box spring(s) to unify the bed and the relationship.

Place the bed so that you can see the room's entrance. Try to avoid placing the bed in a corner; this can make the person who sleeps in the corner feel boxed in and resentful of the relationship. Do not store items under the bed; they will block the flow of chi. If one side of the bed has a nightstand with a lamp, the other side should also have one, to convey equality.

If the bed shares a wall with a toilet, good fortune will drain from the room. The cure is to hang a tapestry on the shared wall to buffer the effect.

The direction in which the foot of the bed points is very important. If the feet are pointing toward the door, the bed is in the "death position," which allows the spirit of the dead to leave the body and home. If the foot of the bed is pointing toward an outside door or the bathroom door, you are more likely to become ill or to have an accident. If one of these inauspicious bed positions is unavoidable, hang a crystal between the door and the bed, and be sure the bed has a solid headboard.

Sleeping under a slanted ceiling or an exposed ceiling beam can cause a split in the relationship or health problems. If you cannot avoid placing the bed in such a position, hang a wind chime, a garland of silk flowers, or a crystal over the bed.

Make sure that the edges of bookshelves, bureaus, and other bedroom furniture are rounded, rather than sharp. Sharp edges can create cutting chi and disturb the comfort and security of those who sleep in the bed. Close closet doors and cover open shelves to avoid such disturbances. If a sharp edge cannot be avoided, hang a five-rod wind chime or a crystal between the bed and the sharp object—or soften the sharp edge by draping a pretty cloth over it or putting a vase of silk flowers above it.

Blankets and Bedsheets

Blankets and bedsheets should be made of natural fibers, not synthetics, so the body can breathe at night. For ultimate comfort, look for cotton sheets with at least a 250-thread count. Bedspreads should be dark in color and plain in design. Do not use bedspreads with abstract or geometric patterns, as their pointed symbols give off cutting chi. Spritz the mattress and pillows with an essential oil solution. (See Chapter 7 for suggestions.)

Bedroom Décor

Décor in the bedroom should focus on pairs; solitary items and images promote independence, rather than harmonious relationships. If you keep one teddy bear on the bed, keep two instead. If you have artwork that depicts living beings on the bedroom walls, the beings should be in pairs. Pairs of birds—especially ducks, geese, peacocks, phoenixes, and swans—carved from precious stones, such as adventurine, jasper, rose quartz, and tourmaline, are especially beneficial feng shui. Two geese flying high is a symbol of togetherness for those already in a relationship; a pair of mandarin ducks attracts new love for those desiring a relationship. For good fortune in marriage, keep an image representing the moon in your bedroom.

If you decorate your home as if it were a goddess sanctuary, you shouldn't wonder why you are unable to attract a man. To attract a relationship with a man, at least one-third of the imagery in your bedroom should represent the masculine. Likewise, to attract a woman, feminine imagery should be featured.

If the bedroom is small, hang wind chimes or a multifaceted or heart-shaped crystal in its center to increase the flow of chi. The symbol of water promotes the healthy flow of chi in many areas of the home, but it is not recommended in the bedroom where it might encourage infidelity. Remove fountains, photographs or paintings of water, and all other water symbols, including sheets with water motifs, from the bedroom.

When you open your eyes in the morning, your first sight should be of beauty. Place a beautiful object in the room in the line of vision that you most often wake up to, so that your days begin with truth, beauty, and goodness.

> Do not keep photos of relatives overlooking the bed. Great Auntie Em does not need to watch you have sex! Also remove mementos of previous relationships, which can create negative energy in the new relationship.

Windows

Weather permitting, during the day open windows to allow the angels of light and air to dance in and bring fresh chi into the bedroom. Hang crystals in the windows to bring rainbows of delight into the boudoir. Use as many crystals as you'd like; you simply can't overdo it.

Closets and Storage

Clutter anywhere in the home encourages one to feel confused, uneasy, stressed, and overwhelmed. As you might imagine, these feelings are particularly undesirable in the bedroom. Keep your bedroom space uncluttered. Organize and clean closets. (To attract a new relationship, leave some space available in closets and drawers as a symbol that there is room for love in your life.) Keep work-related items, such as computers and phones, out of the boudoir, or at least hide them from view.

Color Therapy

Color in the bedroom can have a powerful effect on the psyche and the flow of chi. The most arousing colors are reds, ambers, oranges, and purples. Generally, men find red to be most erotic; women seem to prefer violet. Red, pink, and peach are the best colors for the early years of a relationship. Red symbolizes passion. Pink is a combination of the passion of red muted with the purity of white. Peach blends the passion of red with the wisdom of yellow. However, excess red (such as a room painted red) may be overstimulating and could cause arguments. Blue, yellow, and white are more friendly than sexual.

Different colors can be added to the bedroom in moderation in the form of candles, fresh flowers, pillows, luxurious fabrics, and wall or ceiling hangings.

Lighting

Soft lighting is necessary for romantic occasions. Candles work well. Another option is soft, pink light bulbs, which flatter the body and are easy on the eyes.

Keep one of these bulbs available for a bedside light. Also consider stringing holiday lights in your bedroom for a joyous illuminating effect.

Mirrors

Mirrors create the impression that there are more than two people in the bedroom, interfering with the harmonious energy between the couple. I know that many of us enjoyed mirrored ceilings in the 1970s, but most of those relationships are over, n'est-ce pas? Therefore, there should be no more than one mirror—if any—in the bedroom. If there is a mirror in the bedroom, it should not be visible from the bed.

Televisions should not be kept in the bedroom; they are as reflective as mirrors and can encourage disharmony and infidelity.

Plants

Any of the flowers mentioned on pages 138–140 offer benefits for the feng shui of the bedroom. However, too many plants in the bedroom will produce excess chi and can disturb sleep. Keep it simple with just one or two plants in the bedroom.

According to feng shui tradition, when a mother wants her daughter to find a good husband, she hangs a large picture of peonies in the living room. If you want to attract a man, consider keeping an image of a peony just outside your bedroom door. Once that man is sleeping in your bedroom, however, remove the picture, as the peony energy can cause a man to have a roving eye.

Create a portable love altar so that you can transport your healthy feng shui energy and a sacred space of passion everywhere you travel. Be sure to include a picture of you and your beloved in happy times. My friends Light and Bryan, after many years of marriage, still travel with their wedding picture and have been known to place it on the mantels of Holiday Inns!

11

Massage and Acupressure: An Energetic Connection

ouch is believed to be the first of the senses to develop in the human embryo, and it defines much of our experience of life. The conductor of touch, our skin, is the largest organ of the body, and it is richly endowed with sensitive nerve endings. In fact, it is sometimes described as an external nervous system.

For humans, the awareness of touch is ever-present and overwhelming. Our minds are constantly flooded with sensations such as the feel of our clothing against our bodies or the air against our skin, hot and cold, pain and pleasure. Recognizing this, we can understand that the power of massage— the physical healing resulting from hands-on bodywork—is no small wonder. But while we acknowledge that massage is useful for loosening up sore muscles, soothing aching feet, and rubbing out knots in the back, we often forget that the simple power of touch—the caress of body against body—is itself a potent catalyst for energizing, arousing, soothing, warming, and healing emotionally. Most important, touch is an expression of love.

Massage is a wonderful way to build, support, and express the passion you have for another human being. It stimulates secretion of the hormone oxytocin, which promotes emotional bonding. Furthermore, massage boosts circulation of blood and lymph, stretches muscles and connective tissue, releases physical and emotional tension, stimulates the production of endorphins, and builds the immune system. And when your mate is too tired or tense to make love, massage can be an intimate, tender form of giving yourself to your beloved.

HOW TO GIVE A GREAT MASSAGE

Many people are reluctant to give a massage because they've never done so before and feel that they don't know how to do it properly. Let's set things straight: *Every* massage feels good, whether it's the disorganized rubbing of a novice or the probing bodywork of a professional. That's the beauty of massage; even if you don't do it well, your effort will still be well appreciated.

If you and your beloved make massaging one another a habit, your technique will improve rapidly. Even better, you'll soon learn each other's bodies like you've never known them before. You'll know where your lover carries tension, where he or she tends to develop muscle knots, which spots are particularly sensitive, and which spots inspire arousal. When you're making love, such knowledge can inspire you to new heights of desire and release.

You might not always have the time to give or receive a full-body massage. If that's the case, consider a scalp, facial, hand, foot, buttocks, or back massage; all can give exquisite pleasure and relaxation in a relatively short amount of time.

There are no strict rules for giving a massage; do what seems to feel good to your partner, and try out on your partner those things that feel good to you. The following guidelines will help. For more ideas, take a class on massage or watch an instructional video.

Create a Calming Environment

Because the person receiving the massage will be naked, make sure the room is warm and there are no cold drafts. Use soft lighting; candles are wonderful. Be sure that the surface on which your partner is lying—the floor or the bed—is not covered with a sheet or blanket that you prize. Spilled massage oil sometimes leaves a stain.

Use Oils to Smooth the Way

A light oil enhances the power of massage, allowing the hands to glide over and feel more deeply into the body. The friction of the massage also causes the oil to warm up; the heat is transmitted to the body, encouraging muscles to relax.

The best oils to use for massage are those that are light, do not smell, and moisturize (rather than clog) the skin. My favorites are almond and coconut Do not use heavy, odiferous oils, such as peanut or corn oil, or mineral oil, which is a petroleum byproduct, or oils that have become rancid. Keep your massage oil in a bottle with a flip-top lid; this type of container is easy to close when your hands are full of oil and minimizes the potential for a bottle-tumbling disaster. When you're not using the oils, store them in the refrigerator.

For an aromatherapy massage, you can add a few drops of essential oil to the base oil. See page 120 for more details.

Warm Your Hands and the Oil

Icy-cold hands on a warm back can produce an unpleasant shock. Before touching your beloved, wash your hands in hot water or rub them together briskly to generate some warmth.

It is also important that the massage oil be warm. Place the container of oil in a bowl of hot water for a few minutes before starting the massage. Alternatively, pour just a drizzle of oil into one hand, then rub the oil briskly between the hands. In fact, it's always a good idea to pour massage oil onto your hand first so you can check the temperature.

Let Your Fingers Do the Talking

Before you lay your hands on your lover's body, draw a deep breath and try to center yourself. Call to mind the love, desire, and tenderness you feel for your beloved. Then allow the love in your heart to be transmitted through your hands to your lover's body.

Use a Variety of Strokes

Incorporate a variety of strokes into the massage, such as circles, short strokes, long strokes, squeezing, and tapping. Use your fingers to work at small areas and the entire palm of your hand for rolling, broad strokes. Generally speaking, the left side of the body tends to be more sensitive for women, and the right side for men. When you find a tension spot—a knot or tight muscle—work at it, starting gently and gradually increasing the pressure. Avoid pressing directly on the spine.

Pay attention to your partner's breathing; deep sighs and soft moans signal that you're on the right track. Encourage your partner to give you feedback.

Encourage Quiet

Receiving a massage can bring you to a blissful place where touch rules the senses. It can be hard to think clearly, and even harder to hold up your end of a conversation. As a masseur, you should respect or even encourage that dreamy silence, wherein the only sounds are involuntary sighs and groans drawn forth from a body experiencing true pleasure. If you feel like singing or humming, by all means go ahead, but don't ask for a response from your partner.

Always Stay in Contact

To maintain the bond that has formed between you, don't lose contact with your beloved at any point during the massage. If you have to reach for more oil or shift to a more comfortable position, leave at least a hand on your partner.

End Tenderly

A massage leaves a person emotionally open and physically tranquilized, so it is important to end with tenderness. Give your beloved a soft kiss on the forehead or the back of the neck. Whisper sweet nothings in his or her ear. Lie close and be still.

> Avoid massage during infection, after recent surgery, and when skin is infected or inflamed. Use caution during pregnancy, because massage that is overly deep or centered on particular points can induce labor. If your beloved is pregnant, take a class on prenatal massage so that you can proceed with confidence and give your partner some much-deserved comfort.

REFLEXOLOGY

Reflexology affirms that our feet are a map of the body; they contain points that connect to each of the body's systems. A deep foot massage can stimulate the body's internal organs.

Reflexology aside, our feet carry us to and fro, support our weight all day long, and too often get stuffed into less-than-comfortable shoes. By caring for our feet, we can relax and be more open to bliss.

Foot massages are convenient because they don't require your entire attention. Try giving a foot massage to your partner while you are reading, or trade massages while you are watching television or listening to music.

Don't forget to massage the hollows under the ankle bones, as this helps keep the prostate and uterus healthy. The heel and the center of the arch on the sole of the foot are linked to sexual vitality; massage in these spots nourishes libido. Be sure to massage both feet.

ACUPRESSURE

Acupressure is a noninvasive form of acupuncture. Instead of using needles to tap into pressure points, the practitioner uses finger pressure. Like acupuncture, acupressure is used to strengthen internal organs and move blockages of energy. The finger pressure is increased gradually, allowing the tissues to respond and creating a connection between practitioner and patient. The practitioner and patient can breath in unison to help build a stronger connection. Hold each point for one to five minutes.

For more information about acupressure, take a class, or read *Acupressure for Lovers* by Michael Reed Gach (Bantam Books, 1997).

Sea of Vitality

Location: On the lower back, two to four inches on either side of the spine at waist level, as indicated by the four black dots in the illustration below.

Stroke: The patient should lie on his or her stomach or stand. Squeeze the Sea of Vitality firmly for one minute.

Effect: The Sea of Vitality can help improve many reproductive problems, including erectile dysfunction, premature ejaculation, low libido, infertility, and abnormal vaginal discharge. It also strengthens the immune system and the kidneys and helps relieve trauma. When you wrap your arms around your lover to give him or her a hug, try pressing your hands on this area.

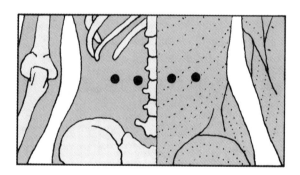

Sea of Vitality

Three Mile Point

Location: Four fingers' width above the inside of the ankle bone and one finger's width to the outside of the leg (the muscle should flex under your finger).

Stroke: Apply deep gentle pressure, gradually increasing the strength of pressure.

Effect: Pressure on this spot, which is also known as Three Yin Meeting, strengthens the reproductive system. If practiced regularly, acupressure here can, over a few months, relieve erectile dysfunction. It also promotes emotional openness and nurturing.

Sea of Intimacy

Location: Two to four fingers' width below the navel, as indicated by the three black dots in the illustration below.

Stroke: Have the receiver lie flat on his or her back with knees bent and feet flat on the ground. Press on the Sea of Intimacy so that your fingers sink at least one inch; maintain pressure for one to two minutes. Alternatively, press the edge of your hand crosswise under the navel, then slide it down toward the genitals. Another effective stroke is to massage the area in a circular motion thirty-six times.

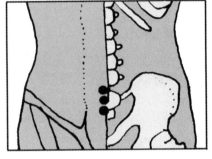

Sea of Intimacy

Effect: This acupressure point helps relieve erectile dysfunction and pre-menstrual syndrome.

MASSAGE AS FOREPLAY

When you are giving a massage that you intend as foreplay, use strokes that move toward the genitals, directing blood flow to, and thus increasing sensitivity in, that area. You needn't touch the genitals directly, nor avoid them, but simply include them in your stroking, without obvious sexual intent. Work from the upper body down, relaxing the neck, shoulders, and back before even approaching the pelvic region.

If you think massage may lead to intercourse and you intend to use a condom, be sure to keep massage oil away from the condom and the genitals. Massage oil and essential oils can degrade the structural integrity of condoms, rendering them ineffective as birth control or as protection against the spread of disease.

A lovely game can be made out of blindfolding your partner for a massage session. During the massage, use not only your hands but also a soft paint brush, silk scarf, or feather to stroke his or her body. Waft under your partner's nose some of the delicate, passion-inspiring essential oils described in Chapter 7. Slip a sweet, sensual food—a strawberry, a sliver of kiwi, or a strip of ripe mango, for example—into his or her mouth. Play soft music, a small chime, or a Tibetan bowl. Turn on all of your beloved's senses to awaken his or her entire being.

12

Hydrotherapy: The Waters of Love

ater, the mother of life, is not only a vital ingredient for life but also a powerful healer and a tremendous aphrodisiac. The sensuous feel of drinking it—water sliding down the throat, penetrating every inch of the body, filling every cell, nurturing the body—or bathing in it—the childlike feeling of weightlessness, the smooth rolling and flowing of it over the skin, the soaking of the skin, water pouring in through the body's outer layer—satisfies the human mind in a way that no other element of daily life can.

Except, perhaps, sex. That may help explain why sex, love, health, and water are such perfect complements of one another.

May you never thirst!

THE SACRED BATHROOM

If the bedroom is a temple of love, the bathroom is the altar of sensuality. Here we cleanse ourselves physically, emotionally, and mentally, so that we enter the sacred bed with washed body, fresh breath, and gentle mind.

The bathroom is so often a neglected space—cramped, cluttered, harshly lit, and often dirty. How much more uplifting and peaceful our homes would feel if the bathroom were, instead, a warm, inviting retreat from the world. Thankfully, it's not difficult to make it so.

First, examine the lighting in your bathroom. The bulbs should emit a warm light, not a harsh glare. If you have a window in the bathroom, leave it open to the air and natural light; if you need to cover the window for privacy's sake, install a light, filmy curtain that allows some natural light to filter through.

Install a night-light with a soft red or yellow bulb in a bathroom outlet within easy reach of the door. If you need to use the bathroom in the middle of the night, a night-light will not offend sleepy eyes to the same degree that bright overhead lights do.

The color of the paint or wallpaper in the bathroom should complement your coloring and complexion. For example, if you think you look good in blue, by all means, paint the bathroom blue. We spend a lot of our time in the bathroom looking in the mirror. Wouldn't it be great if we liked what we saw?

Not many of us actually enjoy cleaning the bathroom, but it's important to keep it impeccably clean. When the bathroom is clean, we are free to relax, refresh, and purify ourselves in it. Keeping the room clean will be much easier if you first reduce the clutter in it. Get rid of all the potions and lotions that you never or hardly ever use. Install doors on all cabinets and shelving so that when it's time to clean, you only have to wipe down the doors, not everything on the shelves.

Keep a small container of bath salts, a bottle of natural bubble bath, some of your favorite essential oils, and soft sea sponges near the tub. Just sitting there, they'll imbue the bathroom with their delicate aromas, and when it's time for a warm soak in the tub, you can add a scoop of bath salts, a splash of bubble bath, or a few drops of essential oil to the bath water for pure bathing delight.

BATHS FOR TWO

Bathing with a lover indulges the senses, but it's also good love-building therapy for a relationship. Bathing together promotes intimacy, erodes inhibitions, and can help partners develop a sense of tenderness and protectiveness toward each other. For new lovers, bathing together is a gentle way to get to know each other.

Time spent together in the bath can encompass much more than washing each other's hair and backs. Try reading to each other, drinking wine, listening to music, practicing deep-breathing exercises, stretching, singing (bathrooms usually have great acoustics), and making love. A joint bath can also be a good time to talk about some of the more difficult issues that you face; it becomes difficult to have an argument with someone when you're lying naked in his or her arms in a warm bath!

Of course, bathing together doesn't have to be limited to the tub. On occasion, comply with the 1960s' slogan "Save water—shower with a friend."

For a truly sensuous break from the everyday hustle and bustle, stay overnight at a spa or hot springs resort. Together indulge in soaking, steaming, and other water-based healing therapies; you'll come back feeling refreshed, invigorated, and thoroughly in love.

FOOTBATHS

If you're in the mood to pamper your partner, consider giving him or her the ultimate of honors: a sensual foot washing with scented waters. The feet are among the most sensitive and erogenous areas of the body, and a hands-on footbath is a lovely way to relax the mind and inspire desire.

Have your partner sit in a comfortable chair and place a towel under his or her feet. Fill a basin with warm water and add a few drops of an essential oil of your choice; if you have small fresh flowers, float a few blossoms in the water. Set the basin on the towel and gently place your partner's feet in the water. Use a soft cloth to gently wash each foot in turn; use a small cup to pour water over each foot from time to time. Linger over each toe and every other part of the foot, taking your time and allowing the experience to unfold leisurely. When you're done, pat each foot dry with a soft towel.

SITZ BATHS

Sitz baths are often recommended to increase circulation to the pelvic region. A sitz bath is nothing more than a shallow bath in which one sits upright. The water should cover the pelvic region but not rise above the navel.

Alternating hot and cold sitz baths can work wonders for the circulation. Take three minutes in the hot water, then two minutes in the cold water. Repeat three times. If you find the baths overheating, try applying a cold compress to your forehead. Afterward, wrap up and keep warm to keep that circulation moving.

A brief soak in a cold sitz bath increases circulation to the genital organs and stimulates the production of sperm and hormones. It is often recommended as a treatment for infertility, fibroids, cysts, and other reproductive problems. If cold water on the sensitive skin of your pelvic area makes you squeal, start with tepid water and gradually build up a tolerance.

Gem Therapy:
The Jeweled Romance

any people categorize gems and crystals as "New Age," but they have been used for thousands of years by a wide range of cultures, including Indian, Chinese, Egyptian, and Native American. Gems and crystals can have powerful healing effects upon the emotional and physical bodies. They've been used as transmitters and receivers in radios, computers, and other electronic equipment. In the same manner, they help humans receive and transmit energy. Granted, no gem by itself is going to save a rocky relationship. However, when combined with other loving ways of living, gems and crystals can be used to attract and reflect love and beauty on many levels.

USING GEMS

Because gems attract energy, they are most powerful when near the body. Hence, humankind has worn jewelry since time beyond recollection. A similar potency can be achieved by placing gems in a place of power, such as the relationship sector of the bedroom or a love altar (see Chapter 10). Gems can also be held during meditation, used as room décor, or placed on the body during healing treatments. Gem elixirs (available at some health food stores) are used in much the same way as flower essences (see Chapter 9).

When your lover must be away for an extended period, give him or her a small pouch containing a lock of your hair, a sprig of rosemary (for remembrance), and a small gem that attracts the energies you wish to bless your beloved with. Anoint the bag with a favorite essential oil, one that will arouse your beloved's memories of you.

May your love reflect the light of the Sun and the Moon!

CHOOSING GEMS AND METALS

We've lost much of our knowledge of the healing power of gems. Today we choose gemstones to match an outfit, to transmit a sense of sophistication, or because tradition dictates that stone *x* is appropriate for occasion *x* and stone *y* for occasion *y*. How much more powerful and evocative would the gift of jewelry be if the gemstone in the setting carried a heartfelt message to the receiver, speaking words of everlasting love, passion, constancy, faith, healing, or lust?

Remember: Gemstones are energy magnets, pulling to them and their wearer powerful earthly and spiritual forces. A gift of jewelry, then, is not simply an expression of generosity but a bestowal of power.

What sort of power do you wish to give to your beloved? Knowing the choices available will help you make a wise decision. Read on!

Agate

Agate opens the heart to love, diffuses anger, and promotes calm. It can help its user be more communicative with loved ones and accepting of difficult circumstances. It ranges in color from blue to turquoise.

Amethyst

Amethyst is governed by Aphrodite and carries a powerful vibration of love. Being violet in color, it combines the energies of blue (wisdom) with red (passion). Amethysts also offer protection from overindulgence and bestow strength and stability. Try wearing an amethyst necklace to bring the stone close to your heart.

Carnelian

Carnelian boosts both confidence and sexual energy, while at the same time counteracting lethargy. A shy lover who is slow to move into a relationship may benefit from carnelian.

Copper

Copper is the metal of Aphrodite. It helps purify the mind and the body. It is a very high conductor of energy and can increase the electrical impulses of the person who wears it. (However, you may wish to wear copper as jewelry only for limited periods, because it tends to discolor the skin.)

Diamond

Diamonds are ideal for solidifying lasting love. They intensify emotions, strengthen unity, and energize a more perfect state of awareness.

Emerald

Emeralds are associated with love and wisdom. They can help heal a heart that has been wounded, and they encourage self-expression and sincerity. Emerald is an excellent stone for healers to wear.

Garnet

This stone is associated with deep love and compassion. It can incite passion, encourage constancy, and help the user strive for higher ideals.

Gold

Gold helps attract, balance, and bring forth beauty. It is usually associated with masculinity and solar energy, and it is a powerful magnetic conductor.

Jade

Jade is used therapeutically to strengthen the kidneys, which govern sexual vitality. In traditional Oriental medicine, jade is used to prolong life and prevent fatigue.

Malachite

This beautiful green stone is used in Ayurvedic medicine to heal and strengthen the kidneys. It can help you purge old, negative emotions and become more open to love. If the emotions become too intense, take a break from wearing malachite.

Obsidian

Jet black obsidian is made from volcanic lava that has cooled very quickly. It aids in the release of stored emotions, particularly those resulting from sexual abuse. To use it, hold a piece of obsidian to the "third eye" at the center of the forehead while practicing deep breathing.

Pearl

Pearl is the stone of femininity and lasting love. Cleopatra herself is said to have drunk pearls dissolved in vinegar. Pearl can help you access deeper levels of emotion. It is associated with lunar energy and represents beauty, purity, and compassion.

Ancient Chinese Practice—Use a Stone to Strengthen Vaginal Muscles

In ancient China, the empress and the emperor's concubines were taught to strengthen their vaginal muscles by clutching a smooth stone within the vagina. This practice not only made the vagina both tighter and more elastic, giving a woman's partner more pleasure during intercourse, but it also made women more orgasmic. Women today can do the same. Find a small, smooth stone (the size and shape of an egg) of obsidian, jade, or rose quartz. Sterilize it in boiling water before the first use; subsequently, the stone can be cleaned with soap and hot water. In the morning, place the "egg" in the vagina, with the wider or larger end inserted first. Hold the egg in the vagina throughout the day. (The act of holding the egg is like a prolonged Kegel exercise.) To increase sexual chi, practice moving the egg to the left and right and up and down. When you tire of this or feel the need to move your bowels, or if the vagina becomes too moist to hold in the stone, remove the stone, rinse it off, and place it in a little medicine bag until you are ready to use it again.

Coughing, sneezing, and vigorous laughing can cause the egg to be expelled, so wear underwear when you are using the egg. The egg will *not* become lost inside you, but if you find it difficult to remove, squatting, bearing down, or jumping up and down should ease its passage. If you still cannot remove it, try simply relaxing your vaginal muscles; eventually the stone will descend.

Note that oddly shaped pearls are not as powerful as perfectly round pearls.

Rose Quartz

Rose quartz calms anger, promotes love, and helps heal grief and emotional wounds. Wear rose quartz (even while sleeping) when you are going through a difficult emotional period.

Ruby

Ruby helps those who lack self-love and enables the timid to have the courage to claim love. It has long been used therapeutically to improve circulation and heart function. It is associated with the sun, vitality, and power. Use this stone to increase energy and intensify love.

Silver

Silver attracts the feminine aspect of lunar energy. It has a calming effect on the heart center and promotes physical healing.

Tigereye

Tigereye has a glassy lustre that attracts attention. It boosts courage and helps strengthen the mind. If two people in a relationship carry a tiger eye, it can help them to connect telepathically.

Part 3

How to Be a Fantastic Lover

14

Improving Your Techniques

h. So you've decided that you *might* be interested in improving your techniques. Well, my friend, you've come a long way just to turn to this chapter. Many people are self-confident that they are already fantastic lovers, and many others are too timid to try experimenting with something new.

Now that you're here, I'll let you in on a little secret. The single best way to inject your lovemaking skills with true finesse and masterful expertise is this: Communicate with your lover. That's it. Really. It's not an earth-shattering pronouncement, but it can be a life-changing realization. Your partner isn't psychic, and even if he or she is psychic, he or she might not be adept at reading your mind. He or she will never learn to please you unless you speak up. Most lovers are too shy to speak openly and frankly with each other about what they do and don't like. Many are so taken with the notion of romantic passion that the thought of a "here's what I like" educational lovemaking seminar would horrify them. But I assure you, twenty minutes taken here and there to point out to your lover your likes and dislikes will be time well spent—and your lover will be forever grateful for the insight.

While you're having these honest discussions, practice tact. Rather than criticizing what you don't enjoy, commend what you do enjoy, and suggest new efforts. If you're trying to pull this information out of your lover, ask pointed questions. Queries such as "Does this feel good?" and "Is this better?" are more likely to get you the advice you want than "Tell me what you want me to do."

Above all, pay attention to your lover's body language. Moans, sighs, and smiles are all signs that your lover is enjoying what you are doing. If your lover pulls his or her pelvis slightly away, jerks, or suddenly tenses, you may need to lighten up.

Likewise, making sounds of delight and approval will encourage your lover to pursue techniques that work for you. Sounds of pleasure can become a signal between you and your partner that all is well. In fact, sounds of pleasure are often both arousing and a form of release. When lovemaking is silent, its pleasure is diminished.

HOW TO BE A GOOD KISSER

If sex can be likened to art, then kissing is like poetry. A kiss is the sweet, symbolic communication of our passion for another person. You might think that the true measure of our intimacy with a lover would be reflected in intercourse. As it turns out, kissing, not sex, is our most emotionally intimate expression of desire and love. Studies have shown that couples having relationship problems are more likely to neglect kissing than sex.

But kissing is far more than a rich emotional connection. It also has the potential to be incredibly arousing. The tongue, lips, and moist walls of the mouth are richly supplied with nerve endings. In Oriental facial diagnosis, the lower lip corresponds to the genitals and the upper lip to the brain's sex center; when the lips are stimulated, so too is sexual desire.

In Oriental tradition, kissing is a way to exchange chi and to encourage compassion. The lips and mouth correspond to the spleen and stomach; using the lips and mouth to kiss stimulates sympathy and compassion. The tongue corresponds to the heart and is highly charged with chi; stimulation of the tongue during kissing inspires joy.

> A flurry of soft, small kisses around the eyes, ears, and forehead make a lover feel adored.

> It takes twenty muscles to form a kiss. To strengthen your kissing ability, practice tongue exercises. Stick the tongue as far out and down as possible. Try touching the tongue to the nose, then the chin. Move it from side to side, reaching as far as you can.

Kiss with Love

The Golden Rule of Kissing: Let your kisses communicate love. When you kiss a lover, even casually, make it an expression of how you feel about him or her.

You don't have to be physically passionate with every kiss, but endowing each kiss with emotional passion will nurture, sustain, and enrich the love in your relationship. This visualization technique will help: Gather all your love, passion, and desire and visualize it radiating through your lips onto and into your partner. You may actually feel your lips tingle a bit! If you're not feeling particularly passionate, pause, breathe, and call up the memory of passion, even if just for a moment.

Let a kiss be a moment unto itself, not necessarily a prelude to sex but a sweet connection nevertheless. In fact, to keep your sex life vibrant, sometimes you have to step back from sex and revert to your "just dating" days. Decide with your partner that you will engage in no sexual activity other than kissing for two or three days. Allow yourself time to just make out. And above all, kiss with feeling. As heartfelt kissing fades to quick pecks on the lips, so, too, does passion in a relationship fade. One of the easiest ways to keep your love alive is to make *every* kiss count, as if it were the last one you'd ever give your beloved. A kiss with feeling takes no more time and just a bit more concentration than a quick peck. The payoff—enduring passion and a strong relationship—is enormous.

Kissing to Arouse

Kissing can be a potent and fun foreplay technique. The trick is knowing where your lover's most sensitive spots are and making good use of them, caressing the body with your lips in a way that promises more to come.

Generally speaking, the human body is most sensitive to stimulation in the following areas:

- Lips
- Ears
- Cheeks
- Eyelids
- Neck
- Palm of the hand

- Chest
- Navel
- Along the spine
- Lower back
- Buttocks
- Genitals

Of course, different people have different sensitivities, and over time those sensitivities can change. Explore your lover's body as if you were on a treasure hunt, mining those areas that elicit soft sighs, goose bumps, and the arching of the back that indicates high arousal.

How you kiss can be just as important as *where* you kiss. Shallow kissing gives the mind space to wander, to fantasize of the lovemaking to come and to feel the warmth and movement of the beloved's body. Deep kissing, also known as French kissing (although, interestingly, the French call it "English kissing"), initiates an escalation of passion. It is a rehearsal for sexual congress and provides an opportunity for a woman to penetrate a man. Deep kissing can be terrifically arousing, but the effect usually wears off quickly, and the longer you keep it up, the more it tends to seem just sloppy, rather than exciting. So use your tongue with delicacy. Don't force yourself into someone's mouth until you know that he or she enjoys—and is ready for—deep kissing.

When you're kissing to arouse, alternate between shallow and deep kisses. Brush your tongue against your beloved's lips. Kiss the upper and lower lips in turn. On occasion, suck gently on your beloved's upper lip, running your tongue over the frenulum, the small membrane that stretches from the inside of the upper lip to the gums just above the front teeth.

Some people enjoy having their lips bitten when they are aroused; ask your beloved whether he or she enjoys being bitten and, if so, whether you should use gentle or firm pressure.

If you're feeling daring, shuffle across a carpet and slowly lean in to your lover, allowing your lips to be the first point of contact. This "electric" kiss will cause sparks to fly, both figuratively and literally. Give hot and cold kisses, taking a sip of a cold or hot drink before pressing your lips to your lover's. In the heat of summer, pass an ice cube from mouth to mouth as you kiss. The cool, slippery surface can incite passion at a time when you might otherwise think it was just too hot to roll around in bed with someone.

When you kiss your lover's body, alternate between soft and vigorous kisses. Barely graze the skin with your lips, then practice deep kissing on the surface of the skin. Gently touch your lips to the skin and hum a little tune; the vibration can be stimulating. Lift your partner's hair and kiss him or her on the nape of the neck. Give a little lick, then pull back and blow warm breath upon it. Warm breath meeting cooling moisture at one of the body's most sensitive spots will have your lover melting in your arms.

Enjoy kissing in the beginning, middle, and end of lovemaking. Drive each other pleasurably wild with kisses!

Sweet Breath Is Essential

Your kissing quota is guaranteed to double if you have the sweetest breath your lover has ever tasted. (The opposite is also true.) Be sure to floss, and brush your teeth (include the tongue) twice a day. Keep a small tin of aniseed, cardamom seeds, cloves, and fennel seeds by your bed; suck on a pinch of this spicy-sweet mixture to freshly flavor your mouth.

If you suffer from chronic bad breath, take three chlorophyll capsules, eat a small handful of fresh parsley, or drink a glass of wheat grass juice every day. Have your teeth examined by a dentist. Monitor your diet; if you have difficulty digesting certain foods (dairy foods are a common culprit), you could develop bad breath after you eat them. And if you can't banish bad breath on your own, enlist the help of your health care provider.

MASTURBATION

Masturbation, or self-pleasuring, is an ideal way to find out what you find pleasing, so that, in turn, you can help a lover please you. Masturbation can help you overcome inhibitions, discover which parts of your body are most sensitive, learn to achieve orgasm, and, perhaps, become multiorgasmic. Masturbation is especially important when you are not in a relationship; not having a partner is no reason not to feel sexually alive and active. It can also be helpful in cases where your partner is absent, feels fatigued, has a lower libido than you, or is ill. For men that ejaculate more quickly than they'd like, masturbating can be an opportunity to practice delaying orgasm, so they can last longer with a partner.

The goal of masturbation is usually orgasm, but there's no need to rush headlong toward it. Masturbation is as much about making yourself feel like a sexually desirable and desiring being as it is about orgasm. Make a ceremony of it, no matter how small. Light a candle. Bathe luxuriously. Create a sacred space that is warm, private, and comfortable. Undress and look at yourself in the mirror. When we look in the mirror, we usually focus on those things that we don't like about our bodies. This one time, at least, focus on those things that you *do* like about your body. See and feel yourself as a desirable being. If you've never examined your genitals closely, do so. Women should use a mirror and part the labia to reveal the clitoris, vaginal entrance, and urethra. Touch yourself. Run your hands over your chest, navel, and hips. Pleasure yourself. Make love to yourself. Breathe deeply. Take your time. Experiment. Practice. Learn. Enjoy.

Over time, vary the methods of self-stimulation, learning to experience pleasure in a multitude of ways. Masturbate slowly, taking fifteen to twenty minutes to reach orgasm. When you are close to orgasm, stop, rest, and practice Kegels (see page 30). Try using lubricant. Most of all, enjoy this time of being available to yourself. Make lots of noise when you orgasm!

Masturbation during Sex

Though it may take some bravery, masturbating in front of your partner, and having him or her do the same, can be a tremendous turn-on. Watching your partner touch his her own body is the best opportunity you will have to find out what really pleases him or her. If your lover feels shy, hold him or her close to you, and help out by kissing and caressing your lover's face, neck, and upper body.

Masturbating while a lover holds and kisses you can be an extremely beautiful and tender form of sex. It is also a wonderful way for a couple to keep their sex life vibrant in times when one person is unable to participate or has a lower libido than his or her partner.

Too Much of a Good Thing

There are a thousand and one myths about the dangers of masturbating: "If you masturbate too much, your penis will fall off." "Nice girls don't masturbate." "You only have so much semen. You'll use it all up if you have too many orgasms." "You'll go blind." If you haven't heard these, I'm sure you've heard others. Most people see them for what they are, silly fabrications cobbled together to inculcate the human psyche with the idea that sex for pleasure is wanton or immoral.

But as with most things, too much masturbation can be harmful. A preoccupation with masturbation doesn't give you much incentive to go out and interact with people. If you feel isolated or shut out from the social world, you may turn to masturbation for relief. This can develop into a progressive downward cycle. Excessive masturbation may also prevent you from devoting energy to creative activities that stimulate the mind and please the spirit. It may also satiate—and thus dampen—your sexual desire, which can undermine the sex life you have with your lover.

According to Oriental tradition, *jing* is life essence in our bodies. It is present in blood, ova, sex hormones, and sex fluids. Menstrual fluid is a physical manifestation of jing in women. Sperm is a physical manifestation of jing in men. For men, excessive masturbation to the point of orgasm can cause a loss of jing and weaken sexual energy.

What's excessive? It depends. Some people have an abundance of sexual energy and may, in fact, need to masturbate every day in order to satisfy it. Others may find that if they masturbate more than once or twice a week, they lose interest in having sex with their lover. Take some time to find and maintain your own balance. Enjoy the pleasure of masturbation without guilt, but avoid excessive indulgence so that your sexual, social, and creative energies remain vibrant.

FOREPLAY

Foreplay is composed of anything that happens before intercourse that gets you "ready." It is truly one of the secrets to great sex. By activating the body's meridians, foreplay, in effect, activates the entire being, both internally and externally, and leads to fuller presence in the moment. Foreplay generates chi, invigorates yin, and calms yang. It also relaxes the body. (You can have much better sex when your body is relaxed than when it holds tension.) It decreases performance pressure, helps men develop stronger erections, and enables women to have better vaginal lubrication.

A Taoist truism says that foreplay "helps bring the waters to a boil while keeping the fire burning slowly." Man is compared to fire, quick to ignite and quickly extinguished. Woman is like water, slow to come to a boil and slow to cool down.

The most common complaint from women is that their partners do not engage in enough foreplay. The key to pleasing a woman is bringing pleasure to her slowly. There is a time and a place for wild, fast, hard sex, but if you're worried about your ability to please a woman, take your time. That includes a long, slow, unhurried session of foreplay.

Foreplay All Day Long

Foreplay can encompass much more than five minutes of heavy petting before intercourse. Indeed, you might say that foreplay is a way of life. Great foreplay constitutes a state of mind that ignores human fault, practices loving kindness, and acknowledges great joy in the everyday presence of a lover.

Foreplay can happen with words, looks, acts of helpfulness, shared activities, and physical affection. It starts when you open your eyes in the morning and look upon your beloved with love in your heart. It continues throughout the day, manifesting as dishes washed because your beloved didn't have time to do them, a smile shared as you head to the bathroom with toddler in tow and your beloved heads to the laundry with a heaping basket, or a hand held on the porch as you watch the evening pass. It does not end when you climb back into bed together, happy to be with this person for whom you care so dearly, but continues through the night, in stray caresses, shared breathing, and the warmth of the bed.

It's true that foreplay is important to sex. But it's also true that foreplay is important to a good relationship. Foreplay is an expression of love and affection that tells your beloved that he or she is an essential part of the joy you find in life.

The "Other" Erogenous Zones

Foreplay is exactly that: *For play.* Instead of having specific goals, play for play's sake. Don't just jump for the genitals! Neglecting foreplay is said to be akin to walking right past the host at a dinner party and helping yourself to the food before it has been served.

The entire body can be a playground for touch and sensuality. Every zone can be an erogenous one. We'll focus on those that are most energetically potent.

The Kidneys

In the tradition of Oriental medicine, the kidneys govern sexual vitality. Strong kidneys contribute to strong libido and sexual ability. To activate the energy of the kidneys, have your partner lie on his or her stomach. Place your hands in the small of his or her back and rock back and forth. This energetic massage can be particularly helpful in encouraging a sexually uptight person to relax.

The Ears

The ears not only are delightfully sensitive but also correspond to the kidneys. An Oriental proverb says, "In order to be a good listener, one must have strong kidneys." Massaging the ears can greatly increase sexual vitality. And as anyone who's experienced it will know, having your ears orally massaged—using the lips and tongue to nibble and delicately lick—can be an incredibly arousing experience.

The Palms and the Soles

The palms of the hands and the soles of the feet are extremely sensitive; the hands alone contain forty thousand nerve endings. The hands and the arms are extensions of the heart meridian. Stimulating them opens both the physical heart and the emotional heart to love.

According to reflexology, the entire foot is like a map of the body, each part of the foot corresponding to a portion of the anatomy. The uterus and the prostate correspond to the inside of the heel. The ovaries and the testicles correspond to the outside of the heel. The Achilles tendon correlates to the reproductive organs. Massaging the feet feels wonderful and can increase circulation to these and other parts of the body.

The Breasts

Women's breasts and men's breasts equally contain several acupuncture meridians, including the pericardium (the tissue surrounding the heart), the liver, and the stomach. They should be touched gently at first; as passion increases, the stimulation can become more vigorous. Many women find having their breasts squeezed, sucked, pinched, or otherwise overstimulated before they are sufficiently aroused to be very agitating. Be aware that a woman's breasts may be especially tender before her menses; approach them more gently at that time.

THE PLEASURES AT HAND: GENITAL MASSAGE

A couple can regularly engage in foreplay just for the joy of building sexual energy, feeling pleasurable sensations, and connecting. Foreplay doesn't always have to end with intercourse. Genital massage can be an erotic alternative. Just relax, enjoy the experience, and be willing to return the favor!

For Her

The golden rule with a woman is patience. Caress her abdomen, hips, and thighs before arriving at the genital area. Touch the inner thighs, mons pubis, and vaginal lips. Stroke the pubic hair. Warm and calm the area by placing your entire hand over the closed lips and rubbing in a circular motion; this also gently stimulates the clitoris.

The labia majora (the fleshy outer lips) are less sensitive than the clitoris but still respond to touch. The hidden inner sides of the labia minor (the inner lips) are richly supplied with nerve endings. Part the labia and tap along the insides of each. Gently pull down on both sets of labia, gradually increasing pressure. As your partner becomes aroused, tenderly part the labia and slide your fingertips up and down over the inner labia, using long, slow movements that just barely touch the clitoris at the top of the stroke. Wait for the woman to part her legs and invite you to touch her before going any further.

Place the three middle fingers over the vagina and gently press and rub in a circular motion. Your partner will let you know when her clitoris is ready to be touched by opening her legs more, raising her pelvis, or pushing against your hand. Wait to be encouraged, as the clitoris is highly sensitive and touching it too soon can cause your partner to pull back from you. The clitoris spends most of its life tucked away behind a hood and protected by the labia, making it supersensitive when it comes out to play. Many women want their clitoris stimulated directly only when they are about to have an orgasm.

Make gradual teasing circles around the clitoris. Draw the circles smaller and smaller until they are about the circumference of a quarter, and occasionally brush against the clitoris. Touch the hood, base, and sides of the clitoris. Because the clitoris is not self-lubricating, overstimulation can cause dryness and pain, so proceed cautiously and use a lubricant if needed. If a circular rubbing motion seems to make your partner uncomfortable, try a gentle pulsing movement. Some women may prefer to have pressure on the inner labia rather than directly on the clitoris.

After your partner is very aroused, roll the clitoris between the fingers, at a pace of about one cycle per second. If she is well lubricated, slide a finger or two inside the yoni while keeping up the clitoral stimulation. If she wants you to lie close to her while you're doing this, you'll have to use just one hand—fingers inside the yoni, thumb stimulating the clitoris. If you find this difficult, ask her to touch herself, while you lie close and continue to stroke inside the yoni.

Use your fingers to create sensuous circles inside the vagina. Massage around, as if the vagina were the face of a clock, stroking at one-hour intervals until you have circled "the clock." Try this at different depths. For many women, twelve o'clock is the most sensitive and six o'clock the least. Begin gently, then stroke more vigorously as orgasm approaches.

For Him

As with genital massage for a woman, begin with foreplay. Touch the man's inner thighs and stomach, building his desire. Tease him. See if you can get him erect and wanting more without making genital contact.

The secret to great manual sex for men is warmth, lubrication, and a snug fit. Use lubrication on both hands. (Botanica Erotica sells several types of lubricants; see Resources.) On occasion, use bubbly mineral water to give a fizzy genital massage.

The most sensitive parts of the penis are the glans (the skin at the tip of the penis) and the rim of the glans, also known as the coronal ridge. The seam of blood vessels on the underside of the penis that runs from the shaft to the scrotum can also be supersensitive. The tiny slit at the tip of the penis, called the urethral meatus, is worthy of attention, as is the sensitive frenulum, also referred to as the F spot, at the underside of the penis where the shaft and the glans meet.

Tap gently over the lingam (the penis) like gentle rain, and tap the head of the lingam against your palm or against your partner's tummy.

Use one hand to hold down the skin at the base of the penis, thus exposing more nerve endings higher up. Work upward with a massaging stroke, making a twisting motion when you reach the head of the penis and continuing to "sculpt" the shaft in an uninterrupted flow. When massaging in a downward stroke, use a more open grip so that the penis isn't shoved into the torso.

The penis is actually rooted two to four inches inside the body. Massage deep and gently into your partner's root. Try rubbing, tapping, and pressing the area.

Make a "fire" by gently rolling and rubbing the lingam between your hands, starting at the base and working upward.

Throughout, avoid choppy, jerky movements. Vary the pressure and speed of hand motion. Stay in contact, leaving at least one hand on the penis if you need to replenish your lubricant.

Try fifteen strokes on the shaft, including the head, then fifteen strokes on the shaft only. As your partner's arousal builds, do thirty strokes on the shaft and five on the head. Start slowly and gently; increase speed and pressure as he becomes more excited.

Most men love having their testicles handled—carefully, of course. Cupping the scrotum while giving a genital massage may add to your partner's pleasure. Try holding the testicles together in the palm of your hand and using the fingers of your other hand to make gentle figure-eight movements over the scrotum. Roll the testicles gently and slowly between the thumb and forefinger of your hand, with a light touch of the fingertip pads.

Another method of testicle massage begins with making a ring with your fingers around the scrotum where it attaches to the groin. Gently squeeze the thumb and forefinger together and pull the scrotal skin taut, though not tight. With the fingertips of your other hand, make small and big circles, using a gentle, tickling touch.

INTERCOURSE

Like other aspects of sex, good intercourse requires good communication between lovers. Instead of performing, be present with yourself and your beloved. Focus on what *is* happening rather than what isn't. If you're thinking "I wish he/she would . . . ," you're missing out on the passion of the moment, the potential for a true connection of souls. If you've communicated well in earlier lovemaking sessions, your lover will know what does and doesn't please you.

Most important, have realistic expectations. Lovemaking isn't designed to give you an orgasm worthy of a fireworks display every single time you have sex. It's a means of connection, of communicating your love to a person, of opening to him or her. Great sex is that which throws open the door to your emotional and spiritual consciousness, draws you deep inside yourself, and lays you bare before your lover, all at the same time. Mind-blowing orgasms are certainly a part of that unveiling. (See Chapter 15 to learn how to improve your orgasmic ability.) But stronger still is the deep connection of love, manifested in the physical joining of two lovers.

Intercourse as Therapeutic Massage

Intercourse is an opportunity to give each other a mutual acupressure treatment. As the yoni and lingam connect, each stimulates the other's internal organs to bring about health benefits. For women, shallow thrusts into the yoni massage the point that corresponds to the kidneys, building sexual vitality. For men, the penis contains more than one acupressure point, each corresponding to a particular body system. (See illustrations below.)

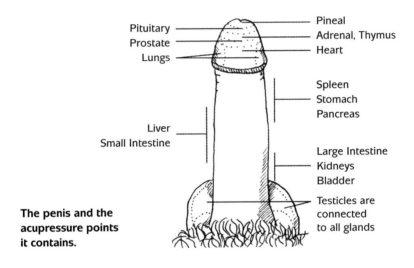

The penis and the acupressure points it contains.

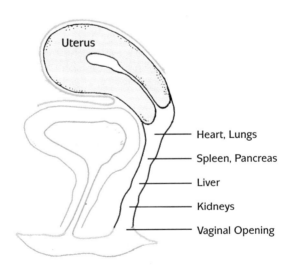

The vagina and the acupressure points it contains.

Sexual Positions

Sexual positions, also known as sexual asanas, ideally enhance genital connection, leading to a deeper union, enhanced pleasure, and a more soulful bonding. The descriptions that follow address the classic sexual asanas. The point is not to instruct you in their usage—I'd guess that most people have tried almost all of them—but, rather, to offer you some ideas for improving your connection in these positions and to encourage you to expand your palette of lovemaking techniques. Being comfortable with four or five different styles allows you to make love in a way that suits your mood and energy at a particular moment. For example, you and your lover may rely on one method of lovemaking when you are tired and another when you want to strengthen your emotional connection.

But more important than any position is the energy that flows between the two people engaged in lovemaking. Without that heart-to-heart connection, it's not possible for any physical configuration, no matter how simple or how contorted, to bring true satisfaction.

Love each other well!

Missionary

This is an excellent position for strengthening an emotional connection, because it allows for verbal communication, eye contact, kissing, deep penetration, and a heart-to-heart connection. Simultaneous orgasm is most likely to happen with this position.

The woman lies on her back and the man lies over her, facing her, with his pelvis between her thighs. Placing a pillow under the woman's hips raises the vagina and allows deeper penetration. To trigger the G spot while making love in the missionary position, press down on the woman's belly just above the pubic mound.

The missionary position impedes manual stimulation of the clitoris. One solution is to have the woman lie with her pelvis at the edge of the bed. The man lies over her but keeps his feet on the floor. This position allows greater freedom of movement between the lovers in the pelvic area.

Woman on Top

The man lies on his back, and the woman straddles him, facing forward. Many women find that this is an excellent method for achieving orgasm; they can control the depth of penetration and stimulate their clitoris against the man's pubis or manually. For good G-spot stimulation, the woman should try sitting on top of the man facing his feet.

Men with large stomachs, men who have trouble maintaining erection, elderly men with heart trouble, and pregnant women will find that the woman-on-top method of lovemaking is easier than most others.

Some men claim that they have more control over ejaculation when their lover is on top of them. Women may tire easily in this position, but men won't. Women must be careful to avoid bending and hurting the erect lingam. To avoid putting too much pressure on the man, the woman may want to support some of her weight with her arms or knees.

Coital Alignment Technique

Coital alignment can be accomplished in the missionary or woman-on-top position. It requires that the man push his body a couple of inches forward over his partner's head. This alignment encourages his pubic bone to rub against her clitoris, creating a greater likelihood of female orgasm. Rock up and down rather than in and out, and maintain constant contact between the pubic bone and the clitoris.

Side by Side

The couple lies side by side facing each other. She has one leg between him and one leg bent over his hips. By turning her hips, she can increase or decrease the depth of penetration. This position requires minimal effort and allows for kissing, facial contact, and heart-to-heart connection.

Spoons

The couple lies side by side with the man spooning the woman's backside and penetrating her from behind. This position allows for a snug fit, and the man can massage the woman's breasts and clitoris to bring her to orgasm. This can be a relaxed way to make love; it's not uncommon to fall asleep this way, still connected.

Worker's Position

The woman lies on her back, and the man lies on his side, facing her. She then lifts the leg closest to her partner and places it over his pelvis, giving the man's penis access to her vagina. This position allows the man to suck on the breast closest to him. It's a low-effort lovemaking position that's useful when couples are exhausted but still want to connect.

X Position

The man and woman sit facing each other, with their legs extended, and hook up (you know what I mean). They clasp hands and move them to their sides, then lie back. They are joined by the hands and genitals and with a bit of movement can sustain delightful pleasures. This is an excellent position for outdoors sex, where you can lie facing the sky.

Wheelbarrow (Butterfly)

This lovemaking method enables deep genital contact. The woman lies on her back. She lifts her buttocks off the bed as far as possible and the man stands as he enters her. Place pillows under the woman's lower back to help support her. She can also wrap her legs around her lover's waist.

Rear Entry

The woman supports herself on her hands and knees. The man kneels behind her and enters from behind, pulling her buttocks toward his pelvis. For deeper penetration, the woman should lift her bottom or lower herself onto her elbows and lower her head.

Another possibility is for the man to sit in a chair with the woman on his lap, facing the same direction, so that his chest is pressed against her back.

This position allows for G-spot stimulation and deep penetration. It also enables the man to manually stimulate the woman's breasts and clitoris during penetration, which can help her achieve orgasm. The rear-entry position is ideal for men who have difficulty inserting their lingam because of weak erection. However, it can make ejaculatory control more difficult.

Woman Lying on Stomach

The woman lies on her stomach with her buttocks raised by pillows, while the man lies over her, laying his chest on her back. This is considered a very easy method of lovemaking. Although penetration is not deep, the couple is connected along the entire length of their bodies.

Sitting in a Chair

An upholstered chair without arms is ideal for this asana. The man sits in the chair, and the woman straddles him, facing him. She sets the pace by lowering and raising herself with her feet.

This position is not strenuous for the male and can help him control ejaculation. It can also be used in cases of male paraplegia.

Standing

Though standing during intercourse can be fatiguing, it increases muscle use and can quickly build excitement. The couple stand facing each other. The woman lifts one leg, turning it slightly outward, to provide the penis access to the vagina. Once the man has entered her, he can lift the woman by putting his hands under her thighs as she holds on to his neck. She can cross her legs behind his back to contribute to her support. If the woman is pressed against a wall for support, thrusting can be more vigorous.

Yab Yum

Yab yum is Sanskrit for "Father Mother" and refers to this position's union of the father and mother aspects of god. The couple sits facing each other, with the woman sitting on top of the man's thighs. The legs can be bent or straight. For comfort, try placing a pillow under the woman's buttocks to help support her.

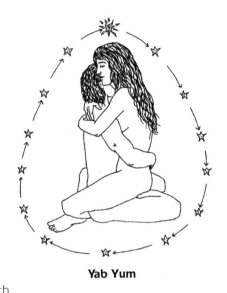

Yab Yum

This position is excellent for building a heart-to-heart connection and practicing synchronized breathing (see page 36). Some people consider it an excellent technique for mystical sexual experiences, because the spines of the lovers are aligned with heaven and earth.

Kneeling *yab yum* is an alternative. The man kneels down and pulls his beloved onto his thighs, facing him. She wraps her legs around him.

New Techniques

Certain lovemaking techniques are known to build sexual energy, increase arousal while delaying orgasm, strengthen orgasms, and nurture the cosmic union between two lovers. Feeling skeptical? Try one. You just might be surprised.

Eye Contact

Staying connected by looking into each other's eyes during intercourse allows for a deep union of souls.

Sets of Nine

Sets of Nine is a delightful technique for providing a restorative massage to the vagina and penis. The man makes nine shallow thrusts into the vagina, using just the head of the penis, then one deep thrust. Next is eight shallow thrusts and one deep thrust. Then seven shallow and two deep, six shallow and three deep, and so on, until he makes nine deep thrusts. Then he reverses the process—one shallow and eight deep, two shallow and seven deep, and so on, making his way back to nine shallow thrusts. At no point should he withdraw the penis completely.

Try doing at least three complete sets of nine before allowing either partner to orgasm. The woman can also deliver Sets of Nine from a position on top of the man.

Kegel Congress

Kegels can add great pleasure to intercourse and possibly strengthen orgasms. To start, both man and woman should perform one Kegel per thrust. (For Kegel instructions, see page 30.) With the inward thrust, both should relax the pubococcygeus muscles. With the withdrawal, both should tighten the pubococcygeus muscles. This is a wonderful way to practice Kegels together!

Kegels can also constitute an alternative to thrusting. The man should thrust forward and then relax as the woman squeezes him with her love muscles. This Kegel exercise helps bring a woman closer to orgasm while giving a man endurance.

Karezza

Karezza (pronounced ka-ret-za) is derived from the Italian word for *caress.* This technique is said to have originated in Persia (now Iran). Also known as *coitus reservatus,* it involves making love without orgasm, thus conserving the male seed. Ahead of time, the couple agrees to avoid orgasm. Intercourse consists of long periods in which the couple is united but passive, mostly lying still. They connect in a relaxed fashion, experiencing calmness and bliss; it is a magnetic connection with love, rather than lust, as its focus, allowing the couple to enjoy the union of their souls.

ORAL PLEASURES

Oral love play can provide special pleasures and deepen intimacy. It can be a prelude or an alternative to intercourse. It can even be a form of birth control, allowing two people to enjoy each other without risking pregnancy. And performing fellatio on a man gives him a unique opportunity to let go of performance anxiety.

As is often the case with other forms of sex, it is best to refrain from jumping right in. Instead, use foreplay to excite your beloved. It is delicious to kiss, lick, and nibble the abdomen, navel, and insides of the thighs, working slowly toward the genitals. Making eye contact as you tease and then begin to give oral pleasure can help build an especially profound sense of connection between you and your lover.

It's best to start out slow and increase the speed of stimulation gradually. Avoid biting or rough play—you're working in a sensitive area! Keep up the same technique for a while, allowing sensations to build, instead of changing your stroke every few seconds.

Receivers of oral pleasure should let their partner know when he or she is on the right path by moving their hips, caressing their partner's hair, and making appreciative sighs and sounds. In the same vein, it's important for givers of oral pleasure to let their lover know that they are enjoying what you are doing. Be demonstrative, showing a desire for and relish in what you are doing.

Many couples enjoy orally pleasuring each other simultaneously. (It's called "69" because of the way the two digits fit together, head curled into the other's tail.) Others enjoy just taking time out to savor the feeling on an individual level. Whatever your preference, be willing to give as well as receive. If you want to get more, give more!

> If you and your partner are not in a monogamous relationship or have not both tested negative for STDs, use dental dams or nonlubricated condoms when performing oral sex.

Playful Dimensions

Hot and cold can add pleasurable dimensions to oral sex. Fill your mouth with ice water or warm it with hot tea before going down on your partner. Or slip a spicy mentholated herbal lozenge into your mouth. Let it dissolve partially so that your mouth is well coated before taking in your beloved. Chewing a pinch of cardamom seeds will yield a similar sensation.

Fellatio

> **Euphemisms for Fellatio**
> * Playing the flute   * Sucking a mango   * Mouth congress

If the man is standing or sitting in a chair, sit, kneel (on a pillow or mat), or crouch in front of him. If he is lying down, stretch yourself out next to or on top of him. Begin with light foreplay, stroking and kissing his belly, thighs, and chest. Give the lingam gentle butterfly kisses with your eyelashes. Roll it against your cheek, your hair, and your breasts.

Start by kissing and licking his belly, thighs, and chest. Make him hunger for you to take his sex into your mouth. Sucking on the lingam when it is soft gives you the opportunity to feel it grow in your mouth. Use your lips to cover your teeth so you don't scratch or bite the penis.

When you're ready to begin, flick the head of the lingam lightly with your tongue. Gradually progress to longer strokes of the tongue, as if you were licking an ice cream cone. Use both the top and underside of the tongue. Swirl your tongue around the head, first clockwise, then counterclockwise.

Try giving gentle "lip pinches." Use your teeth to gently comb over the glans. Lick. Nibble. Suck, moving the lingam in and out of your mouth. In general, short intense sucks are better than long ones. When taking the lingam in your mouth, try twisting your head in a gentle corkscrew motion to give even more stimulation. Try humming with the lingam in the mouth to create stimulating sound vibrations. Run the tip of your tongue over the little hole at the top of the penis. If your man has been circumcised, pay special attention to the scar that marks where the foreskin used to be. If your mouth becomes tired, use your hands for a while.

The thick cord running the length of the penis's underside is an important erogenous zone. Try lightly flicking your tongue over this ridge; this is called the "butterfly flick."

To perform the vacuum technique, which most men find extremely pleasurable, take in as much of the lingam as is comfortable. Make a seal around the shaft with your lips and then pull your head back, creating a vacuumlike effect.

You can hold the base of the lingam with one hand to keep yourself from taking it too deep in your mouth and setting off the gag reflex. If you can, hold the lingam so that your knuckles point downward; this brings extra stimulation to the sensitive underside. Use your free hand to caress the root of the lingam, the scrotum, the perineum, the buttocks, and the area from the navel to the pubic bone.

It's been scientifically proven that men are especially turned on by visual stimulation. Of course, the long and successful history of "men's" magazines could have told us that. In any case, when performing fellatio on a man, keep in mind that visual stimulation can be as important as physical stimulation. Don't hide what you're doing. Consider performing in front of a mirror. And try giving oral pleasure in various states of undress. You might be surprised by what really turns on your man!

Overcoming the Gag Reflex

Many people have a difficult time taking the penis into their mouth without gagging. If this is your situation, try breathing through your nose and keeping the penis to the side of the mouth, rather than the center, where it is more likely to stimulate the gag reflex. Make a fist around the base of the lingam, with your little finger resting on the pubic bone, to give yourself a buffer zone against gagging.

Another quick trick is to gargle beforehand with 1 cup of warm water to which 1 teaspoon of salt has been added. The salty mixture has an astringent effect, temporarily tightening the loose tissue at the back of the throat that initiates the gag reflex.

It's Not a Marathon

When a couple is having intercourse, a man often tries to pace himself, wanting to last long enough to please his partner. However, during oral sex, the giver can tire easily, so this is not the ideal time for a man to show off his endurance.

If you're the giver and your jaw becomes fatigued, rest your head on your lover's thigh or encourage him to lie on his side so that you can curl in a semi-fetal position near his hips, where the penis is at mouth level. Take brief breaks and kiss his thighs and abdominal area. Prolonged sucking and caressing can be fatiguing for muscles unused to such work. When you need a rest, use gentle tongue and lip stimulation on the ridge along the underside of the shaft, where the penis is particularly sensitive.

Ejaculation

When a couple is familiar with each other, a man's partner may be able to tell when he is about to ejaculate by his body language. One giveaway, for example, is that a man's testicles ascend when orgasm is imminent. A man can also let his partner know when he is close to orgasm through some prearranged signal.

A man should not take it for granted that his partner wants ejaculate in the mouth. Some people simply don't enjoy it, and a man should restrain himself and ejaculate outside the mouth until the invitation is extended. In addition, unprotected oral sex puts the giver at high risk of STDs; it should not be undertaken until both partners are sure that they are free of disease. Very arousing oral sex can be had while using a nonlubricated condom.

If the relationship is monogamous and the partners have taken reasonable measures to determine that they will not transmit STDs to each other (see Chapter 22 for more information), then barrier-free fellatio becomes a possibility. If you don't want to swallow your man's ejaculate, keep a towel close by, so that you can spit the ejaculate into it. If you do want to swallow the ejaculate, your man may feel thrilled that you would lovingly accept his fluids. For a woman, swallowing ejaculate is a wonderful opportunity to receive yang fluids as a chi tonic. As your man is erupting, place your lips as far down the shaft as possible, and stay there calmly until orgasm is complete.

The average ejaculate contains between five and thirty-six calories. It is composed mainly of protein and fructose but it also contains vitamins C and B_{12}, potassium, sulfur, and zinc. Sperm makes up only 2 to 5 percent of semen.

The flavor of a man's ejaculate can be a reflection of his health. Normal semen tastes sweet. If a man's ejaculate tastes excessively sweet, he may be eating too much sugar. A bitter flavor may indicate the presence of toxins, drugs, or other chemicals in the body.

If the ejaculate tastes truly unpleasant, the man should eliminate coffee and alcohol from his diet for several weeks and stop or reduce smoking, as well. He should add to his diet plenty of celery, pineapple, strawberry, mango, and citrus fruits. If the semen continues to taste unpleasant, the man should consult with a health care provider, because he may have an undiagnosed infection.

Cunnilingus

Euphemisms for Cunnilingus
- Sipping at the vast spring
- Drinking from the jade fountain

For women who have difficulty achieving orgasm, oral sex may be the answer. However, the technique of performing pleasurable oral sex on a woman is often considered one of the Great Mysteries. It's actually not that difficult, provided you know where to look and have the patience to be persistent.

You may find that cunnilingus is most pleasurable when the woman lies on her back, while you lie with your head between her thighs. Your woman may also enjoy kneeling over you, again with your head between her thighs.

Patience, Patience, Patience

The vagina is primarily an internal organ. All that's left outside the body are the lips, or labia. Even the clitoris, the most sensitive part of the vagina, is hidden under a hood. All this tucking away is done for a reason: A woman needs to be approached slowly and gently. In most cases, she needs to be warmed and teased and aroused before she can even come close to orgasm. So reread the section on foreplay, beginning on page 173, and put some of those tips into practice.

Gently separate the outer and inner labia with your tongue. Use your tongue to massage the sensitive inner sides of these lips, moving up and down as well as in and out. In general, the woman will derive more pleasure when you use your entire tongue than when you use just the tip, although you may want to switch back and forth occasionally.

Once a woman is aroused and has become "wet" (her vagina has started to secrete sexual fluids), the clitoris should become the focus of your attention. The clitoris is the primary vehicle of pleasurable sensation, but you must be careful not to overstimulate it, because it can be very sensitive. The tip and underside of the clitoris tend to be the most sensitive areas; some women find oral stimulation in that area orgasmically divine, while others cannot tolerate it. If your partner suddenly jolts, it may be that you have stimulated her too intensely. If this happens, retreat for a bit, using your lips rather than tongue until your woman warms up again.

Using one type of pressure for a minute or so, rather than switching from spot to spot and stroke to stroke every five seconds, often yields better results. Some women prefer hard pressure, others soft pressure, and still others variations of the two. There's no way to tell for sure unless you just flat-out ask. Your beloved will most likely be glad to tell you.

Orgasm Secrets

If you're having trouble bringing a woman to orgasm while giving oral pleasure, try the following:

- Push up on the mons veneris, the mound atop the pubic bone. This can expose the underside of the clitoris at a new angle.

- Insert one or two fingers into her vagina; simultaneous stimulation from outside and inside the vagina can often bring a woman to orgasm.

- Use a free hand to stimulate your lover's nipples. There is a direct nerve connection between the nipples and the clitoris, and taking advantage of it can bring a woman great pleasure.

Eliminating Vaginal Odor

The vagina normally smells slightly musky and tastes somewhat salty. If a woman's vagina has an unpleasant odor or taste, she should eliminate coffee, alcohol, and dairy products from her diet for several weeks and stop or reduce smoking, as well.

The woman should consider adding chlorophyll, which is a natural deodorizer, to her diet. Wheat grass juice is loaded with chlorophyll; taking a shot of it daily may help eliminate odor. She should also eat plenty of dark green, leafy vegetables. Acidophilus capsules used as a vaginal suppository could also help. (See page 331 for more details.)

As further treatment, the woman should bathe regularly in a tub; add 7 drops of lavender essential oil to the bath water. Lavender essential oil is not only pleasantly fragrant but also mildly antiseptic and antiyeast. In addition, it's very mild, which makes it safe to use in close proximity to the delicate mucous membranes of the yoni.

If the unpleasant odor or flavor persists, the woman should consult with her gynecologist to rule out a possible infection.

ANAL PLEASURES

There's a certain "taboo" surrounding anal sexual pleasures. For some, anal stimulation is highly erotic; for others, it's uncomfortable and deflates arousal. Whatever your preference, it's important to recognize that no person should be coerced into anal sexual pleasures if he or she isn't comfortable with them. If you haven't experienced anal sex but would like to try it, talk to your lover about it. If he or she seems open to the idea, read through this chapter so that you're both comfortable with the precautions anal sex requires.

Anal pleasuring can make lovers more open, trusting, and receptive to each other. It also can be very opening emotionally, if it is done slowly and respectfully. For some people, it is just as likely to bring up fears or tears as it is to bring arousal. In this case, use the intimacy created by anal pleasuring to support your lover. Hold your beloved close, remind him or her that you are there, and allow him or her to undergo the cleansing of stored negative emotions in the safety of your arms.

> Anal sex carries a much higher risk of disease and infection than vaginal and oral sex do. It may expose you to fecal matter, which can be a risky business. In addition, the walls of the rectum are made of very thin tissue that tears easily, exposing you to blood. Therefore, safety precautions are a top priority for anal sex. Any item—penis, finger, sex toy, and so on—inserted into the anus must be washed before it is introduced to the mouth, the vagina, or any other part of the body. For anal stimulation and intercourse, latex gloves and condoms, respectively, are imperative.

Anal Stimulation

The body becomes aroused from front to back, so wait until your lover is very aroused before attempting to stimulate the anal area. Unless you and your partner engage regularly in anal pleasuring, it's usually a good idea to ask him or her for permission before approaching the anal area. Always allow your lover to feel in control of what you're doing.

Begin by moistening a finger with lubricant. Press or massage around the perineum (the area between the anus and the genitals) and over the outside of the anal opening. Imagining the anus as the face of a clock, press gently yet firmly at all the hourly positions. Ask if any of these areas feel sensitive. Most people find that the regions around ten o'clock and two o'clock are the most sensitive.

Stimulation of the outer rim may satisfy your lover, so that you will not proceed any further. But many people find anal penetration to be highly erotic. Ask permission to enter your beloved's vulnerable place. If he or she assents, replenish the lubrication on your finger. Insert it just slightly into the anus. Hold it still until the area becomes relaxed before proceeding.

For most people penetration itself is not a means of stimulation. Some movement is required. Initially, practice only circular and front-to-back, "come hither" motions inside the anus, avoiding in-and-out and side-to-side motions until your lover is quite comfortable with anal stimulation. If your initial stimulation is well tolerated, try using the fingertip to gently stretch the anal entrance. Keep the heel of the hand gently pressed against the perineum.

To put your lover at ease, try simultaneously touching a familiar place of pleasure, such as the penis, vagina, or clitoris.

When you are ready to exit the anus, your lover may find it more comfortable to ease away from your finger slowly, rather than having you pull it out.

The Male G Spot

The male version of the G spot is sometimes identified as the prostate gland stimulated from the back of the upper wall of the anus. It feels like a firm mass about the size of a walnut. Stimulation of the prostate gland in this manner can trigger a rapid and intense orgasm, particularly if the stimulation takes place during intercourse or oral sex.

Anal Intercourse

Before attempting anal intercourse, practice finger penetration until the receiver is quite comfortable with it. Thrusting of the penis in the anus should not be as deep or as rapid as it is in the vagina; remember, anal tissue is quite thin and fragile, and with rough play it can tear. Be sure to use plenty of lubricant on the penis to avoiding damaging the anal tissue.

To protect against the spread of disease, a condom *must* be used for anal intercourse. Use an extra-strength condom, which is better suited to the rigors of anal sex, and spread lubricant over the outside of it.

Above all, when having anal sex, be kind, be patient, and be safe.

AFTERPLAY

After lovemaking, men and women may have a refractory period during which additional stimulation can be uncomfortable. This period can last from thirty seconds to several minutes to an hour or more.

I believe that this hypersensitivity is a physical defense against the reawakening of passion. After orgasm, the body is suffused with sexual energy. Blood is flowing freely through the circulatory system, endorphins are sweeping through the body, and the mind is released of tension. To fully absorb the influx of energy, the body must rest.

After love, indulge in this time of sweetness. Allow your mind and body to relax and soak up the sexual energy of your beloved. Enjoy the feeling of peace. Sleep if you can, for lovemaking often calls forth the bliss of deep slumber. If you don't want to sleep, recognize that the urge to sleep will pass in a few minutes, and you will soon feel invigorated.

Some people feel energized after orgasm and may need to expend some creative energy before they can rest. Others cry after experiencing a powerful release, and they may be frightened by a perceived loss of control. Be there for your lover, supporting the emotions and energies that arise. If lovemaking has taken your beloved to a distant emotional place, speak tenderly, using his or her name, calling him or her back to you. Stay together with your beloved, maintaining physical contact.

If you must get up, sustain the mood and the flow of energy by sharing an activity. Eat together. Go for a walk. Enjoy some music. Garden. Rejoice in a blessed soul connection with your partner. Allow your lovemaking to be an opportunity to create more love and bliss. Bask in the afterglow!

15

Controlling and Intensifying Orgasms

he word *orgasm* is derived from the Greek *orgasmos,* meaning "to grow ripe, swell, or boil over." The French refer to orgasm as *le petit mort* or "the little death." In Sanskrit, orgasm is referred to as *urja,* meaning "power" or "nourishment." It has been described as an altered state of consciousness, resplendent with waves, colors, light, warmth, and energy. It is said that the first mystics had glimpses of enlightenment at the moment of orgasm.

Sounds like pretty powerful stuff, right? Not sure whether you've ever experienced an orgasm quite that cosmically altering? With a little help, you could. Read on.

ORGASM FOR WOMEN

As a woman becomes aroused, blood begins to circulate more quickly through the body. Her face and chest may flush. Her muscles may tense, her breasts swell, and her nipples become erect. Blood engorges the labia, which become red, swollen, and sensitive. The labia secrete mucus and become moist and slippery. The clitoris becomes hot and swollen.

At the point of orgasm, muscles in the lower third of the vagina, which is suffused with blood, contract involuntarily in intense, rhythmic, pleasurable waves of spasm. For most women, the contractions take place at a rate of about one every 0.8 seconds. Muscles in the rectum may contract in sync with the vaginal muscles. Veins and arteries in the pelvic area constrict. Her entire body may become rigid as the spasms continue, then totally relax as they subside and pulse, circulation, and breathing slow down.

ORGASM FOR MEN

As in a woman, arousal in a man causes blood circulation to speed up. Increased blood flow to the penis combined with the constriction of arteries and veins that allow outflow of blood from the area causes the penis to become engorged with blood. Muscles in the penis contract, causing it to become erect. The man may become flushed on the lower abdomen, face, neck, chest, forearms, and thighs. He may sweat. The testicles draw closer to the torso as orgasm approaches. The glans may darken.

The prostate and Cowper's glands may secrete a few drops of pre-ejaculate, a clear alkaline fluid that lubricates the urethra, easing the passage for sperm, and neutralizing any acid that may remain from the passage of urine.

When ejaculation is inevitable, the prostate contracts rhythmically, squeezing out the alkaline fluid that forms the base of semen. The seminal vesicle empties its contents into the urethra, also contributing to the seminal fluid. Sperm travels from the epididymis through the prostate and into the urethra. A series of powerful muscular contractions causes the forcible ejection of 2 to 5 ml of semen, which spurts from the tip of the penis.

Ejaculate that dribbles rather than shoots out may indicate a weak prostate. Ejaculation of only a very small amount of semen may indicate digestive or muscle weakness. Semen that is clear may indicate a digestive disorder.

After ejaculation, the muscles at the base of the penis relax. Blood flow from the penis is restored, and penile tissue once again becomes flaccid.

INTENSIFYING ORGASMS: THE SIX-STEP PROGRAM

Achieving great orgasms involves a commitment to good health, a few simple techniques, and an awareness of how to use sexual energy. Many of the sexual techniques outlined in Chapter 14 and the love therapies presented in Part 2 will carry you a long way on the path to intensifying orgasms. The six steps outlined here, if undertaken with goodwill and patience, can help speed your progress.

1. **Support sexual energy.** Read through Chapters 4, 5, and 6, which deal with supplements, nutrition, and herbs that can be used to build and support radiant sexual health. Work with your lover to make some of the practices suggested in these chapters a part of your daily life. Try the recipes. Live healthfully. Great sex will soon be yours—naturally.

2. **Exercise the love muscles.** Practice Kegels to strengthen the muscles that control orgasm. See page 30 for more information.

3. **Be patient.** Allow yourself (or your lover) to achieve a high level of arousal before permitting orgasm. Approach and pull back from orgasm at least three times.

4. **Relax.** Let the orgasm come to you; don't force it by tightening up your muscles.

5. **Stimulate the nipples.** In women, the nipples share a nerve response with the clitoris; stimulating the nipples just before orgasm brings an almost leaping response of arousal from the clitoris. Men's nipples are also very sensitive to arousal just before orgasm. For either gender, try rolling the nipples between your fingers or taking them into your mouth.

6. **Visualize.** Just before orgasm, visualize sexual energy building in the genitals, radiating up the spine, and streaming into all the cells of your body. You may see that energy as a current of light or a stream of color. Breathe deeply, and direct the energy in and around your connected bodies. See yourselves enveloped in dazzling rainbow light!

Beyond these simple tricks, recognize that having great sex involves an opening of the mind. In order to be more orgasmic in love, we should be more orgasmic in life—laugh more, love more, and experience the rush of life!

CONTROLLING ORGASM

In order to approach and then pull back from orgasm (step 3 of "Intensifying Orgasms"), we must learn to control orgasm.

The normal heart rate is 70 beats per minute; during orgasm, heart rate reaches 140 to 180 beats per minute. Breathing rate also increases, from an average of 12 breaths per minute to thirty or forty. One of the best ways to establish control over orgasm is to breathe more deeply and fully. Slowing down the breath promotes calmness and increases sexual stamina.

When you get to the brink of orgasm and want to pull back, you need to disperse the highly charged energy that suffuses your body. Try doing Kegels while pressing the tongue to the roof of the mouth. (In the tradition of Oriental medicine, touching the tongue to the soft spot of the palate helps delay ejaculation by causing energy to flow down the front of the body to the navel.) Look up or roll your eyes several times in each direction.

To delay ejaculation in a man, reach between his legs and grasp his testicles. Circle the top of the sac with your thumb and forefinger while gently tugging the testicles down, away from the torso.

Men should relax enough to allow an erection to deflate somewhat at least once every twenty minutes. This allows healthy circulation of blood to move into the genitals.

PREMATURE EJACULATION

Premature ejaculation, also referred to as rapid ejaculation or involuntary ejaculation, is sometimes defined as the inability to delay ejaculation long enough to satisfy one's partner 50 percent of the time. Other sexologists define it as ejaculating within thirty seconds, not being able to maintain vaginal contact for at least two minutes, or not being able to endure fifty strokes. Many definitions!

In fact, research has shown that the biological response of most men is to ejaculate within two minutes of vaginal penetration. Because few women can reach orgasm within that time, most men could be qualified as having premature ejaculation and could please their partner by learning to delay ejaculation. As an alternative solution, if a man learns to please a woman by oral or manual stimulation (see Chapter 14) before initiating intercourse, she may not care how long he lasts, which can relieve the pressure on him.

Causal Factors

Stress can often be a factor in premature ejaculation. Do your best to slow down in other aspects of your life and you may find that you'll slow down in the bedroom as well.

Premature ejaculation can also be related to diet. Excess consumption of salt and animal products (meat, dairy, and eggs) can be excessively stimulating, contributing to overexcitement. Try cutting down on salt and switching to a vegetarian diet. Prostate malfunction may also be a contributing factor. See "Improving the Health of the Prostate" on page 349 for tips on supporting healthy prostate functioning.

In traditional Oriental medicine, premature ejaculation is considered a deficiency of the kidneys and can be aggravated by chronic fatigue (yin deficiency), stress, and digestive problems. If yin is deficient, the body cannot retain yang and sex will be completed quickly. Herbs that can help nourish the kidneys include cubeb, damiana, dendrobium, hops, ho shou wu, nutmeg, oatstraw, and saw palmetto; look up these herbs in the Herbal Compendium in Chapter 6 to find out how to use them.

Delaying Ejaculation

A good exercise to practice delaying ejaculation is to masturbate with a dry hand. Concentrate on the sensations. Stop before you lose control and ejaculate. Breathe. Continue, starting and stopping as needed, for fifteen minutes. Get a sense of what strokes and rhythms affect you. Have a goal of being able to arrive at the brink of orgasm without going "over the edge" three times within one fifteen- to twenty-minute session. When you can masturbate in this fashion reasonably well, try it with lubrication.

Because a second erection generally lasts longer than the first, some men masturbate two to four hours before intercourse. Other preintercourse tricks include urinating (a full bladder will increase the desire to ejaculate) and practicing the Taoist exercise called The Deer (see page 31) just before making love.

During intercourse, try to keep your buttock and pelvic muscles relaxed. When you feel the urge to ejaculate, breathe deeply and contract the abdominal muscles. Exhale deeply after the urge passes. A female partner can help you survive the moment by minimizing or stopping movement and relaxing the vaginal muscles.

Also useful in preventing premature ejaculation is for the man to practice Kegels, both during intercourse when the urge to ejaculate occurs and as a general endurance-building exercise. Kegels have an effect similar to that of the squeeze technique (see below) and are totally safe as you are in control.

Another simple technique is to dip the lingam in a bowl of cold water until the erection decreases by about half. As you do this, continue to caress your partner to keep the momentum of sexual energy flowing.

Some men find wearing one or two condoms decreases sensation enough to prevent premature ejaculation. You could also try applying Clove Anesthetic Balm (see below).

Clove Anesthetic Balm

Combine 1 or 2 drops of clove essential oil with 1 or 2 ounces of sesame oil. When massaged onto the genitals, this aromatic oil brings a warm glow and has a pleasant numbing effect, which can allow for prolonged lovemaking.

Highly regarded is the "squeeze technique," which helps retrain the brain to control ejaculation. Before the man reaches ejaculation, either thumb is placed firmly on the frenulum (the area underneath the head of the lingam). The first and second fingers are placed on the ridge of the glans, on the lingam's upper side, or pressing back to front at the base of the lingam. This must be done firmly enough and with constant pressing, until the urge to ejaculate has passed. Repeat for up to twenty minutes. The man must have an empty bladder before engaging in the squeeze technique. Though this is a well-known practice, it is not a first choice and is potentially dangerous.

ORGASM WITHOUT EJACULATION

Orgasm is defined by contraction rather than fluid release. For men, it can be achieved without erection or ejaculation. In some cases, those who have experienced nerve injuries and lost genital sensation may still experience orgasm in other parts of their bodies, including the face, lips, necks, chest, arms, and back. A whole-body orgasmic experience might include the back, legs, toes, neck, face, and brain.

Though ejaculation is often referred to as "coming," "going" might be a more appropriate term for it. Ejaculation moves energy outward and can leave a man fatigued, both physically and emotionally. In the Taoist tradition, one drop of semen is considered to have the life force of one hundred drops of blood. By not ejaculating, a man can conserve the powerful energy that orgasm produces and turn it toward the development of creativity and spiritual growth. This is also an important tenet of Tantrism, a religious practice that, simplistically put, combines meditation and sex.

> Some Oriental traditions encourage avoiding ejaculation one time to strengthen essence, two times to improve vision and hearing, three times to cure diseases, and more than that to have a religious experience.

A plant that does not go to seed outlives the other plants in its surroundings. Likewise, a man who conserves his seed may stay healthier than he otherwise might. This is particularly true for older men or men with a weak constitution; for them, having orgasm without ejaculation can provide a reservoir of energy and vitality to draw from. In general, strong, young men can ejaculate freely without risk of harm to their health. Even these strapping men, however, would benefit from occasionally drawing in the strength of orgasm, rather than sending it out with ejaculation.

It's important to ejaculate after vigorous sex to avoid undue stress to the prostate gland. However, when lovemaking is relaxed, avoiding ejaculation should not be stressful.

If a man does not ejaculate, semen is broken down and reabsorbed by the body. It is not a waste product that needs to be eliminated. In fact, semen contains many hormones and proteins that can stimulate the pituitary gland and other creative brain centers. When analyzed, semen and brain matter have many similarities, including a rich supply of magnesium, phosphorus, sodium, and chlorine. If not ejaculated, the nutrients from semen are carried to every part of the body, including the brain.

Preventing ejaculation during orgasm requires practice. One of keys is breathing more slowly, through the nose and into the belly, which will slow down heart rate. Feel the sexual energy released by orgasm being drawn up the spine, into the brain, and throughout the entire body.

To learn more about ejaculatory control, take a tantra workshop.

INABILITY TO ORGASM

Inability to orgasm during sex is a common female complaint; it is rarely experienced by men except when they have a physical dysfunction. Between 10 and 15 percent of women claim that they have never reached orgasm, and a great majority of women have had difficulty with it at one time or another. If you have never had an orgasm, don't give up hope! Consider yourself preorgasmic, rather than nonorgasmic.

Most women experience their first orgasm through self-stimulation. Learning to orgasm by masturbation can teach a woman what brings her pleasure so that she can better inform and help her partner please her. If you've never had an orgasm, make a commitment to practice self-stimulation every day for two to three weeks. (See page 171 for advice.) If after this time you still haven't experienced masturbation, try using a vibrator. If that, too, doesn't help, consider consulting with a sex therapist. The American Association of Sex Educators, Counselors, and Therapists (see Resources) can help you find one in your area.

If you can experience orgasm through masturbation but have trouble achieving it consistently or during sex, read on.

Identifying Anti-Orgasm Factors

There are a variety of physical and emotional factors that can impede orgasm. Most can be resolved through lifestyle changes or natural therapies or with the help of a sex therapist.

Histamine Deficiency

People who have a hard time achieving orgasm may suffer from inadequate histamine release. Most of us recognize histamine release as the result of an allergic reaction. However, histamines are also contributors to the intensity and frequency of orgasms. They cause dilation of capillaries and contraction of smooth muscles. Supplementation with niacin may contribute to histamine production. See Chapter 5 for more details.

Dietary Imbalances

A diet that is overly rich in saturated fats may make a person less sensitive physically, which can have a detrimental effect on orgasmic ability. Fats have a tendency to insulate the body and decrease nerve sensitivity. They also impair circulation, which is vital to arousal and orgasm. Try eating more fruits, vegetables, and whole grains; avoid fatty meats, fried foods, and heated oils.

Supplementation with niacin has the opposite effect of a high-fat diet. It increases circulation and sensitivity to touch and can, in some cases, intensify orgasms. See Chapter 5 for more information.

Emotional Armoring

Be sure you are not withholding enjoyment in bed as a way of having power over your lover, or because you feel resentment toward your lover or fear losing control of yourself. Make sure you feel entitled to pleasure and are comfortable with your body. Communicate openly with your partner about your feelings and physical needs.

If you have doubts about your emotional openness and suspect it might be having a negative effect on your orgasmic ability, consider consulting with a sex therapist.

Intellectual Distancing

You may have difficulty reaching orgasm if you pay too much attention to the process instead of becoming lost in the connection. That's a tough challenge for women who have difficulty achieving orgasm; of course you're going to be concerned about the process if you're concerned about your potential for orgasm. Try to relax into the lovemaking. Follow the advice given in the next section, but when it comes to the time of stimulation, do your best to enjoy the pleasure of connection rather than worrying about the outcome.

With the strength of their dual connection to body and mind, flower essences may be able to help those who experience emotional armoring and intellectual distancing. See Chapter 9 for more information.

Achieving Orgasm during Sex

If you know that you're able to achieve orgasm but your lover is unable to bring you to orgasm, it's time to step up to the plate. Be responsible for your own orgasm. Stimulate yourself, or show or tell your partner how to do it. Wonderfully intimate lovemaking *with orgasm* can be had if a woman will take the initiative to touch herself during intercourse.

In fact, most women need clitoral stimulation to achieve orgasm, and it may be difficult for a lover to provide that, depending on the position, during lovemaking. Only about 30 percent of women are able to achieve orgasm from penetration alone, and many of those find that the orgasm is intensified if the vaginal pressure is accompanied by clitoral stimulation.

It may be that only certain positions can bring orgasmic release. During intercourse, consider woman-on-top (see page 179) or rear entry (see page 181) positions, which offer G-spot stimulation. If you're most comfortable in the missionary position, try the coital alignment technique (see page 180), which can bring the man's pubic bone in contact with the clitoris. Many women find that the only method by which their lovers can bring them to orgasm is oral sex. If you are lying on your back, try placing pillows under your pelvis to arch the clitoris toward better stimulus. Find out what works and communicate with each other about it.

Try massaging your breasts, or having your lover do so, when you have reached a just-preorgasmic state of arousal. Bear down with the vaginal muscles upon your man's penis or fingers. Make sounds of pleasure as you approach orgasm; sometimes they can help you reach it.

Women are often more orgasmic around ovulation. If you're tired of trying and failing to reach orgasm, you may want to designate the week or so after menstruation ends, when ovulation usually happens, for the lovemaking sessions in which you make a real effort to achieve orgasm. And remember: It's not necessary to experience orgasm every time you have sex. Expecting to do so is unrealistic and sets you up for disappointment. Whether or not orgasm occurs, we can still experience extreme levels of pleasure and a deep connection with a lover.

FEMALE EJACULATION

When deeply stimulated, some women emit a fluid that is called, technically, female ejaculate but that is more poetically named in various traditions *amrita* (Sanskrit for "immortal"), moon flower medicine, or female nectar. In the Hindu tradition, female ejaculation stimulates a tremendous release of kundalini, or life force, which travels up the woman's spine and down to her yoni, blessing the woman, her lover, and the planet.

About one in ten women are able to achieve female ejaculation. The ejaculate is a spurt of fluid released through the urethra. It is believed to originate from the ductus paraurethrales, also known as the Skene's glands, which are vestigial organs located behind the vaginal wall. (Not all women have them.) The liquid is similar to prostatic fluid, containing high levels of glucose and acid phosphatase.

Female ejaculation seems to occur more frequently with the second or third orgasm. It is most likely to be achieved when a woman's G spot is stimulated.

THE G SPOT

The G spot is named after Ernest Grafenberg (1881–1957), a German gynecologist practicing in the United States who published a paper about it in 1950. Yet long before Dr. Grafenberg's time, the G spot was known to Indian, Chinese, Roman, and Japanese cultures, as well as many others, I'm sure.

The G spot can be felt from inside the vagina, 1½ to 2 inches up on the front of the vaginal wall. The tissue there is spongy and has many tiny folds that causes the skin to feel bumpy. A woman can reach inside herself to feel it, but it's usually a stretch, so it can be difficult to stimulate the G spot during masturbation.

This G-spot area is richly endowed with nerve endings, ducts, and glands. Stimulation of the G spot can contribute to a woman's arousal, and when a woman is aroused, it swells to about the size of a dime. The swelling appears to help protect the bladder and urethra from injury and stress during intercourse.

To find a woman's G spot, have her lie on her back, knees apart and slightly elevated. Insert a finger into her yoni, with the pad of the finger facing up, and feel for the pubic bone at the front of the vaginal wall. There's a small "ledge" of sorts there, and the G spot is just above it. Fold the finger forward in a "come hither" motion and you'll find it. You'll know you have it when the pressure of your finger causes the woman to feel an urge to urinate, even if she has just urinated. If you keep up the pressure and the woman relaxes into it, the urge to urinate will pass, transformed into sexual pleasure.

The most effective way to stimulate the G spot manually is to apply prolonged steady pressure and to stroke gently from left to right over the spot, to pulse against the spot, or to massage the spot in a circular motion. Gently pushing down on the mound of Venus (mons veneris) with your other hand can enhance your lover's pleasure.

To stimulate the G spot through intercourse, the best positions are rear entry, man on top (with the woman's feet on his shoulders), *yab yum,* woman on top, or woman lying on her stomach. (See "Sexual Positions" on page 179 for explanations.)

It is not unusual for G-spot stimulation to trigger a release of emotions or memories. Be there to comfort and support your partner if this occurs. Allow the surfacing of old emotions to be healing and cleansing.

THE A SPOT

Stimulation of the A spot, more formally known as the anterior fornix or fornix vaginae, can trigger women to have copious vaginal lubrication and also, as has been reported, multiple orgasms. The A spot is located above the G spot on the front wall of the vagina, between it and the cervix. To locate the A spot, moisten two fingers, insert them into the vagina, and find the G spot (see previous section). Continue upward until you find the cervix, which feels like the end of a nose sniffing down into the vagina. Bring your fingers back down to a spot about one-third of the way down from the cervix to the G spot. If you can find a smooth area of the wall here that your lover says feels sensitive, you've found the A spot. Try stimulating this spot in a circular or up-and-down motion.

16

Adapting to Special Circumstances

During a lifetime, many special circumstances arise that can affect sexuality. Menstruation, pregnancy, illness, and disabilities can all challenge the sexual habits you and your lover are accustomed to. You may sometime find yourself with a lover whose large or small build must be accommodated. And as you grow older, you'll find that your sexual needs and abilities also grow and change, requiring new ways of thinking about sexuality.

Humans are sexual beings. Thankfully, we are also amazingly adaptable. When we find ourselves faced with circumstances that challenge our sexual comfort zone, we figure out a way—usually with great speed—to handle them. This chapter offers ideas for handling some of the more common "special" circumstances.

LOSING YOUR VIRGINITY

You will always remember your first time, so do your best to create a moment worth remembering, with someone worthy. If you and your lover are both virgins, learning together and teaching each other can be one of the sweetest pleasures on earth.

An intact hymen is an indicator of virginity for a woman, but a woman who is a virgin may not necessarily have an intact hymen. Athletic pursuits and even tampon use can stretch and even break the hymen. If the hymen has not been broken, the woman may experience some pain and bleeding the first time she has intercourse. If you're concerned about the potential for bleeding and staining the sheets, place a thick towel underneath you.

Allow for plenty of time, privacy, and freedom from interruptions. The missionary position is a good choice for your first time, because it allows good eye contact and verbal communication. Make sure that the woman is sufficiently aroused and has good vaginal lubrication before penetration. Penetration itself should be slow and gentle, and thrusting should also be gentle. Prolonged pressing and pushing can be painful for a woman during her first experience with intercourse.

Women may not experience orgasm during their first time, though most men will. Men tend to orgasm very quickly their first time.

Do all you can to make the experience of losing your virginity safe and pleasant. It can color how you feel about sex for years to come.

SEX DURING MENSTRUATION

Many people enjoy making love during a woman's menstrual time. However, sex during menstruation is considered taboo by Native American, Jewish, and Arab cultures, among others. And traditional Oriental medicine cautions that having intercourse during the menses "brings illness to both men and women."

These warnings come for a reason. Having sex during menstruation does carry risks, although they are relatively low. The vagina is normally acidic, which helps destroy invading bacteria. During the menses, it becomes more alkaline, which can leave a woman susceptible to infection. In addition, menstrual blood washes away some of the naturally occurring mucus that covers the cervix, making it easier for infection to penetrate her reproductive system.

Intercourse during menstruation can push menstrual flow back into the uterus and fallopian tubes, which can be a contributing factor to endometriosis. For this reason, those who are prone to reproductive disorders or who have been diagnosed with endometriosis should avoid intercourse during menstruation. If you do engage in intercourse, the woman–on–top position has a lesser likelihood of pushing blood back inside the woman's uterus.

But you'll notice that these warnings apply only to intercourse, in which the penis penetrates the vagina. Manual stimulation does not offer any risks to the woman, nor does oral sex. (If you practice oral sex, use a dental dam or other barrier device to prevent oral-blood contact.)

Beyond sex, it's a loving gesture to be especially considerate of a woman just before and during her menstrual time. For many women, menstruation causes cramps, bloating, fatigue, and mood swings. So treat your beloved with extra kindness, speak softly, do your best to minimize stress, and try to avoid being demanding yourself.

SEX DURING PREGNANCY

Kidney chi works to support pregnancy and can give women a healthy, beautiful glow. Some women also experience an increase in libido due to increased blood flow to the pelvic region. Others experience a decrease in libido due to hormonal changes, fatigue, morning sickness, and the body's desire to conserve kidney chi.

Sex during pregnancy is a given. It's nine months, after all! However, there are some precautions. Women who have a history of miscarriage may be cautioned to refrain from intercourse in the early months, until the pregnancy is well established. Some physicians may suggest that lovers use a condom during pregnancy, because hormonelike substances in ejaculate may trigger contractions and pose a risk of infection for the woman. And when a woman is late in her pregnancy, intercourse should be approached gently; recent research indicates that rough, vigorous intercourse late in a pregnancy may be linked to premature labor and respiratory disease in newborns. Approached gently, sex generally will not induce labor unless it is already about to begin.

Avoid intercourse if you experience uterine bleeding or vaginal pain, or if your water has broken—that is, the membrane enclosing the amniotic fluid has ruptured.

Massage, oral sex, and manual sex can all become a greater part of lovemaking during pregnancy. Anal intercourse is not recommended during pregnancy because it causes the rectum to be pushed against the vagina, which could initiate labor.

Sexual positions that can accommodate a woman's belly during the later stages of pregnancy include woman on top, rear entry, and spooning. Of course, no position is prohibited; you just have to get creative.

Most women can resume intercourse six weeks after giving birth; healing after a cesarean section may take longer. When you do resume lovemaking, go very slowly and gently and use lubrication.

Breast-feeding does inhibit fertility, but it doesn't prevent it. If you have sex while you're breast-feeding, use contraception. When my husband was only six weeks old, his mother became pregnant with his brother! Are you ready for two babies in diapers?

New parents must work hard to find alone time and keep flourishing the love that brought them together in the first place. Make an effort to show and share love for each other.

SEX FOR SENIORS

So long as you're in good health, sexual activity need never end. Despite the physical changes that accompany aging, sex and orgasm can feel as pleasurable as ever for older folks. Some couples say that the older they get, the better sex gets. Indeed, sex itself can ease the aging process. Research has shown that humans are likely to die at younger ages if they are deprived of touch. And practicing nonejaculatory sex (see page 198) can help a man build sexual chi and improve his energy level.

As men age, they often are able to extend the duration of erection, experience longer periods of high sexual excitement, and become more emotionally open with others. They will also experience viropause, the male version of menopause; sperm production normally ends while men are in their seventies.

Older men may need longer and more direct stimulation to achieve erection. Their erection may be less firm and less upright. The scrotal sac may not bunch up during arousal as much as it used to, and testicle size may diminish. There may be less ejaculate and less ejaculatory force. Frequency and desire for masturbation may also decrease. A man's refractory period (the time needed between ejaculations) may also become longer. As throughout their lives, however, men's sex drive will be highest in the morning; that's often a good time for older couples to make love.

For women, fear of pregnancy ceases to be an issue after menopause. However, women can become pregnant during menopause, so be sure to use contraception for twelve months following a woman's last period. After the menopausal drop in estrogen levels, blood flow to the vagina may diminish, and vaginal walls may become thinner and less elastic and may take longer to produce lubrication. The vagina may shorten in width and length. However, these changes do not equate to changes in sensitivity or orgasmic ability. In fact, women often become more orgasmic as they age.

Staying physically fit can help older men and women stay sexually active. At this stage of life, exercise and a healthy diet are more important than ever. Avoid habits such as smoking and heavy drinking. Be aware of the side effects of any medication you are taking. Many prescription drugs decrease libido and sexual ability; if your health care provider prescribes one of these medications for you, ask him or her if there are alternative treatments that do not diminish libido as a side effect.

When you do make love, spend some extra time on foreplay, allowing the woman adequate time to accumulate sufficient vaginal lubrication. Use a lubricant if necessary. Mutual masturbation and oral sex may become increasingly easier than intercourse. Laugh and play together to keep your love alive.

SEX DURING ILLNESS OR WITH DISABLEMENT

Like everybody else, people with a disability have a fundamental need for intimacy. Whether a disability is temporary or permanent, it does not preclude the possibility of being sexual with a lover. If you have any particular concerns, discuss them with your health care provider. Otherwise, get creative and experiment!

It's important to let go of the belief that sex must be spontaneous. A love exchange with a person who is ill or disabled often requires some planning. At the very least, you'll need to discuss what hurts and what can and cannot give pleasure. You may also need to gather props to help minimize discomfort and maximize the connection and pleasure that you feel. The stronger partner should take the more dominant role, although the disabled partner may need to take the responsibility of communicating his or her needs.

If your lover is in pain, allow him or her to lie, sit, or stand in a position that is most comfortable, and find a lovemaking position that accommodates it. (See "Sexual Positions" on page 179 for suggestions.) Use chairs, pillows, or whatever else is needed to cushion vulnerable areas such as the knees, neck, or back. Make love slowly, while the stronger partner visualizes sending healing energy into his or her beloved.

A person with heart disease should avoid lying facedown or on his or her left side. These positions increase pressure on the heart.

If a disability is new, begin slowly with manual pleasuring and work up to intercourse only when you feel ready. If illness or an accident has caused loss of sensation in the genitals, it is very possible that other areas of the body will increase in sensitivity and enjoy stimulation. If intercourse isn't the ticket, there are plenty of other possibilities. Pleasure can be experienced by all parts of the body! Keep communication open, and share with each other your thoughts on what hurts and what feels good. The council of a marriage or sex therapist may be helpful.

A loving, open-minded partner is a true blessing for anyone, but especially for a person with a disability. Let your partner know that you appreciate his or her help and patience. Allow your inner radiance to shine.

SIZING DIFFERENCES

Men and women come in all different shapes and sizes. Many men take great pride in the size of their penis, but the size of one penis compared to others matters little. All that matters is the fit of penis and vagina together. Vaginal tissues are elastic and can accommodate almost any size. In certain situations, however, couples have to make some adjustments to ensure a pleasurable fit. Finding ways to fit together is part of the challenge—and delight—of a loving relationship!

When the Penis Is Larger than the Vagina

When the lingam is much larger than the yoni, engage in plenty of foreplay and use plenty of lubricant. If possible, bring the woman to orgasm with manual or oral stimulation before penetration, so that the vaginal passage is naturally lubricated.

The man should insert the lingam in stages and proceed slowly until the woman is receptive. She should breathe slowly and relax. If the penetration becomes uncomfortable, the man and woman should lie motionless for a few seconds, until the vagina has adjusted to the penis. The woman may enjoy the woman-on-top position, because it gives her greater control of the penetration.

If the lingam is too long rather than too wide, try having intercourse with the woman lying on her back, with her legs straight and close together, and the man on top, with his legs placed outside hers. This position prevents overly deep penetration. The side-by-side position may also be comfortable.

When the Penis Is Smaller than the Vagina

In this situation, both the man and the woman should practice Kegels (see page 30). For her, the Kegels will strengthen the muscles that contract around the penis, holding it to her. For him, the Kegels will increase endurance, allowing him to last longer and maximizing his ability to please the woman through intercourse.

As always, penetration is not the best method for bringing a woman to orgasm, and in this situation, especially, it rings true. The man may wish to pleasure the woman with manual or oral stimulation before intercourse.

To encourage a tight fit during intercourse, employ sexual positions in which the woman's legs are kept close together. For the missionary position, place pillows under the woman's back to allow the man deep access in the pelvis. The woman might try wrapping both legs over the man's shoulders, which will constrict the yoni and allow for deeper access. Other beneficial positions include rear entry and woman on top, leaning slightly backward.

17

Practicing Safe Sex

irth control has become a ubiquitous symbol of Western civilization. Condoms are available at every corner store. The Pill, as it's called, is covered under some health care plans. Even the Roman Catholic Church, known for its firm stand against birth control, advocates and teaches "fertility awareness," a natural method of avoiding pregnancy. The pregnancy rate in the United States is dropping, and it's not because we're having less sex. Contraception enables family planning, and more and more people are choosing to have fewer children, and to have them later in life.

But pregnancy isn't the only risk of sex. Sexually transmitted diseases (STDs) are among the most contagious diseases known to afflict humankind. They are widespread and often asymptomatic (meaning that they don't produce symptoms), and their effects range from irritating to debilitating to deadly.

Certain types of contraception are supposed to safeguard users against these infectious diseases. But if contraception is so widely available, why, then, do STDs continue to spread so quickly? Hepatitis C and HIV—each a very scary disease—have infected vast populations of people. Genital herpes affects one-sixth of all sexually active persons. The numbers are staggering.

The answer is twofold:

1. Most sexually active persons don't know enough about STDs. They don't know how they're spread, what their symptoms are, or which activities can and cannot put them at risk of contracting an STD.

2. Most sexually active persons resist using contraception to its full potential.

They focus on preventing pregnancy rather than STDs, even if they are having sex with multiple partners. Many pursue this reckless path because they believe that "safe" equates to "boring." Not so, my friends. Proper use of contraception can be as much a part of foreplay and arousal as kissing. You just have to open your mind to it.

PROTECTING YOURSELF AGAINST STDS

There are two categories of contraception: contraception that protects you against pregnancy alone, and contraception that protects you against STDs and pregnancy. If you are not having monogamous sex, you must employ the latter.

If you and a partner want to have a monogamous relationship, get tested together. Practice safe sex for six months, using STD-prevention contraception, and remain monogamous. Get tested again. If the results are negative, then enjoy each other freely and delightfully, using a non-barrier method of contraception if you wish to avoid pregnancy.

No method of contraception, whether against pregnancy or STDs, is absolutely foolproof. But it sure does cut down your risk. Remember: It takes only one unsafe sexual encounter to expose yourself to a disease that could stay with you for life.

Minimizing Risk

Risk-free activities include:

- Abstinence;
- Hugging;
- Massage (see page 150);
- Kissing, so long as neither person has gum disease or open sores in the mouth;
- Genital massage (see page 175), so long as your partner does not have any genital sores;
- Masturbation.

Low-risk activities include:

- Monogamous sex with a partner who is free of disease.

High-risk activities include:

- Vaginal intercourse without use of a condom;

- Anal intercourse without use of a condom;
- Sexual activity in which semen, vaginal secretions, or blood are exchanged;
- Oral-anal contact;
- Moving an item (including a finger) directly from anal to genital contact, without washing it first;
- Oral sex without use of a barrier, such as a condom or dental dam;
- Sharing sex toys or douching supplies;
- Sexual activity with an infected partner without use of proper safeguards to prevent transmission of the disease.

Safeguards against STDs

The only sure way to eliminate your risk of contracting an STD is abstinence, plain and simple. For most of us, that's not an option. The following methods, however, can substantially reduce the STD risk.

STD Testing

Before engaging in unprotected sex, you and your partner should undergo a thorough physical, including examination and testing for STDs. Practice safe, STD-prevention sex for six months and go through another round of testing before abandoning your concerns about potential STD infection.

Condoms

Condoms, including female condoms, are key to STD prevention. They should be used for vaginal, anal, and even oral sex. (Condoms designed for oral sex come in many flavors.) They should be used once and then discarded.

Dental Dams

Dental dams are small squares of latex used by dentists that have been appropriated as an effective barrier for vaginal-oral and anal-oral contact. In a pinch, household plastic wrap can also be used. They should be used once and then discarded.

Spermicides

Spermicidal creams, foams, and jellies were designed to reduce the risk of pregnancy, but they have also been shown to kill herpes, syphilis, gonorrhea, and Trichomoniasis organisms. The active ingredient in most spermicides sold in the United States is nonoxynol-9. In laboratory studies, nonoxynol-9 has been shown to kill HIV; however, whether it can offer increased protection against HIV in the vagina has yet to be proven. The compound does sometimes irritate vaginal tissue, which can make a woman susceptible to HIV infection.

Diaphragms

Diaphragms are rubber vaginal inserts that cover the cervix, denying sperm access to a woman's ova. They can offer some protection against diseases that tend to affect the cervix, such as chlamydia and gonorrhea. They are best used in combination with a spermicide. They can be reused, provided that they are removed and washed after each use.

CONTRACEPTION

Both men and women need to be responsible for taking measures to ensure safe sex. In most heterosexual relationships, the responsibility for contraception falls to the woman. That's unfortunate, because the best prevention against STDs is a condom. Men may complain that the condom barrier reduces the pleasurable sensations of intercourse, but honestly, that's a lousy excuse for exposing a partner to possible STD infection. If lovers want to engage in barrier-free sex, they should get tested and begin a monogamous relationship, as described earlier in this chapter.

Once barrier-free sex is possible, heterosexual lovers have two choices: try for pregnancy, or use birth control. The latter is described here.

Methods of contraception vary in effectiveness; each method's rate of success as a means of birth control is given in the descriptions that follow.

Condoms

Success rate as a method of birth control: 85–98 percent

Condoms are designed to sheath an erect penis. To be effective, they must be put on before the penis comes in contact with the vagina, because even pre-seminal fluid can contain sperm. For maximum effectiveness, they should be used in combination with a spermicide; the spermicide should be placed in the vagina before intercourse.

Condoms are available just about everywhere—pharmacies, grocery stores, convenience stores, and so on. They're even available in some public bathrooms, although I wouldn't recommend taking advantage of this convenience unless the condom dispenser offers high-quality, name-brand condoms. Condoms of unknown origin are of unknown quality and, therefore, unknown effectiveness.

If you keep condoms in stock, store them away from extremes of hot and cold, and honor the expiration date posted on the packaging.

Lubrication on the outside of the condom can help prevent it from breaking. An additional drop of lubricant placed on the head of the penis before the condom is rolled on can create a soft, moist, pleasant sensory experience. Some condoms are prelubricated; with others, you have to add the lubrication yourself. Use only water-based lubricants. Oil-based lubricants, including lotions, mineral oil, and petroleum jelly, can quickly degrade the latex barrier. You can purchase water-based lubricants at most pharmacies and at any store that sells "sensuality" supplies.

Putting on a condom can be worked into foreplay. A man's partner can help him slip one on, giving him a genital massage at the same time. If the man is uncircumcised, gently push the foreskin back first. Then expel the air from the tip of the condom and place it over the head of the penis. Slowly unroll the condom down over the shaft of the penis. Leave just a pinch of space in the condom at the tip of the penis, so that when the man ejaculates, there is room for the ejaculate in the condom. (Otherwise, the condom may burst.) When unrolled completely, the condom should fit smoothly over the penis and extend almost to the base of the shaft.

After ejaculation, the condom must be removed carefully, before erection has completely subsided, to prevent semen from leaking into the vagina. The man should withdraw from the vagina while holding the condom securely at the base. Take care that any semen that may end up on the fingers or hands is not transferred into the vagina. Do not flush the used condom down the toilet; it is not biodegradable and can cause the plumbing to back up.

> Don't suggest that you and your partner use a condom; assume that you will. Both men and women should carry condoms. Just imagine—if someone tries to convince you to have unprotected sex, he or she will likely have convinced others. And that means that he or she has been at risk of contracting an STD.
>
> A common male rationale for not using a condom is that it isn't big enough to fit him. There's a quick fix for that situation. Open the condom and unroll it over your hand, wrist, and arm, being careful of your fingernails. Most condoms are quite stretchy and can reach your elbow. Ask your "big" man how much bigger than that he is.

Alternatives to Latex

Many people have a sensitivity to latex. In that case, lambskin and polyurethane condoms are options. Many people feel that lambskin condoms offer a man greater penile sensitivity than do latex or polyurethane condoms.

However, lambskin is more porous than latex and may not prevent transmission of HIV. If a man is sensitive to latex, he can apply a lambskin condom first, then a latex one over it. If a woman is sensitive to latex, her partner can apply a latex condom first, then a lambskin one over it.

Polyurethane condoms have a porosity similar to that of latex. They are also safe to use with any kind of lubricant, including those that are oil based.

If a Condom Breaks

If a man senses that a condom has broken or is coming loose, he should pull out immediately. If the condom has broken or come loose before the man has ejaculated, simply remove it and apply another one. If the malfunction occurs during or after ejaculation, the woman should urinate immediately. Do not douche or insert spermicidal creams into the vagina, as they may actually push sperm along in their journey. Wash with soap and water, apply some spermicide to your outer genitals, and consider taking emergency contraception ("the morning-after pill"), especially if you are near ovulation.

Female Condoms

Success rate as a method of birth control: 76 percent

A female condom looks like an enlarged, unrolled male condom. It has a ring at either end; one end is open, and one end is closed. The ring at the closed end is inserted into the vagina and helps hold the sheath in place during intercourse. The ring at the open end provides passage for the penis. Female condoms are made of polyurethane, are usually prelubricated, and do not need to be used in combination with a spermicide. They are excellent protection against both pregnancy and STDs, and they're available just about everywhere male condoms are sold.

The female condom can be inserted up to eight hours in advance of intercourse. You may wish to apply a drop or two of a lubricant (oil- or water-based) to the closed end to ease the insertion. Squeeze the ring at the closed end and insert it into the vagina, pushing it up just about as far as it will go. When the ring is let loose, it springs back into shape and covers the cervix. The other end of the sheath remains outside the vagina, partially covering the labia.

To remove the condom after intercourse, twist the outer ring to trap semen inside the sheath and gently pull it out. Female condoms are designed for one-time use, so dispose of the used condom. They are less effective than the male condom at preventing pregnancy. Do not flush it down the toilet, because it can clog up the plumbing.

Diaphragms and Cervical Caps

Success rate as a method of birth control: diaphragm, 80–94 percent; cervical cap, 74–91 percent

Diaphragms and cervical caps are soft, rubber cups that fit over the cervix and prevent sperm from passing through the cervical opening. A diaphragm looks like a small saucer; a cervical cap is the size of a large thimble. Each comes in different sizes and must be fitted to the user; your gynecologist or a practitioner at a family planning clinic will assist you in choosing one and learning to insert it. Diaphragms and cervical caps must be used with a spermicide. They offer some protection against STDs that affect the cervix, such as chlamydia and gonorrhea.

A diaphragm or cervical cap can be inserted up to eight hours before sex. Spread a layer of spermicide over the inside of the cup. Squeeze the sides of the cup together and, while squatting or standing with one leg raised, insert the cup into the vagina, pushing it up and back toward the cervix. You should feel it lock into place. Confirm that the diaphragm or cervical cap is in the correct position by reaching in and making sure you can feel the cervix behind the rubber cup. A properly fitted cup should not cause any discomfort.

The diaphragm or cervical cap should be left in place for at least eight hours after intercourse to give the spermicide time to do its work. If intercourse is repeated, use of a diaphragm will require that you first insert more spermicide into the vagina, without removing the cup. With a cervical cap, additional spermicide is not necessary for repeated intercourse.

A diaphragm should be removed within twenty-four hours; if it's left in for longer than forty-eight hours, toxic shock syndrome becomes a risk. A cervical cap can be left in for up to forty-eight hours.

To remove a diaphragm or cervical cap, simply reach inside the vagina and gently pull it out. Wash the device carefully in warm, soapy water. Check for tears or holes. If you don't find any, let it dry, and store in a cool place. If you do find perforations in the cup, discard it, and see your gynecologist for a replacement.

The fit of a diaphragm or cervical cap should be reexamined by your gynecologist in the event that you gain or lose twenty pounds or more or after miscarriage, childbirth, or pelvic surgery.

Diaphragms and cervical caps have very few negative side effects. Some women report an increased rate of bladder infection. Others report a sensitivity to the rubber material. And, of course, the cups are not foolproof. They may shift around during intercourse and are not a guaranteed method of birth control. They are best used in combination with a condom. They should not be used during the menses, as they can contribute to toxic shock syndrome. Note that the cervical cap has a high failure rate in women who have given birth but a very low failure rate in women who have not.

Vaginal Contraceptive Film (VCF)
Success rate as a method of birth control: 90 percent

VCF is a fairly recent arrival in the U.S. marketplace, although it has been around for years in Europe. It's a thin film that contains spermicides. Simply fold the film in fourths and insert it into the vagina, pushing it up as close to the cervix as possible. The film must be applied at least ten minutes before intercourse, and a new film should be applied if intercourse is repeated. The film dissolves; it does not need to be removed. This method of birth control is less messy than some other spermicide methods, but frequent use may cause vaginal irritation.

Emergency Contraception
Success rate as a method of birth control: 76–99 percent

Emergency contraception is often referred to as the "morning-after pill," but in fact it can be an effective method of birth control up to seventy-two hours (three days) after unprotected sex. It should be reserved for emergency situations in which a woman has forgotten to use birth control, the chosen method of birth control did not work properly, or a woman was raped.

Emergency contraception consists of a concentrated dose of hormones that stops the ovary from releasing the egg and changes the lining of the uterus so that the egg cannot implant there. Two doses are taken, the second dose coming twelve hours after the first.

Do not use emergency contraception if you are pregnant. Possible side effects include nausea, vomiting, dizziness, headache, and spotting. Taking the pill with food will minimize the side effects. If you suffer from nausea, drink ginger tea to settle your stomach. If you throw up within thirty minutes of a dose or become too sick to complete the second dose, seek the guidance of the clinic from which you obtained the contraception.

For information on health care practitioners in your area who can provide emergency contraception, contact the Emergency Contraception Hotline: 1-800-584-9911.

Fertility Awareness
Success rate as a method of birth control: 80–95 percent

Fertility awareness is a method of natural birth control effective only for the disciplined, organized woman. It involves tracking the fertility cycle and practicing abstinence or using contraception during the times when a woman is able to conceive. There are three signs to keep track of: basal body temperature, cervical mucus, and the menstrual "rhythm." Monitoring all three signs can offer a very effective means of birth control. As a side benefit, women practicing fertility awareness will become more familiar with their body's cycle.

To avoid pregnancy, a woman should not have unprotected sex from seven days before to three days after ovulation.

Basal Body Temperature

Basal body temperature is the temperature of the body at the beginning of the day. (*Basal* means "of the base" or "of the foundation.") To monitor your basal body temperature, you can use a basal body thermometer, which can measure temperature in tenths of a degree. A regular thermometer is fine, however, and less expensive. Take your temperature every morning, before you even get out of bed. Keep track of your body's temperature over the course of a few cycles. Most women's basal body temperature rises slightly, just less than one degree Fahrenheit, two days before ovulation. It remains elevated until ovulation begins, and then it slowly drops back down to the preovulation temperature.

Cervical Mucus

Women normally experience a vaginal discharge—mucus produced by the cervix—at different times in their fertility cycle. The fluid varies in texture and quantity depending on the stage of the fertility cycle. Monitoring cervical mucus, then, is an excellent way to monitor a woman's fertility. This method is sometimes called the Billings or ovulation method.

Cervical mucus is thought to be an expeditor of sorts for semen; it smoothes the passage of sperm from the top of the vagina to the traveling ovum.

1. **Menstruation begins.** Menstruation generally signals the end of a fertile cycle. The endometrium is being shed, and a new egg is developing in several follicles. For many women, particularly those who often or occasionally experience short cycles, menstruation is not a safe time for intercourse. Sperm can survive for several days inside a woman, and sperm ejaculated during the time of menstruation can fertilize the egg of a woman who ovulates quickly after menstruation. In regard to the mucus theory, some women begin to discharge cervical mucus toward the end of menstruation; the mucus may not be noticed until menstruation stops.

2. **Menstruation ends.** Most women experience several "dry" days after menstruation, when no cervical fluid is present. A woman is not fertile during a dry period.

3. **Mucus appears.** The first sign of cervical fluid is a sign of approaching ovulation. The mucus will grow in volume and become more slippery over the course of the next few days. A woman is fertile during this time and should refrain from intercourse if she does not wish to become pregnant.

4. **Mucus disappears.** When slippery cervical fluid becomes dry or tacky and opaque and gradually disappears, a woman's time of fertility has ended. From this point until the time of her next menses, she cannot conceive.

The Rhythm Method

The Rhythm Method (sometimes called the Calendar Method) involves keeping close track of menstruation. Generally speaking, the period of fertility is assumed to fall halfway between the first bleeding day of one menses and the first bleeding day of the next menses. The woman assumes she is fertile from four days before to four days after the halfway point. For this method to work, of course, you must be reasonably certain of when your next menses will occur, and so your menses must be regular. Chart your cycles for six to twelve months to establish the pattern before relying on this method.

> If these natural methods of birth control appeal to you, find a competent fertility awareness counselor who can offer instruction and guidance. The techniques I've described here are only a brief sketch; successful fertility awareness requires further training in the methodology.

Injectable Contraceptives

Success rate as a method of birth control: 99 percent

There are two types of injectable contraceptives currently available in the United States. One, currently marketed under the trade name Depo-Provera, is a progestin (a progesteronelike hormone). The other, marketed under the trade name Lunelle, contains both progestin and estrogen. They are very effective methods of birth control. However, they do not offer any protection against STDs.

There are several other injectable contraceptives that are not currently approved for use in the United States. They can be classified in either the progestin or the progestin-and-estrogen category.

If, after reading the descriptions that follow, you think you'd like to use injectable contraceptives, consult with your gynecologist.

Depo-Provera (Progestin)

Depo-Provera contains depot-medroxyprogesterone acetate, a man-made hormone that greatly resembles progesterone. This progestin prevents ovulation and also thickens cervical mucus so that sperm can't penetrate it. It gives no protection against STDs. The injection is given once every three months; you'll need to schedule an appointment with your gynecologist for each injection.

More than 80 percent of women who use Depo-Provera stop menstruating after three to four injections. When you stop using Depo-Provera, it can take nine to eighteen months for menstruation and fertility to return.

Depo-Provera should not be used if you are pregnant, have unexplained vaginal bleeding, have or have had breast cancer, are taking certain medications, or have diabetes, liver dysfunction, high blood pressure, heart disease, or serious depression.

Side effects can include depression, weight gain, irregular menses, absence of menses, headache, breast tenderness, nausea, appetite change, skin rash, hair loss or growth (on the face or the body), dizziness, abdominal distress, nervousness, and change in libido.

Lunelle (Progestin and Estrogen)

Lunelle contains both progestin and estrogen. The progestin, like that found in Depo-Provera, prevents ovulation and thickens the cervical mucus. The estrogen promotes a monthly menstrual cycle. The Lunelle injection must be received every month. Lunelle holds an advantage over progestin-only methods of contraception in that fertility is recovered quickly after the contraception is discontinued. Ovulation and predictable menstrual cycles begin one to two months afterward.

Lunelle should not be used if you are pregnant, have abnormal vaginal bleeding, are taking certain medications, have a history of breast or uterine cancer, or have high blood pressure, elevated cholesterol levels, heart disease, liver dysfunction, or diabetes. Women over the age of thirty-five who smoke heavily are also discouraged from using Lunelle.

Side effects include nausea, breast tenderness, skin changes, and fluid retention. Women who use a contraceptive method containing estrogen, such as Lunelle or the Pill, are at risk of developing blood clots. The risk is low, but it must be recognized. Symptoms of a blood clot include: sudden, severe chest pain; unexplained shortness of breath; sudden vision problems; numbness or weakness in the extremities; and severe pain in the calf or thigh. If you experience any of these symptoms, get to a health center immediately.

Intrauterine Devices (IUDs)

Success rate as a method of birth control: 97–99 percent

An IUD is a small plastic or metal device inserted into the uterus via the cervical opening. One or more strings hang down from the IUD and can be felt in the upper vagina. IUDs are usually available from and inserted by a family planning practitioner.

Some IUDs contain copper, which is thought to cause inflammation in the uterus. As a result, the immune system kicks into gear, and the resulting overflow of white blood cells, enzymes, and prostaglandins interferes with a sperm's ability to fertilize an egg. IUDs with copper can be left in place for years at a time.

Other IUDs contain progestins, which cause the cervical mucus to thicken so that sperm cannot pass through it. These IUDs must be replaced yearly. Mirena is a newer progestin IUD that lasts five years.

Neither type of IUD offers protection against STDs.

The most common problem with IUDs is expulsion—that is, sometimes they fall out. The danger here is that a woman may not know that she expelled an IUD, which can lead to an unplanned pregnancy. IUD expulsion is most likely to take place in the first three months after insertion and most common in women who have not given birth. Check weekly to make sure that your IUD is still in place by reaching up into the vagina. You should be able to feel the IUDs strings. If you cannot, schedule a visit with the practitioner who made the insertion.

IUDs should not be used if you have abnormal vaginal bleeding, a recent genitourinary infection, a recent abnormal Pap smear, any immune-compromising disease (such as AIDS), an artificial heart valve.

Possible side effects include pain, discomfort, bleeding, fever, and discharge. There have been cases of pelvic inflammatory disease, resulting in sterility. If a women does contract an STD, the danger of the infection traveling deeper into her reproductive organs is greater if she has an IUD. There have also been cases in which IUDs have perforated the uterine wall, requiring a surgical repair. Seek medical attention if you have severe abdominal pain, fever and chills of unknown origin, pain or bleeding during intercourse, or a foul-smelling vaginal discharge.

The long list of side effects may cause concern about the safety of this method of birth control, but it is important to note that most of these side effects are rare. The World Health Organization considers the IUD a safe, effective means of birth control.

If an IUD fails and you become pregnant, seek medical attention immediately. Having an IUD in place during pregnancy puts you at risk of serious infection or tubal pregnancy.

Contraceptive Implants

Success rate as a method of birth control: 99 percent

Contraceptive implants are hormone-containing capsules that are inserted under the skin; the hormone is slowly released from the capsules and affects the user's reproductive system. Norplant is the most common contraceptive implant. It is designed for use by women and is implanted in the fleshy skin on the underside of the upper arm. Its active ingredient is the progestin levonorgestrel, which causes the cervix to thicken, prevents the ovaries from releasing eggs, and thins the endometrial lining so that it cannot support egg implantation.

If the implants are removed and not replaced (which can take place at any time), ovulation and menstruation generally begins anew within the next month. Implants do not offer any protection against STDs.

Side effects of contraceptive implants vary depending on the mechanism that they employ to prevent pregnancy. Consult with the practitioner who provides you with the implant for information about side effects. In general, you should not use implants if you are pregnant, are taking certain medications, or have a history of unexplained vaginal bleeding, blood-clotting problems, breast cancer, stroke, heart disease, or liver disease.

Seek medical attention if you experience extreme vaginal bleeding, absence of menses (if you are accustomed to having them regularly), or severe abdominal pain; if you spot pus or infection at the site of the implant; or if an implant comes out.

Oral Contraceptives

Success rate as a method of birth control: 95–99 percent

The oral contraceptive known as "the Pill" contains both progestin and estrogen. The progestin thickens cervical mucus so that sperm cannot penetrate it and also prevents proper development of the endometrium, so that if, by chance, an egg is fertilized, it will not be able to implant in the endometrium. The estrogen is at a high enough level that it stops the pituitary gland from producing follicle-stimulating hormone (FSH). FSH triggers the follicles in the ovaries to begin developing. If there's no FSH, there's no follicle development and, thus, no egg.

There are many different kinds of combination (containing both estrogen and progestin) oral contraceptives; your health care provider can help you select the type that is best suited for you. Another type of oral contraceptive is the mini-pill, which contains only progestin. As a means of birth control, it is generally not quite as effective as combination pills, but it can be useful for women who are sensitive to estrogen therapy.

The Pill must be taken faithfully every day, preferably at a set time. If you miss one pill, take it as soon as you remember. If you miss two pills, take two a day until you are caught up, and use a backup method of contraception. If you miss three or more pills, call your health care provider. He or she will probably suggest that you use another form of birth control until after your next period, at which time you can begin the Pill cycle anew.

The Pill may increase, but often decreases, a woman's sex drive and can cause vaginal dryness. Other side effects may include headache, nausea, breast tenderness, weight gain, bleeding between cycles, and depression. Positive side effects include menses that are lighter, less painful, and more regular. Some oral contraceptives also help to clear acne.

There may be more risk in taking the Pill if you are obese, if you are a smoker (particularly if you are over thirty-five), or if you have a history of diabetes, liver disease, cancer, heart disease, or blood-clotting disorders. If you are taking antibiotics or medications for treating epilepsy or tuberculosis, consult with your health care provider to make sure that they won't interfere with the Pill's effectiveness. Seek medical help immediately if you experience sudden chest, arm, or abdominal pain; severe headache; shortness of breath; blurred vision; severe depression; or swelling or pain in the legs. As this goes to press, birth control patches worn on the skin have recently become available. Also new are intravaginal rings that contain hormones.

Spermicides

Success rate as a method of birth control when used on its own: 74 percent

Spermicidal creams, jellies, foams, and suppositories contain sperm-killing chemicals, most notably nonoxynol-9. They are inserted directly into the vagina before intercourse. They should not be used on their own as a means of birth control, but they make a powerful partner for other methods of birth control, such as diaphragms, cervical caps, and condoms. They also offer some protection against syphilis, gonorrhea, and trichomoniasis.

Each spermicidal product has unique properties and applications. Read the product label for instructions.

About 5 percent of women who use spermicides experience a localized allergic reaction that manifests as vaginal irritation, soreness, or discharge.

Tubal Ligation

Success rate as a method of birth control: 99 percent

Tubal ligation is a surgical procedure for sterilizing a woman. It is an option only for women who are positive that they do not want to conceive children in the future. It does not offer any protection against STDs.

There are five different surgical procedures for tubal ligation. All, in one way or another, seal off the fallopian tubes (from which comes the colloquialism, "getting your tubes tied").

In rare cases, a woman becomes pregnant after tubal ligation. (Her fallopian tubes may have reconnected.) Pregnancy in this situation is likely to be tubal, and dangerous. If you have had tubal ligation and experience severe abdominal pain, or miss a period and test positive for pregnancy, contact your health care provider immediately.

Vasectomy

Success rate as a method of birth control: 99 percent

Vasectomy is a surgical procedure for sterilizing a man. It involves sealing off the vas deferens, which carries mature sperm from the epididymis to the seminal vesicle ducts. It does not offer any protection against STDs.

A vasectomy can be a simple outpatient surgery that takes about twenty minutes. It does not alter a man's sex drive or the appearance of his semen. There may be short-term bruising or swelling near the testicles. Small lumps may form near the testicles, occasionally requiring medical treatment. In rare cases, the vas deferens may recover, making a man fertile again.

After a vasectomy, some sperm may remain in the man's testes, and he must be considered fertile for at least the next fifteen to twenty ejaculations. He should be tested before engaging in unprotected sex to determine for certain that he is not ejaculating sperm.

Part 4

Achieving and Maintaining Sexual Health

18

Menstruation and Menopause

n our time, menstruation and menopause are often treated as diseases. Superdrugs and invasive medical techniques have been designed to "treat" them. They're considered to be disabilities of a sort, something to be gotten over as quickly as possible.

However, menstruation and menopause are not health problems but, rather, simply part of the natural rhythms of life. Rather than placing the responsibility for your health into the hands of the medical establishment, learn to nurture and care for yourself. Take back control of your own body. Go with the flow.

> **Herbal Dosages**
> You'll find many recommendations for herbal therapy in this chapter. Unless stated otherwise, the therapeutic adult dosage for a recommended herb is:
>
> - 1 cup of tea three times daily;
> - 1 or 2 capsules three times daily; or
> - 1 dropperful of tincture three times daily.

MENSTRUATION

The process of menstruation is driven by hormones released from the brain and from the organs of the reproductive system. A woman has two ovaries, and each contains millions of follicles—tiny balls of cells surrounding a germ cell, or egg. At the beginning of every cycle, the pituitary gland releases folli-cle-stimulating hormone (FSH), which stimulates the development of ten to twenty follicles. Usually only one of the follicles develops into a true ovum, or egg. The developing follicles secrete estrogen, which stimulates growth of the endometrium, the lining of the uterus. When the egg is released from the fol-licle, it is swept into one of the fallopian tubes; over the course of several days, it will travel along the fallopian tube to the uterus.

The leftover cells of the follicle, called the corpus luteum, now begin to secrete progesterone in addition to estrogen. The pituitary gland secretes luteinizing hormone (LH), which, in combination with the progesterone from the corpus luteum, stimulates tiny endometrial arteries to keep blood circu-lating through the endometrium.

If the egg becomes fertilized (which, in most cases, happens along its journey through the fallopian tubes), it implants in the endometrium and begins to grow, and a whole new round of hormonal production is set off. If the egg does not become fertilized, the corpus luteum is eventually absorbed into the ovaries, shutting off the supply of estrogen and progesterone and, consequently, shutting off the tiny arteries that feed the endometrium. The endometrium is starved of blood, and eventually detaches from the uterus and is shed. We call that shedding process menstruation. The body then begins preparing for a new cycle by releasing FSH into the bloodstream. And so the cycle perpetuates, over and over.

Menstrual flow is composed of blood, endometrial tissue, and mucus. The unique odor of menstrual flow is caused by vaginal bacteria interacting with the blood. Blood loss averages between $1/4$ and $3/4$ of a cup. A loss of more or less than that can signal a larger health problem.

Menstruation can be a time of healing, rest, and regeneration. Many women experience it as a time of increased awareness. Unfortunately, many other women experience it as a time of great tension and pain; their bodies are unequipped to deal with the physical demands of menstruation, and their schedules don't permit them to slow down for a day or two. Imagine what it would feel like to be able to spend that first day of menstruation resting, meditating, pursuing quiet activity and inward thought. Glorious!

Research suggests that a woman's immune system is at peak strength dur-ing ovulation and begins to decline after the egg is released. It has been pro-posed that this decrease in strength keeps the immune system from attacking the fertilized egg. The wider implication is that surgery, vaccina-tions, and other medical procedures may be safest during the ovulation phase of a woman's cycle.

Whether or not you're able to gear down on the first day of menstruation, normalizing the menstrual cycle, regulating menses, eliminating cramps, and reducing premenstrual tension will help make the passage easier. I hope this chapter will help.

Feminine Hygiene Products

Until the 1920s, marketing feminine hygiene products was considered immoral. There were no commercial products available. Women had to make do on their own, and in my opinion, that may have been for the best.

In the 1930s, tampons became commercially available and wildly popular. For decades they were made primarily of cotton. In the early 1980s, four new, highly absorbent materials—carboxymethyl cellulose, polyacrylate rayon, viscose rayon, and polyester cellulose—were combined with the cotton to increase its absorption power. Soon after, toxic shock syndrome (TSS) became a household word.

Toxic Shock Syndrome

TSS is a life-threatening blood infection caused by the bacterium *Staphylococcus aureus.* Although researchers are not yet able to explain the connection between this Staph infection and tampons, we do know that using high-absorbency tampons, cervical caps, and other intrauterine birth control devices increases a woman's risk for developing TSS. The use of all-cotton tampons has *not* been linked to TSS.

Warning signs of TSS include:

- Sudden fever (usually over 102°F)
- Diarrhea
- Vomiting
- Faintness
- Rash

If you exhibit any of these symptoms while you are using a tampon, remove the tampon immediately. Seek medical help.

Because of the risk of TSS, tampon use should be restricted to brief periods when menstrual pads are impractical, such as while a woman is swimming, receiving a full-body massage, traveling, and so on. Avoid overnight use. Use only all-cotton tampons.

Because cotton is not a food crop, there are no governmental restrictions on how many chemicals can be used in its production. As a result, most commercial brands of cotton tampons contain some pesticide residue. In addition, cotton is often bleached, giving it a dioxin residue. So if you're going to use all-cotton tampons, I highly recommend that they be organic and unbleached.

Alternatives to Tampons

Tampons can alter the balance of vaginal flora, can release irritating fibers into the vagina, and if they're used when flow is minimal, can make tiny tears in the vaginal wall. As a result, tampons can expose a woman to infection. In addition, tampons are themselves an internal blockage, which can impede the flow of energy. A woman using tampons may even experience exacerbated cramping as the menstrual flow backs up.

I encourage all women to go with the flow and don't block the energy. It only makes cramps worse. Most of us recognize the environmental impact of thousands of plastic baby diapers in our landfills. We must consider also the impact of thousands of feminine hygiene products.

Reusable cloth menstrual pads are effective sanitary devices, comfortable, and, in the long run, less expensive than disposable tampons. You can find them at most health food stores or make them from pieces of absorbent flannel. Line your underwear with a pad, and replace it with a fresh one when necessary. Soak the used pads in a bucket of water to get rid of excess blood before running them through a washing machine. Pour the water from the bucket over the roots of a tree. Menstrual flow is, after all, the sacred blood intended to nourish an unborn child. As a fertilizer, it can't be beat!

If you need to use an internal sanitary device from time to time, consider a sea sponge, which is highly absorbent and reusable. Before each use, boil the sponge in water for five minutes. Then let air dry. After each use, rinse the sponge well, soak it in apple cider vinegar, and rinse again. Dispose of the sponge after a few menses.

Premenstrual Syndrome

Premenstrual syndrome (PMS) is a major emotional and physical health concern for many women. Common emotional symptoms include depression, crying spells, irritability, anger, agitation, and even being more prone to accidents and absentmindedness. In severe cases, withdrawal and suicidal tendencies can emerge. In France, PMS has been accepted as grounds for pleas of temporary insanity. Common physical symptoms include water retention, weight gain, a feeling of heaviness in the abdomen, and tenderness in the breasts.

Causes of PMS

PMS is usually linked to abnormally high levels of estrogen; women who suffer from PMS tend to have higher levels of estrogen in their blood five to ten days before menstruation than women who do not have PMS. Estrogen production is initiated at the onset of ovulation and continues to increase until the corpus luteum disappears. Once the follicle has ruptured and the egg has been released, the corpus luteum produces progesterone, which counteracts the effects of elevated estrogen levels. However, if progesterone levels are insufficient, then estrogen dominates and the symptoms of PMS are likely to intensify.

This is a simplified explanation of a complicated problem. There are a wide variety of hormonal imbalances that contribute to PMS, and while only a small percentage of women suffer from extreme PMS, many women experience some of its symptoms, in varying degrees. If you suffer from extreme PMS, consult with your health care provider for diagnosis and appropriate treatment. If you experience only moderate symptoms, consider some of the natural therapies suggested below.

> In traditional Oriental medicine, liver stagnation is thought to be a major contributing factor in menstrual difficulties. The liver governs the amount of menstrual flow and the regularity of the cycle. It also breaks down excess hormones, including estrogen. Therefore, treatments for PMS often focus on strengthening liver function.

PMS can be broken into several categories, each with a particular set of symptoms and causes.

1. PMT-A is characterized by emotional difficulties, such as anxiety, mood swings, and tension. It is associated with elevated estrogen levels and decreased progesterone levels in the luteal phase of ovulation.

2. PMT-B is characterized by breast soreness, bloating, and weight gain. It is associated with increased levels of aldosterone, an adrenal hormone that causes water and sodium retention. Increased levels of prolactin, a hormone released when the pituitary is stressed, can be a contributing factor to the breast tenderness. Stagnation in the liver often contributes to PMT-B.

3. PMT-C is characterized by food cravings, hypoglycemia, headache, and physical shakiness; in severe cases, it can result in fatigue, fainting, and heart palpitations. It is associated with blood sugar imbalances and, in some cases, low levels of prostaglandin.

4. PMT-D manifests as depression, lethargy, insomnia, crying, withdrawal, and forgetfulness. It is associated with increased levels of aldosterone and progesterone and low levels of estrogen. In extreme cases, PMT-D can stimulate suicidal tendencies and require psychiatric care.

Chart your cycle on a calendar so that you can see if there is a pattern to the changes you experience. For a diagnosis of PMS, you must experience the symptoms from one to fourteen days before the menses begin and then be free of symptoms for at least seven days after the menses end. On the chart, keep track of your emotional state, physical health, sexual vitality, dreams, and diet. After a few cycles, you may discover some interesting correlations. Once you identify the patterns, you can use your energy in ways that support your body to best effect.

Relieving PMS

Some women would swear that PMS stands for "Please, more sweets." However, giving in to sugar cravings will only make mood swings more severe and more erratic. Avoid salty foods, which contribute to bloating and weight gain, and hydrogenated oils (found in fried foods, margarine, and shortening), which impair liver function and prevent it from breaking down excess estrogen. To improve liver and kidney function, drink a lot of water, and add a squeeze of fresh lemon juice to the water. Also eat plenty of green, leafy vegetables.

Relaxation therapies can do wonders for PMS. Take aromatherapy baths. Get massages. Drink the "I Got the PMS Blues" tea described on page 248. Practice deep breathing. Play relaxation tapes. Take long walks. Undertake some sort of a creative outlet, such as writing, drawing, or singing. Above all, do your best just to nurture yourself during your "moon" time.

For advice on how to use any of the natural therapies suggested for PMS and the other menstrual dysfunctions discussed on the following pages, see "Natural Therapies for Healthy Menstruation" (page 238).

Dysmenorrhea

Dysmenorrhea is the term for difficult, painful menstruation. After ovulation, the uterine lining (endometrium) prepares itself for a fertilized egg. Tiny arteries feed it blood and embryo-nourishing substances. If fertilization does not occur, those tiny arteries shut down, and the lining starts to deteriorate. The arteries may spasm as the lining dies off. The cramping usually ceases sometime during menstruation, because the menstrual blood helps clean out the area.

Causes of Dysmenorrhea

Dysmenorrhea can be caused or exacerbated by a variety of hormonal and reproductive dysfunctions.

Constipation. Constipation can cause pressure on the uterus and contribute to cramping.

Inflammatory prostaglandins. Prostaglandins are hormonelike derivatives of unsaturated fatty acids that act as chemical messengers in the body. There are several types. An overabundance of prostaglandin E_1 is thought to contribute to premenstrual inflammation; its production can be controlled by evening primrose oil, zinc, and vitamin E.

Magnesium deficiency. A magnesium deficiency can cause cramping and spasms during menstruation.

Calcium deficiency. Calcium is important not only for the bones and teeth but also for the muscles. Cramping and other symptoms of dysmenorrhea are similar to the symptoms of a calcium deficiency; maintaining adequate levels of calcium can prevent those symptoms from occurring.

Pelvic congestion. Dysmenorrhea can also be caused by ischemia (lack of blood flow) in the pelvic area. Pelvic ischemia is most common in young women who have not yet given birth. The herb blue cohosh can offer relief in this situation.

Spinal misalignment. If the spine is out of alignment, nerves may be pinched, causing cramping. Yoga, bodywork, and chiropractic adjustments can all be of service in this case.

Relieving Dysmenorrhea

Physical tension or tightness can worsen dysmenorrhea, so do your best to stay warm and loose. Practice deep breathing (see page 35). Wear loose clothing. Stay warm. Avoid cold drinks and icy foods, which can cause muscle contractions. Apply a hot water bottle over the kidneys to relieve pain. A castor oil compress (see page 292) over the abdomen might also be helpful.

To prevent constipation, stick to a high-fiber diet. Be sure to include sources of omega-3 and omega-6 fatty acids, such as fish, flaxseed oil, and evening primrose oil, which can help control prostaglandin levels. Drink plenty of water. If you still need help, chew a handful of flaxseeds daily, or grind them up and sprinkle them on your food.

To reduce the occurrence and severity of cramps, eat plenty of foods that are rich in magnesium and calcium. As you're in the process of improving your diet, you may also wish to take magnesium and calcium supplements. See Chapter 5 for more information.

The herbs black cohosh, chamomile, cinnamon, cramp bark, ginger, peppermint, red raspberry, and yarrow and the essential oils anise, carrot seed, clary sage, jasmine, and rose can all help relieve cramping.

Some women have found that crushing a bromelain tablet, mixing it with a bit of cocoa butter, and inserting it vaginally can help relieve severe cramps. Bromelain has an anti-inflammatory effect on the uterine tissues.

Leg lifts are a tremendously beneficial exercise. You may feel as though you couldn't possibly move an inch, but if you give it a try, you'll find that cramps become less severe. Massage of the Achilles tendon can also help.

Menorrhagia

Menorrhagia is either excessively long or excessively profuse bleeding during menstruation. Before attempting at-home treatment, consult with your health care provider; he or she will most likely give you a thorough examination to make sure that a cyst, tumor, or complication in pregnancy is not causing the bleeding.

Causes of Menorrhagia

Menorrhagia is often a result of insufficient levels of progesterone; the tiny arteries that feed the endometrium aren't signaled to stop. In traditional Oriental medicine, excessive menstrual bleeding is thought to result from excess heat, deficient chi, or blood stagnation. Profuse dark clots of blood may indicate a liver imbalance. Blood that is profuse and light red may indicate a spleen imbalance (the spleen governs the passage of blood through the proper channels of the body).

Relieving Menorrhagia

To stop alarmingly excessive bleeding, drink a glass of water to which you've added 1/8 teaspoon of cayenne pepper or the juice of a lemon. However, don't rely on this "Band-aid" approach. Pay attention and focus on correcting the imbalance causing the excess bleeding.

To compensate for blood loss, eat plenty of blood-building foods, such as beets and dark green, leafy vegetables. To help normalize hormone production, eat plenty of cold-water fish, such as salmon, herring, sardines, and mackerel, and supplement with sources of essential fatty acids, such as flaxseed oil, evening primrose oil, and black currant seed oil. Nourish the thyroid gland, which helps regulate all the cycles of the body, by incorporating seaweeds into your diet. Iron-rich adzuki beans, lentils, and amaranth tea are excellent foods for women who bleed too much.

Herbs that can decrease the flow of blood include cinnamon, lady's mantle, nettle, red raspberry, shepherd's purse, uva ursi, and yarrow. Also consider supplementing with vitamin C (with bioflavonoids) to help strengthen your capillaries.

Amenorrhea

Amenorrhea is characterized by lack of menstruation in a woman who has experienced puberty but not yet menopause, and who is not pregnant or lactating. It is not uncommon in women who exercise excessively, such as professional athletes; their bodies may focus less on estrogen production or reproduction.

Causes of Amenorrhea

There are many possible causes of amenorrhea, some of them quite serious. They include hormonal imbalances, infertility, tumors, nutritional deficiencies, glandular dysfunctions, weight imbalances, exposure to environmental toxins, and stress. Some pharmaceutical medications can cause amenorrhea. Before attempting at-home treatment, consult with your health care provider. He or she will probably recommend a thorough physical examination to determine the cause and the appropriate treatment.

Correcting Amenorrhea

Correcting any nutritional deficiencies is imperative. Incorporate into your diet blood-building foods, such as beets, blueberries, parsley, raspberries, and nettles, and iron-rich foods such as apricots, blackstrap molasses, bran, carrots, chicken (dark meat), eggs, fish, green, leafy vegetables, green peppers, Jerusalem artichokes, millet, miso, oatmeal, parsley, persimmons, prunes, pumpkin seeds, raisins, seaweeds, sesame seeds, squash, sunflower seeds, and turkey (dark meat).

Herbs that can help amenorrhea by building the blood and improving circulation to the pelvis include angelica, basil, blue cohosh, burdock, cinnamon, licorice, mugwort, nettle, and red raspberry.

Also consider supplementing with vitamin B complex, vitamin E, and a multimineral supplement to correct potential nutritional deficiencies.

Essential oils to use topically include clary sage, fennel, lavender, and rosemary. See Chapter 7 for suggestions.

Hot sitz baths can also help increase circulation to the reproductive organs. See Chapter 12 for details.

Metrorrhagia

Metrorrhagia is the term used to describe menstrual bleeding that occurs at irregular intervals or outside the duration of normal menses. As with other menstrual dysfunctions, it can be a side effect of other, more serious health problems. Consult with your health care provider before beginning at-home treatment to rule out conditions such as endometriosis, fibroids, cancer, or cysts.

Causes of Metrorrhagia

In Oriental tradition, excessively early or late menses are said to be caused by a chi deficiency or by stagnation in the blood or liver. If the menses are very light, coldness and deficiency are suspected.

From a Western perspective, menses that come early may be due to an insufficiency of either estrogen or progesterone. Menses that are delayed more than eight or nine days in the average twenty-eight day cycle could be a symptom of a cyst, late ovulation, or lack of ovulation.

Correcting Metrorrhagia

A common, often unrecognized factor in the regulation of menses is light. Too often, we go to work in darkness, return home in darkness, spend our days under fluorescent lights, and spend our nights bathed in the artificial lights of street lights, night lights, and digital clocks. Light has a powerful effect on hormones, and aberrant patterns of light exposure can result in aberrant hormonal behavior. If you are suffering from metrorrhagia, try sleeping in total darkness—pull all the shades, close the door, and unplug all electrical appliances. And be sure to spend some time outdoors every day, enjoying natural, full-spectrum light.

Consider supplementing with vitamin C (with bioflavonoids) to strengthen the capillaries, iron to strengthen the blood, and vitamin K to improve the blood's clotting factor.

Herbs that can help regulate the menstrual cycle include dandelion root, false unicorn, and vitex. If the menses tend to come too early, try rose hip and sage teas. If the menses tend to be delayed, try red raspberry leaf.

Essential oils that can be used topically to help regulate the menses include basil, clary sage, cypress, geranium, hops, nutmeg, oregano, parsley, peppermint, and savory.

Natural Therapies for Healthy Menstruation

Natural therapies for normalizing and supporting the menstrual cycle focus on four main goals:

1. **Blood.** Improving circulation and building the blood help normalize the menstrual cycle.

2. **Blood sugar.** Controlling blood sugar levels helps reduce food cravings and minimize mood swings.

3. **Hormones.** Regulating hormone production helps moderate emotional states and normalize the menstrual cycle. Strengthening the liver enables the expedient breakdown of excess hormones.

4. **Muscles.** Relaxing the muscles helps reduce cramping and enables smoother menstrual flow.

Exercise

Women who exercise regularly are less likely to have menstrual difficulties than those who don't. Exercise improves circulation, strengthens the liver, and stimulates the production of "feel good" endorphins. Brisk walking and swimming are especially helpful for menstrual dysfunctions; they stimulate the body's systems without taxing the body's joints and muscles.

Diet

Keep blood sugar levels stable by eating small, frequent meals. And resist that sweet tooth; when we give in to sugar craving, we're likely to get raving! Sugar raises glucose levels in the blood, making us feel temporarily energetic, but as soon as the sugar is burned up, we crash. Menstruation offers enough emotional difficulties on its own, without us adding a sugar-induced emotional roller coaster to them.

To build the blood, eat plenty of green, leafy vegetables and seaweeds. Seaweeds can also help regulate erratic menstrual cycles, as can carrots.

To normalize estrogen levels, incorporate into your diet cruciferous vegetables, such as broccoli, cabbage, and cauliflower. Soy is often promoted as a good source of phytoestrogens, which can help normalize the body's production of its own estrogen. However, soy can be difficult to digest and is a common allergen, and soy products are often manufactured from genetically modified soybeans. For these reasons, the best forms of soy are tempeh and miso (from organically grown, non-genetically-modified soybeans); they are fermented and easy to digest. Eating less meat, or eating only meat from animals that were raised without hormone treatments, can also help. Many farm animals are fed estrogenlike drugs to promote earlier maturity and weight gain; traces of these estrogenlike substances can be found in the meat from these animals. These synthetic hormones, some of which are known carcinogens, overburden the liver.

Cutting down on salt will help prevent water retention and bloating. To further the "no bloating" cause, eat foods that are naturally diuretic, such as artichokes, asparagus, watercress, and watermelon (including the seeds). Drinking more water will also help the body excrete sodium and excess fluids.

Herbal Therapy

When reviewing the herbs that are beneficial for menstruation, keep in mind that those plants listed as phytoestrogenic are best used during the first phase of the cycle (from the first day of menstruation until ovulation). Plants with phytoprogesteronic activity are best used during the second phase of the cycle (from ovulation until the first day of menstruation).

Agrimony (*Agrimonia eupatoria*). The herb encourages the coagulation of blood, which can help reduce excessive menstrual flow. It also relieves cramps. It is an analgesic, anti-inflammatory, antispasmodic, astringent, diuretic, emmenagogue, hemostatic, and hepatic. Avoid during pregnancy and in cases of constipation.

Alfalfa (*Medicago sativa*). The leaf supports clotting of the blood, which can help women who bleed heavily during menstruation. It is also rich in nutrients that build the blood, and it is often recommended in treatments for anemia. It also relieves fatigue and normalizes estrogen production. It is an anti-inflammatory, diuretic, nutritive, and phytoestrogenic.

The Plant-Human Hormone Connection

The study of hormones is a relatively new science, and we are still learning about the connection between plant and human hormones. Plants that are phytoestrogenic, for example, contain within them estrogenlike compounds. These compounds do not themselves have an estrogenic effect on the body. However, the body is thought to be able to use them to manufacture estrogen. Phytoestrogenic compounds also can occupy receptor sites in the body that normally are used by estrogens. As a result of this dual service, phytoestrogenic compounds may have a normalizing effect on estrogen levels in the body. If the body has inadequate estrogens, it can convert phytoestrogenic materials to estrogens. If the body has excess estrogens, then the phytoestrogenic materials are not converted to estrogens; instead, they compete with the estrogens for receptor sites.

Angelica (*Angelica archangelica, A. atropurpurea*). The root helps build the blood, increases menstrual flow, and can normalize the menstrual cycle in women who tend to have delayed menses. It also relaxes the muscles and improves liver function. It's often recommended in treatments for amenorrhea, anemia, dysmenorrhea, migraine, and nausea. It is an anti-inflammatory, antispasmodic, diuretic, emmenagogue, nervine, phytoestrogenic, tonic, and uterine stimulant. Avoid during pregnancy and in cases of heavy bleeding or diabetes. In rare cases, the root causes photosensitivity.

Anise (*Pimpinella anisum*). The seed relieves bloating, dysmenorrhea, and nausea. It may curb a sweet tooth. It is antispasmodic and phytoestrogenic.

Basil (*Ocimum basilicum*). The leaf can help calm anxiety and clear mental fogginess. It also increases circulation to the pelvic region. It is an antidepressant, antispasmodic, circulatory stimulant, and sedative.

Black cohosh (*Actaea racemosa*). The root can soothe irritation and break up congestion in the uterus, cervix, and vagina. It's often recommended in treatments for amenorrhea, dysmenorrhea, moodiness, and PMS. It is an alterative, anti-inflammatory, antispasmodic, astringent, diuretic, emmenagogue, phytoestrogenic, muscle relaxant, nervine, and uterine stimulant. Avoid during pregnancy, except in the final stages, and then only under the guidance of your health care provider. Avoid while nursing and in cases of high blood pressure or pressure in the inner eye. Consult with your health care provider before use. This herb is endangered in the wild; do not use wildcrafted supplies.

Black haw (*Viburnum prunifolium*). The bark (including the bark of the root) helps smooth muscles in the uterus relax. It's often recommended in treatments for amenorrhea, dysmenorrhea, and menorrhagia. It is an analgesic, antispasmodic, astringent, and uterine sedative.

Blessed thistle (*Cnicus benedictus*). The herb strengthens the spleen, liver, and reproductive system. It's often recommended for amenorrhea.

Blue cohosh (*Caulophyllum thalictroides*). The dried root can stimulate menstrual flow. It relieves uterine inflammation and cramping due to insufficient blood flow. It's often recommended in treatments for dysmenorrhea and PMS. It is an anti-inflammatory, antispasmodic, diuretic, emmenagogue, oxytocic, and uterine stimulant. Avoid during pregnancy, except in the final stages, and then only under the guidance of your health care provider. Make sure the root is dried, not fresh. This herb is endangered in the wild; do not use wildcrafted supplies.

Bupleurum (*Bupleurum chinense, B. falcatum*). The root relieves pain and relaxes the muscles. It also boosts blood circulation and helps improve liver function. It is an alterative, anti-inflammatory, and tonic. Avoid in cases of fever, headache, or high blood pressure.

Burdock (*Arctium lappa*). The root is a great liver cleanser. It builds the blood and can reduce tenderness in the breasts. It also helps dispel the irritability of PMS. It is an alterative, anti-inflammatory, diuretic, nutritive, and rejuvenative.

Cayenne (*Capsicum annuum*). The fruit improves circulation and can also help decrease menstrual flow when the menses are excessively profuse. It is an alterative, astringent, and hemostatic. Avoid contact with eyes and mucous membranes. Avoid therapeutic doses during pregnancy and while nursing.

Chamomile (*Matricaria recutita*). The flower relieves cramps caused by stagnation in the pelvic region. It also has a potent effect on the psyche, calming anxiety, hysteria, and nervousness. It is often recommended in treatments for amenorrhea. It is an anti-inflammatory, antispasmodic, and analgesic. In rare cases, individuals exhibit an allergic response to this herb.

Cinnamon (*Cinnamomum cassia, C. verum*). The bark can reduce excessive menstrual bleeding. It is often recommended in treatments for dysmenorrhea, headache, and nausea. Avoid in cases of hemorrhoids, dry stools, bloody urine, or excess heat, such as fever and inflammation. It may exacerbate premature ejaculation. Avoid therapeutic dosages during pregnancy.

Codonopsis (*Codonopsis pilosula*). The root builds the blood and tonifies the spleen. It can stabilize blood sugar levels, boost energy, and increase the time between menses. It is a chi tonic and nutritive.

Cotton root (*Gossypium hirsutum, G. herbaceum*). The bark constricts blood vessels and is often recommended for menorrhagia that is caused by fibroids, as well as for dysmenorrhea, endometriosis, uterine fibroids, and uterine inflammation. It is an emmenagogue, hemostatic, nutritive, oxytocic, and uterine tonic. Avoid during pregnancy. Large doses may cause nausea and vomiting. Avoid in cases of urogenital irritation.

Cramp bark (*Viburnum opulus*). The bark relieves cramps, headache, and hysteria. It is an analgesic, anti-inflammatory, antispasmodic, astringent, diuretic, nervine, tonic, and uterine sedative.

Dandelion (*Taraxacum officinale*). The root is a cholagogue and liver tonic; it improves liver function and can relieve tenderness in the breasts. The leaf is an alterative and diuretic; it can relieve edema and is often recommended in cases of anemia.

Dong quai (*Angelica sinensis*). The root helps regulate estrogenic activity. It improves circulation to the pelvis, increases menstrual flow, and can normalize the menstrual cycle in women who tend to have delayed menses. It is often recommended in treatments for amenorrhea, anemia, dysmenorrhea, and headache. It is an alterative, anticoagulant, antispasmodic, blood tonic, emmenagogue, muscle relaxant, and nervine. Avoid during pregnancy, except under the guidance of your health care provider. Do not use in cases of diarrhea, heavy menstrual flow, poor digestion, bloating, or in conjunction with blood-thinning medications such as ibuprofen.

False unicorn (*Chamaelirium luteum*). The rhizome is a uterine tonic and increases circulation to the pelvic area. It is often recommended in treatments for amenorrhea, dysmenorrhea, endometriosis, hormonal imbalance, infertility, leukorrhea, and uterine prolapse. It is a diuretic and phytoestrogenic. The bitter taste of this herb can cause vomiting. Excessive amounts may cause kidney and stomach irritation, blurred vision, and hot flashes. Do not use without employing birth control during sex unless pregnancy is desired. Discontinue use during pregnancy. False unicorn is endangered in the wild; do not use wildcrafted supplies.

Fennel (*Foeniculum vulgare*). The seed increases menstrual flow and helps dispel liver congestion. It may curb an excessive desire for sweets. It is antispasmodic, diuretic, and phytoestrogenic.

Ginger (*Zingiber officinale*). The root improves circulation and relieves the type of cramps that improve with warmth. It is recommended when menses are delayed and produce scant dark blood. It is also helpful in cases of amenorrhea and nausea. It is an analgesic, anti-inflammatory, and anticoagulant. Avoid large doses in cases of acne and eczema. Discontinue use if heartburn results.

Hops (*Humulus lupulus*). The strobile calms anxiety and relieves cramping and headache. It can improve the temperament of those who have a quarrelsome nature. It is an anodyne, antispasmodic, diuretic, emmenagogue, muscle relaxant, nervine, phytoestrogenic, sedative, and soporific. Avoid during pregnancy and in cases of depression. The fresh plant may cause dermatitis in some individuals.

Horsetail (*Equisetum arvense*). The herb helps prevent breakthrough bleeding (bleeding that occurs outside of the menstrual period) and excessive bleeding. It encourages blood coagulation, reduces edema, and relieves cramping. It is an alterative, anti-inflammatory, astringent, diuretic, hemostatic, and nutritive. Use horsetail that has been collected in spring.

Lady's mantle (*Alchemilla xanthochlora*). The herb relieves congestion in the liver and encourages blood coagulation. It is often recommended in treatments for excessive or irregular bleeding and dysmenorrhea. It is an anti-inflammatory, astringent, diuretic, emmenagogue, hemostatic, and tonic. Avoid during pregnancy, except in the final stages, at which point you should seek the guidance of your health care provider.

Licorice (*Glycyrrhiza glabra, G. uralensis*). The root normalizes ovulation and inhibits the production of prostaglandin E_2 production. It is often recommended in treatments for amenorrhea caused by chi deficiency. It can help stabilize and calm the emotions. It is an anti-inflammatory, antispasmodic, chi tonic, and phytoestrogenic. Avoid during pregnancy and in cases of edema, high blood pressure, or diabetes. Do not use in combination with digoxin drugs. Excessive use can cause sodium retention and potassium depletion.

Marijuana (*Cannabis sativa, C. indica*). Though cannabis has been used medicinally for thousands of years, it is currently illegal to grow or possess it in some parts of the world. Claims have been made that the herb can help relieve premenstrual anxiety and dysmenorrhea. It is an anti-inflammatory, analgesic, antispasmodic, muscle relaxant, and sedative. Dry mouth and eyes are common side effects. Certain individuals may experience paranoia, perceptual disorders, and personality deviations. Do not drive while under the influence of marijuana. Excessive use can lower androgen production and, thus, libido. It can also lead to short-term memory loss. Avoid during pregnancy.

Meadowsweet (*Filipendula ulmaria*). The herb can help relieve the pain of cramps. It is an analgesic, anti-inflammatory, antispasmodic, astringent, diuretic, progesteronic, and sedative. Avoid if you are allergic to salicylates.

Motherwort (*Leonurus cardiaca*). The herb dilates uterine blood vessels and thus eases pressure that can contribute to cramping. It is often recommended in treatments for amenorrhea, dysmenorrhea, and menses that are scanty when they begin. It is an antispasmodic, astringent, circulatory stimulant, muscle relaxant, emmenagogue, nervine, and vasodilator. Avoid in cases of heavy menstrual bleeding and during pregnancy, except during the final stages, and then only under the supervision of your health care provider.

Mugwort (*Artemisia vulgaris*). The herb is often recommended in treatments for amenorrhea and dysmenorrhea. It is an anti-inflammatory, antispasmodic, bitter tonic, emmenagogue, hemostatic, muscle relaxant, and uterine stimulant. Do not use for more than a month at a time. Avoid in cases of nervous system disorders and during pregnancy, except during labor, and then only under the supervision of your health care provider. Use only five drops of tincture of $\frac{1}{4}$ cup tea no more than three times daily.

Nettle (*Urtica dioica, U. urens*). Nettle is a good herb to use for almost anything! It can reduce bloating, relieve tenderness in the breasts, prevent anemia, help control excessive menstrual bleeding, and clear stagnation from the liver or kidneys. It is an alterative, astringent, cholagogue, circulatory stimulant, diuretic, hemostatic, nutritive, and thyroid tonic. Contact with the fresh plant will irritate the skin. Use only dried herb. Wear gloves when collecting. Nettle may cause some irritation to the kidneys.

Oregon grape (*Mahonia aquifolium*). The root can relieve edema, clear liver stagnation, and correct menorrhagia. It is an alterative, anti-inflammatory, astringent, cholagogue, diuretic, hepatic, and thyroid stimulant. Avoid during pregnancy, and do not exceed the recommended dosage.

Parsley (*Petroselinum crispum*). The leaf helps regulate menstrual cycles. It can relieve tenderness in the breasts, edema, and is often recommended in treatments for amenorrhea, anemia, and dysmenorrhea. It is an antispasmodic, diuretic, emmenagogue, nutritive, and sedative. Avoid therapeutic doses during pregnancy and in cases of kidney inflammation.

Partridge berry (*Mitchella repens*). The herb is often recommended in treatments for amenorrhea and dysmenorrhea. It is an astringent, diuretic, emmenagogue, nervine, and uterine tonic. Dosages in excess of what is recommended can irritate the mucous membranes. This herb is endangered in the wild; do not use wildcrafted supplies.

Pennyroyal (*Hedeoma pulegioides, Mentha pulegium*). The herb can help counteract amenorrhea that is caused by blood stagnation. It is often recommended in treatments for dysmenorrhea, headache, and nausea. It is an antispasmodic, diuretic, emmenagogue, and uterine vasodilator. Avoid during pregnancy.

Peony (*Paeonia lactiflora*). The root helps bring menses closer together. It is often recommended in treatments for amenorrhea and dysmenorrhea. It is an alterative, anti-inflammatory, antispasmodic, blood tonic, diuretic, emmenagogue, hepatotonic, sedative, uterine astringent, vasodilator, and yin tonic. Avoid during pregnancy and in cases of diarrhea.

Peppermint (*Mentha piperita*). The leaf can relieve cramping, fatigue, headache, migraine, and nausea. It is an analgesic, anodyne, antispasmodic, cholagogue, diuretic, and vasodilator. It is among the safest of herbs, even for people who are very ill, with its only side effect being occasional heartburn.

Red clover (*Trifolium pratense*). The herb and flower build the blood and can resolve blood clots. They are alterative, anti-inflammatory, antispasmodic, diuretic, nutritive, and phytoestrogenic.

Red raspberry (*Rubus idaeus*). The leaf contains phytosterols. It strengthens the reproductive system and relaxes smooth muscles in the uterus. It is often recommended in treatments for amenorrhea, anemia, dysmenorrhea, and menorrhagia. It is an alterative, antispasmodic, astringent, hemostatic, hormonal regulator, kidney tonic, nutritive, and uterine tonic.

Rehmannia (*Rehmannia glutinosa*). The root tonifies and detoxifies the blood. It is often recommended in treatments for amenorrhea and menorrhagia. It is an alterative, diuretic, hemostatic, kidney, and liver tonic. Avoid in cases of loose stools, poor appetite, bloating, or a coated tongue.

Rose (*Rosa* spp.). The hips contain vitamin C and bioflavonoids, which can strengthen capillaries and help relieve cramping. They are often recommended in treatments for menses that come too early and for deficient kidney chi. The hip is an astringent, diuretic, and hormonal regulator.

Sage (*Salvia officinalis*). The leaf helps control excessive menstrual flow and delay menses that come too early. It can relieve cramping, depression, and migraines. It is an anti-inflammatory, antispasmodic, astringent, emmenagogue, hormonal tonic, and phytoestrogenic. Avoid therapeutic dosages in cases of vaginal dryness, during pregnancy, and while nursing.

Sarsaparilla (*Smilax* spp.). The root is both phytoprogesteronic and phytoestrogenic. It is often recommended in treatments for leukorrhea and ovarian cysts. It is an alterative, anti-inflammatory, antispasmodic, diuretic, and tonic.

Shepherd's purse (*Capsella bursa-pastoris*). The herb strengthens capillaries and is often used to control excessive menstrual bleeding and spotting between menses. It is an alterative, astringent, diuretic, hemostatic, and vasoconstrictor.

Skullcap (*Scutellaria lateriflora*). The herb helps draw menses farther apart. It can also help dispel anger and anxiety. It is often recommended in treatments for dysmenorrhea and headache. It is an alterative, anodyne, anti-inflammatory, antispasmodic, astringent, diuretic, nervine, sedative, and yin tonic. Avoid during pregnancy.

Tribulus (*Tribulus terrestris*). The fruit helps draw menses farther apart. It is often recommended in treatments for dysmenorrhea, headache, and leukorrhea. It is an alterative, analgesic, anodyne, antispasmodic, nervine, and bone, liver, and kidney tonic.

Trillium (*Trillium* spp.). The root curbs excessive menstrual bleeding and helps relieve dysmenorrhea. It is an alterative, antispasmodic, astringent, emmenagogue, and uterine tonic. Avoid during pregnancy, except under the guidance of your health care provider. This herb is endangered in the wild; do not use wildcrafted supplies.

Uva ursi (*Arctostaphylos uva-ursi*). The leaf reduces blood flow to the pelvic area and can relieve edema. It is an astringent, diuretic, and vasoconstrictor. Avoid during pregnancy.

Vitex (*Vitex agnus-castus*). The berry helps regulate the menstrual cycle by normalizing the function of the pituitary gland. It helps control menses that are excessively profuse and too frequent, and it is often recommended in treatments for amenorrhea, breast tenderness, dysmenorrhea, metrorrhagia, and PMS. It also can dispel headaches and acne caused by menstruation. It is both phytoestrogenic and phytoprogesteronic.

White willow (*Salix alba*). The bark inhibits prostaglandin production, which reduces uterine inflammation. It can relieve headaches, migraines, and dysmenorrhea. It is alterative, analgesic, anodyne, anti-inflammatory, astringent, and phytoestrogenic. Avoid if you are allergic to salicylates.

Wild yam (*Dioscorea opposita, D. villosa*). The root relieves dysmenorrhea, ovarian pain, and glandular imbalances. It is an anti-inflammatory, antispasmodic, cholagogue, diuretic, nutritive, and phytoprogesteronic. Avoid therapeutic doses during pregnancy, except under the guidance of your health care provider. The *Dioscorea villosa* species is endangered in the wild; do not use wildcrafted supplies.

Yarrow (*Achillea millefolium*). The herb reduces blood flow to the pelvic area. It is often recommended in treatments for amenorrhea, dysmenorrhea, and menorrhagia. It is an anti-inflammatory, antispasmodic, astringent, cholagogue, diuretic, hemostatic, and sedative.

Yellow dock (*Rumex crispus*). The root improves liver function. It is an alterative, astringent, blood tonic, cholagogue, and diuretic.

I GOT THE PMS BLUES TEA

When your emotions are down, savor a cup of this sweet,
uplifting, aromatic herbal tea.

1 quart water

½ teaspoon burdock root

½ teaspoon dandelion root

1 teaspoon basil herb

1 teaspoon fennel seed

1 teaspoon nettle leaf

Bring the water to a boil. Add the burdock and dandelion root, cover, and simmer for twenty minutes. Remove from heat and add the remaining herbs. Cover and let steep for ten minutes. Strain. Store in the refrigerator. Drink 1 quart daily.

CRAMPS BEGONE TEA

When cramps make every move an effort, slow down
and rest awhile. Sip this nourishing, relaxing,
mineral-rich brew to calm the spasms.

1 quart water

1 teaspoon dandelion root

½ teaspoon cramp bark

1 teaspoon oatstraw

1 teaspoon chamomile blossom

1 teaspoon red raspberry leaf

1 teaspoon skullcap herb

½ teaspoon ginger root

Honey (optional)

Bring the water to a boil. Add the dandelion root and cramp bark, cover, and simmer for twenty minutes. Remove from heat and add the remaining herbs. Cover and let steep for ten minutes. Strain. Add honey to sweeten, if desired. Store in the refrigerator. Drink 1 quart daily.

NORMALIZE THE FLOW TEA

If your menstrual bleeding is excessive, the blood-building,
astringent, tonifying herbs in this formula will soon
have you feeling like yourself again.

6 cups water

1 teaspoon vitex berries

1 teaspoon wild yam root

¼ teaspoon licorice root

2 teaspoons alfalfa herb

2 teaspoons nettle herb

2 teaspoons red raspberry leaf

Bring the water to a boil. Add the vitex berries, wild yam, and licorice root. Cover and simmer for twenty minutes. Remove from heat and add the remaining herbs. Cover and let steep for ten minutes. Strain. Store in the refrigerator. Drink 1 quart daily.

Nutritional Therapy

Although the most effective way to maintain nutrition is by incorporating into your diet natural sources of the nutrients your body needs (see Chapter 5), supplementation can also be helpful.

Vitamin B complex. The B-complex vitamins offer great support to the liver. Vitamin B$_6$, in particular, can help prevent fluid retention and assist in the metabolism of estrogen. Choline helps prevent the buildup of fat, which can impair liver function. Take 50 mg of vitamin B complex daily.

Vitamin C. Vitamin C with bioflavonoids can help strengthen the capillaries. Bioflavonoids can also control estrogen levels. Take 1,000 mg of vitamin C with 500 mg of bioflavonoids three times daily.

Vitamin E. Vitamin E can help relieve tenderness in the breasts and control prostaglandin levels. Take 400 IU daily.

Magnesium. Magnesium is a natural diuretic and can help satisfy cravings for chocolate, relieve tenderness in the breasts, and control weight gain associated with PMS. Usually twice as much magnesium as calcium is recommended. Look for magnesium in a citrate form; it's easier to assimilate when citric acid is used as a carrier. Take 500 to 750 mg daily. An excess of magnesium may cause diarrhea.

Zinc. Zinc, like vitamin E, can help control prostaglandin levels, an overabundance of which can contribute to dysmenorrhea. Take 25–50 mg of chelated zinc daily.

Aromatherapy

Essential oils have a variety of healing applications for menstrual dysfunction, depending on the symptoms that need to be addressed. The oils recommended here can be used in massage, in the bath, and in inhalations. (See Chapter 7 for more information.)

To control emotional upheavals before and during the menstrual cycles, try jasmine, lavender, and Roman chamomile essential oils.

To bring physical and emotional comfort during the menses, use basil, chamomile, clary sage, fennel, hyssop, juniper berry, lavender, marjoram, myrrh, peppermint, rose, and rosemary essential oils.

To relieve cramping, use anise, carrot seed, clary sage, jasmine, and rose essential oils.

To stimulate menstruation in cases of amenorrhea, try clary sage, fennel, lavender, and rosemary essential oils.

Homeopathic Remedies

When the symptoms of menstrual dysfunction match one of the descriptions below, try the suggested homeopathic remedy. The usual dosage is four pellets, or as many liquid drops as the package label recommends, taken under the tongue four times daily. Rather than swallowing the pellets whole, allow them to dissolve slowly.

Aconitum Napellus. The patient is experiencing amenorrhea or menorrhagia. She is cold, has a frail constitution, and is nervous. She may have an excessive fear of death.

Aletris Farinosa. Menstruation is profuse, early, and filled with large blood clots. The patient feels weak from loss of fluids and has no appetite.

Apis Mellifica. The patient skips periods regularly, feels a stinging pain in the vagina, and exhibits cloudy thinking.

Belladonna. The patient has amenorrhea, dysmenorrhea with irregular cramping, or menorrhagia with profuse, foul-smelling, bright red blood. Urination and the pelvic area are painful, and the face is flushed. Symptoms are worsened by noise and excitement.

Byronia. The patient's breasts are tender for two or more weeks before menses. She has amenorrhea and may have frequent nosebleeds. Motion and rising suddenly worsen symptoms.

Calcarea Carbonica. The patient had delayed menarche (first menses), and her head sweats easily. She has a bloated abdomen and sore breasts. She has menorrhagia with copious, bright red blood. Symptoms are initiated by emotional shock.

Carbo Vegetabilis. The patient has menorrhagia with long, early, copious bleeding.

Caulophyllum Thalictroides. The patient has dysmenorrhea and has suffered from intense cramps since puberty.

Chamomilla. The patient has amenorrhea or cramps that are relieved by heat. She is stressed, impatient, and irritable about everything. One cheek may be red while the other is pale.

Cimicifuga Racemosa. The patient suffers from depression, cramps, pains that shoot down the hips, and headaches. The menses are profuse.

Cocculus Indicus. The patient has dysmenorrhea with nausea. She feels too weak to stand. Dark clots of blood appear in the menstrual flow.

Colocynthis. Menstruation is painful, but pressure applied to the area in pain brings relief. The patient is irritable.

Dulcamara. The patient suffers from emotional ups and downs and tender, engorged breasts. She has amenorrhea caused by cold, damp conditions. She may have warts.

Ferrum Metallicum. Menarche was delayed because of debility. The patient has puffy ankles and poor complexion. She suffers from menorrhagia that is early, profuse, and weakening. The menstrual flow is watery and pale.

Hamamelis Virginiana. Menstruation is profuse.

Ignatia. The menses are delayed because of emotional distress.

Kali Carbonicum. The patient suffers from exhaustion and feels a pain in her left side. She is overweight and exhibits fear and anxiety. This remedy can also be used for amenorrhea if *Natrum Muriaticum* fails.

Lachesis. The patient suffers from dysmenorrhea with severe headaches that abate as soon as menstrual flow begins. Wearing tight clothing worsens symptoms. This remedy may also be used for amenorrhea that is caused by fear, if menarche has not happened by eighteen years of age, and for menorrhagia with a heavy, painful flow containing dark blood clots.

Lycopodium. The patient has vaginal dryness, bloating, and pain in the right ovary. She feels weepy, craves sweets, and suffers from premenstrual depression. Headaches may occur in the temples in late afternoon and early evening.

Magnesium Phosphate. The patient has dysmenorrhea. The pain is worse on the right side. Symptoms are worsened by cold and improved by warmth and bending over.

Natrum Muriaticum. The patient has PMS or amenorrhea. She craves salt, feels tired and weak, and suffers from bloating and fluid retention. She wants to be alone and cries.

Phosphorus. The patient has metrorrhagia caused by fibroids.

Pulsatilla. The patient feels weepy and gentle. She faints easily. She suffers from migraines, backache, and diarrhea, and her endocrine system is unbalanced. Use this remedy for amenorrhea caused by wetness, dysmenorrhea accompanied by sore breasts, excessively delayed menarche, and menstrual irregularity caused by anger and overwork.

Sabina. The patient has early, long, and heavy periods. The menstrual flow may contain red blood clots, and cramping may be intense. She has menorrhagia; bleeding may occur without stopping until the next menses.

Senecio Aureus. The patient has amenorrhea that causes digestive upset.

Sepia. The patient has amenorrhea; she discharges leukorrhea instead of menstrual flow. She has intense headaches and a delicate constitution. She may suffer from a general feeling that every action requires tremendous effort.

Silicea. The patient suffers from general weakness. She is underdeveloped and has cold extremities. Her menses are excessively heavy and her breasts are tender.

Sulfur. The patient has amenorrhea, and all other remedies have failed. She may also suffer from acne, itchy rashes, irritability, and forgetfulness. She may crave sweets and have headaches.

Viburnum Opulus. The patient experiences sudden uterine pain, backache, and late, light menses. Symptoms worsen at night.

Xanthoxylum. The patient suffers from dysmenorrhea, with pain felt down the thighs. The menses are early and profuse. Menstrual flow is thick and blackish. Before menstruation, the patient develops a headache over her left eye. She has a nervous, frail constitution.

Flower Essences

Flower essences for women with menstrual difficulties include the following. The usual dosage is 7 drops under the tongue, or taken with a glass of water three or four times daily.

Evening Primrose. This essence helps balance hormonal cycles and can be used in treatments for amenorrhea, dysmenorrhea, and metrorrhagia. It helps heal painful emotions picked up from our mothers.

Fairy Lantern. Fairy Lantern can help adolescent girls, who are not developing physically or emotionally, integrate better into the world and develop into responsible adults.

Impatiens. Impatiens can relieve nervous tension, calm emotional outbursts, and ease cramps.

Mugwort. This essence can help clear old, negative emotions and control hysterical, irrational behavior.

Pomegranate. Women who have a difficult time balancing their career and their family will find that this essence encourages creativity and a feeling of nurturing. It's especially helpful when psychological stress is affecting the reproductive system.

Star Tulip. Women who seem to have a protective wall around their emotions will find that Star Tulip helps them tune in to their inner voice and become more sensitive and receptive.

MENOPAUSE

Menopause is defined as the cessation of menstruation. It can happen as a natural cycle in a woman's life or as the result of a hysterectomy. It usually begins about forty years after menarche; if it occurs before the age of forty, it is considered premature. Menopause may pass through a woman's life very quickly or may persist for several years. When a woman has not had a period for thirteen months, it is time to celebrate her graduation from menopause and her entrance into the age of wise womanhood.

> Of all the mammals, only humans experience menopause. Other mammals are capable of reproducing until they die. Perhaps this is part of the Great Plan, that women can have babies and be there to take care of them until they are all grown.

Though menopause may bring some discomfort, it is not an illness. It is, instead, a rite of passage. It is by no means the beginning of the end. After menopause, many women experience renewed energy, new creative potential, and self-empowerment. And they continue to live healthy, productive, joyous lives.

During perimenopause—the five to ten years preceding the end of the menses—the ovaries become sluggish and produce inconsistent amounts of hormones, which can cause menstruation cycles to become unpredictable. Anovulation (a menstrual cycle in which a woman fails to ovulate) becomes more common, even though thousands of immature follicles remain in the ovaries. Estrogen and progesterone levels vascilate, although the pituitary gland continues to produce follicle-stimulating hormone (FSH) and luteinizing hormone (LH).

Hormonal changes during perimenopause can have opposite menstrual results: very heavy bleeding and very light bleeding. These are early signs of menopause. Heavy bleeding (on par with menorrhagia) can occur when progesterone levels drop but estrogen levels do not. Although more common in African-American women, heavy bleeding is not experienced by all women. Eventually estrogen levels drop as well, resulting in light bleeding and missed periods.

Most women experience the gradual cessation of menstruation, unless it occurs abruptly through surgery or other circumstances. Other signs of menopause may include hot flashes, vaginal dryness, and thinning vaginal walls; these are thought to be triggered by sudden drops in estrogen levels.

In the tradition of Oriental medicine, menopausal difficulties are often associated with a blood, liver, or kidney deficiency. If blood and yin fluids are imbalanced, night sweats, excessive menstrual bleeding, irritability, dizziness, headaches, and insomnia can occur. The liver is responsible for breaking down and eliminating excess hormones; if the liver is exhausted, depression, anger, restless sleep, and hot flashes can occur. The kidneys govern sexual vitality and mental energy; when the kidneys are deficient, lower back pain, decreased libido, and incontinence may result.

Menopause can be a good time to clear stored-up negative emotions. Are there people in your life to whom you owe an apology, a letter, flowers, or money? Are there people whom you need to confront to clear your mind, such as a parent or an old lover? And if you've ever thought about recording your life and all the history of your family that you can remember, now is a good time to get started, while you're entering the introspective years of wise womanhood.

Enjoy this time of change and growth!

One of my favorite books about menopause is *New Menopausal Years, The Wise Woman Way: Alternative Approaches for Women 30–90* by Susun S. Weed (Ash Tree Publishing, 2001). If you're interested in learning more about menopause from a self-help, natural-healing standpoint, I wholeheartedly recommend this book as an excellent resource.

Hot Flashes

Researchers have yet to pinpoint why menopausal women experience hot flashes, although they believe them to be linked to sudden drops in estrogen levels and elevated levels of FSH and LH. Hot flashes are characterized by a sudden feeling of intense warmth, often accompanied by heart palpitations, anxiety, faintness, flushing, headache, and sweating. On average, hot flashes last about three minutes, but they can persist for up to an hour.

When you're experiencing a hot flash, there's not much you can do but ride it out. If you're having hot flashes regularly, get prepared. Set a fan near your desk or wherever you spend most of your time. Drink plenty of cool beverages. Wear light clothing in layers, so that you can strip down if you need to. Avoid hot and spicy foods. Prepare an aromatic spritzer by mixing 8 ounces of water and 20 drops of peppermint essential oil; when you experience a hot flash, spritz this cooling mixture onto your face and neck (keep eyes and mouth closed). Furthermore, express your feelings. Bottled-up emotions can cause you to heat up and blow your top!

Hydrotherapy can also help with hot flashes. Fill a tub with cold water to a depth of six inches. Walk barefoot in the tub, pacing back and forth for about three minutes. Then dry your feet, put on shoes, and go for a short walk. You'll quickly feel cooled and energized.

Natural Therapies for Healthy Menopause

Natural therapies for encouraging health and minimizing discomfort during menopause focus on building the blood, supporting the liver and kidneys, promoting vaginal elasticity, strengthening the bones, and normalizing estrogenic activity.

Diet

During menopause, eat plenty of foods that build the blood and strengthen the liver, such as barley, beets, beet greens, black beans, black sesame seeds, fish, green, leafy vegetables, jujube dates, lycii berries, millet, mulberries, mung beans, pomegranates, string beans, walnuts, and yams. Also incorporate into the diet seaweeds, which are rich in minerals and help promote elasticity of the vaginal tissues.

Soy is gaining recognition as a beneficial food for menopause because of its normalizing effect on the body's production of estrogen. In addition, soy is rich in calcium, which helps build the bones, and isoflavone antioxidants, which can reduce hot flashes. However, remember that soy can be difficult to digest and is a common allergen. The best forms of soy are tempeh and miso (from organically grown, non-genetically-modified soybeans), which are fermented and easy to digest.

Dairy products are often touted for their calcium content. Of all these products, yogurt is the most beneficial for women. It not only provides bone-strengthening calcium but also supports and replenishes friendly vaginal bacteria.

Minimize your intake of alcohol, sugar, caffeine, carbonated beverages, fried foods, and high-fat foods. When eaten in large quantities, they can worsen hot flashes.

Exercise

Weight-bearing exercise such as walking, jump roping, dancing, or light weight lifting can help build bones, increase muscle mass, and control the tendency to gain weight. Be sure to stretch both before and after exercising to encourage flexibility along with strength.

To keep the reproductive organs in good tone, practice Kegel exercises daily. (See page 30 for instructions.)

Herbal Therapy

For best effect, an herbal protocol should be continued for at least three menstrual cycles. Some may become partners in health for years.

Alfalfa (*Medicago sativa*). The herb helps build the blood and normalize estrogen levels. It is a diuretic, nutritive, phytoestrogenic, and tonic. Avoid in cases of heavy menstrual bleeding.

Angelica (*Angelica archangelica, A. atropurpurea*). The root relieves muscle spasms and tension headaches. It has a gladdening effect on the emotional state. It is a diuretic, emmenagogue, nervine, phytoestrogenic, and uterine stimulant. Avoid during pregnancy and in cases of heavy bleeding or diabetes. In rare cases, the root causes photosensitivity.

Asparagus (*Asparagus officinalis, A. cochinchinensis*). The root is particularly helpful for women who have had hysterectomies, because it helps relieve vaginal dryness. It also can improve libido and reduce irritability. It is an aphrodisiac, cardiotonic, demulcent, diuretic, nutritive, and kidney tonic.

Black cohosh (*Actaea racemosa*). The root can soothe irritation of cervix, uterus, and vagina, calm hysteria, and reduce FSH levels. It is often recommended in treatments for edema, hot flashes, and headaches. It is an antispasmodic, cardiotonic, emmenagogue, smooth muscle relaxant, phytoestrogenic, and sedative. Avoid during pregnancy, except in the final stages, and then only under the guidance of your health care provider. Avoid while nursing and in cases of high blood pressure or pressure in the inner eye. Consult with your health care provider before use. This herb is endangered in the wild; do not use wildcrafted supplies.

Black haw (*Viburnum prunifolium*). The bark is a tonic and sedative for the reproductive organs and nervous system. It also can reduce heart palpitations. It is an antispasmodic, hypotensive, and sedative.

Blessed thistle (*Cnicus benedictus*). The herb strengthens the liver and reproductive organs. It is a bitter, meaning that it stimulates natural digestive secretions, and it is often recommended for menopausal women who have difficulty with digestion. It is an antidepressant, bitter tonic, and cholagogue.

Blue cohosh (*Caulophyllum thalictroides*). The root promotes estrogenic activity and can tonify a weak uterus. It is an anti-inflammatory, antispasmodic, diuretic, emmenagogue, and uterine tonic. Avoid during pregnancy, except in the final stages, and then only under the guidance of your health care provider. Make sure the root is dried, not fresh. This herb is endangered in the wild; do not use wildcrafted supplies.

Bupleurum (*Bupleurum chinense, B. falcatum*). The root supports liver function and promotes blood circulation. It can help dispel anger, grief, moodiness, and fatigue. It is an alterative, anti-inflammatory, chi tonic, choleretic, hepatic, muscle relaxant, and tonic. Avoid in cases of fever, headache, or high blood pressure.

Burdock (*Arctium lappa*). The root helps improve liver function, cleanse the kidneys, and relieve lymphatic congestion. It also tonifies the uterus. It can cool hot flashes and clear anger from the body. It is an alterative, aphrodisiac, diuretic, nutritive, phytoestrogenic, and rejuvenative.

Chickweed (*Stellaria media*). The herb cools hot flashes and can help relieve vaginal dryness. It is an alterative, anti-inflammatory, demulcent, nutritive, and refrigerant.

Cramp bark (*Viburnum opulus*). The herb can calm heart palpitations. It is an anti-inflammatory, antispasmodic, cardiotonic, diuretic, nervine, sedative, uterine sedative, and tonic.

Dandelion (*Taraxacum officinale*). The root improves liver function; the leaf improves kidney function. The leaf is also rich in potassium. The root and leaves are cholagogues, diuretics, and hypotensives.

Dong quai (*Angelica sinensis*). The root helps build the blood and clear blood stagnation. It can relieve anxiety, depression, and hot flashes and help restore moisture to dry vaginal tissues. It is an alterative, anticoagulant, emmenagogue, and uterine tonic. Avoid during pregnancy, except under the guidance of your health care provider. Do not use in cases of diarrhea, heavy menstrual flow, poor digestion, or bloating. Do not use in conjunction with blood-thinning medications such as ibuprofen.

Elder (*Sambucus nigra, S. canadensis*). The flower helps the body regulate its temperature, discouraging hot flashes. The berry has a restorative effect for women who have had heavy menstrual bleeding. The flower and berry are alteratives, antispasmodics, and diuretics.

False unicorn (*Chamaelirium luteum*). The rhizome is a tonic for the reproductive organs and helps normalizes ovarian function. It is often recommended in treatments for hormonal imbalance. It is a diuretic and phytoestrogenic. The bitter taste of this herb can cause vomiting. Excessive amounts may cause kidney and stomach irritation, blurred vision, and hot flashes. Do not use without employing birth control during sex unless pregnancy is desired. Discontinue use during pregnancy. False unicorn is endangered in the wild; do not use wildcrafted supplies.

Fennel (*Foeniculum vulgare*). The seed clears congestion from the liver and is a natural appetite suppressant. It has mild phytoestrogenic effect and is also antispasmodic and diuretic.

Fenugreek (*Trigonella foenum-graecum*). The seed boosts kidney chi and contains phytosterols. It is an alterative, anti-inflammatory, aphrodisiac, demulcent, nutritive, rejuvenative, and restorative. Avoid during pregnancy. If you have diabetes, consult with your health care provider before use.

Ginger (*Zingiber officinale*). The root reduces the risk of stroke, invigorates the reproductive system, can inhibit blood clots, and lowers blood pressure. It is often recommended in treatments for amenorrhea, dysmenorrhea, and hypertension. It is an antioxidant, anticoagulant, and circulatory stimulant. Avoid large doses in cases of acne and eczema. Discontinue use if heartburn results.

Ginseng, American (*Panax quinquefolius*). The root can relieve both vaginal dryness and hot flashes. It is often recommended in treatments for adrenal deficiency and menorrhagia. It is an adaptogen, aphrodisiac, chi tonic, digestive tonic, rejuvenative, and restorative. Avoid in cases of excess heat, such as inflammation, fever, and high blood pressure. Since ginseng can be energizing, avoid taking it within four hours of bedtime. Avoid during pregnancy. American ginseng is at risk of becoming endangered in the wild; use only cultivated—never wildcrafted—supplies.

Hawthorn (*Crataegus* spp.). The leaf, flower, and berry lower blood pressure and can relieve heart palpitations and insomnia. They are high in flavonoids and function as cardiotonics, diuretics, hypotensives, and vasodilators. The flowers can also help cool hot flashes.

Ho shou wu (*Polygonum multiflorum*). The root tonifies the blood, the liver, and the kidneys and can help strengthen the bones and muscles. It also calms the nerves. It is an alterative, antispasmodic, aphrodisiac, chi tonic, and rejuvenative.

Hops (*Humulus lupulus*). The strobile can relieve heart palpitations, induce sleep, and calm feelings of anxiety, hysteria, and restlessness. It is an antispasmodic, phytoestrogenic, emmenagogue, muscle relaxant, nervine, and soporific. Avoid during pregnancy and in cases of depression. The fresh plant may cause dermatitis in some individuals.

Horsetail (*Equisetum arvense*). The herb is a muscular and skeletal tonic that can help reverse bone loss. It is often recommended in treatments for menorrhagia. It is an alterative, anti-inflammatory, diuretic, hemostatic, and nutritive. Use horsetail that has been collected in spring.

Lady's mantle (*Alchemilla xanthochlora*). The herb promotes blood coagulation and tissue healing. It is often recommended in treatments for menorrhagia and for hot flashes that are accompanied by an itchy feeling. It also helps clear congestion from the liver. It is an anti-inflammatory, diuretic, emmenagogue, tonic, phytoprogesteronic, and vulnerary.

Licorice (*Glycyrrhiza glabra, G. uralensis*). The root is phytoestrogenic and can improve adrenal function. It can be helpful after a hysterectomy. It is an adrenal tonic, anti-inflammatory, chi tonic, demulcent, nutritive, and rejuvenative. Avoid during pregnancy and in cases of edema, high blood pressure, or diabetes. Do not use in combination with digoxin drugs. Excessive use can cause sodium retention and potassium depletion.

Linden (*Tilea europaea, T. americana*). The leaf and flower cool hot flashes, calm anxiety, and relieve headache, insomnia, and stress. They are antispasmodic, choleretic, diuretic, hypotensive, nervine, sedative, and tonic.

Motherwort (*Leonurus cardiaca*). The herb cools and reduces the frequency of hot flashes and night sweats. It can relieve uterine pain associated with stress, cramps, feelings of emotional upheaval, and heart palpitations. It also clears stagnation from the blood and nourishes the mucous membranes of the vaginal walls. It is a heart and uterine tonic. Avoid in cases of heavy menstrual bleeding and during pregnancy, except during the final stages, and then only under the supervision of your health care provider.

Nettle (*Urtica dioica, U. urens*). The leaf is a muscular and skeletal tonic. It strengthens the kidneys and adrenals and can be used to clear chi stagnation from the liver and kidneys. It boosts the body's metabolism of fat and helps build the blood. It can curb excessive menstrual bleeding. It is an astringent, circulatory stimulant, diuretic, nervine, nutritive, and thyroid tonic. Contact with the fresh plant will irritate the skin. Use only dried herb. Wear gloves when collecting.

Oat (*Avena sativa, A. fatua*). The spikelets and herb reduce the severity and frequency of night sweats and improve vaginal moisture. They nourish the nervous system and help strengthen the bones. They also strengthen the adrenals. Oat is an antidepressant, aphrodisiac, and a cerebral, endocrine, nutritive, rejuvenative, and uterine tonic.

Peony (*Paeonia lactiflora*). The root clears stagnation from the blood. It is often recommended in treatments for irregular menses, cramps, and emotional upheaval. It improves liver function and encourages elasticity of skin. It is a diuretic, emmenagogue, rejuvenative, sedative, and yin tonic. Avoid during pregnancy and in cases of diarrhea.

Poria (*Poria cocos*). The fungus is calming to the spirit and quieting to the heart. It is often recommended in treatments for anxiety, edema, headache, insomnia, or tachycardia. It is an antitumor, cardiotonic, chi tonic, diuretic, restorative, sedative, and tonic.

Red clover (*Trifolium pratense*). The herb is an excellent tonic for general health. It is an alterative, antispasmodic, antitumor, diuretic, nutritive, phytoestrogenic, and vulnerary.

Red raspberry (*Rubus idaeus*). The leaf helps regulate the menses and cool hot flashes. It can relax smooth muscles in the uterus and is often recommended in treatments for anemia, cramps, heavy bleeding, and spotting. It is an astringent, adrenal tonic, kidney tonic, nutritive, and uterine tonic.

Rose (*Rosa* spp.). The hips are rich in flavonoids and can strengthen the nails and hair. They are antispasmodics, aphrodisiacs, blood tonics, cholagogues, kidney tonics, nutritives, and phytoestrogenics.

Sage (*Salvia officinalis*). The leaf helps restore emotional balance and can relieve anxiety, hot flashes, migraines, and night sweats. It is an anaphrodisiac, antioxidant, antispasmodic, cerebral tonic, choleretic, nutritive, phytoestrogenic, and rejuvenative. Avoid therapeutic dosages in cases of vaginal dryness, during pregnancy, and while nursing.

Sarsaparilla (*Smilax* spp.). The root has a mildly stimulating effect on endocrine activity. It also purifies the genitourinary tract and tonifies the reproductive organs. It is often recommended in treatments for hot flashes and after a hysterectomy. It is a diuretic and nutritive.

Saw palmetto (*Serenoa repens*). The berry prevents atrophy of the reproductive organs. Use after a hysterectomy to help normalize the function of the remaining sexual organs. It is a mild aphrodisiac, diuretic, nutritive, rejuvenative, tonic, and urinary antiseptic.

Shepherd's purse (*Capsella bursa-pastoris*). The herb can control menstrual hemorrhage, minimize midcycle bleeding, and reduce varicose veins. It is an alterative, anti-inflammatory, astringent, hemostatic, hypotensive, urinary antiseptic, and vasoconstrictor.

Siberian ginseng (*Eleutherococcus senticosus*). The root (including the bark) can cool hot flashes. It is often recommended in treatments for depression, high cholesterol, hypertension, infertility, and insomnia. As an adaptogen, it protects health during times of stress. It is also an anti-inflammatory, antispasmodic, aphrodisiac, cardiotonic, and chi tonic.

Suma (*Pfaffia paniculata*). The root relieves fatigue and stress. It is often recommended in treatments for anemia. It is an adaptogen, aphrodisiac, chi tonic, demulcent, and nutritive.

Violet (*Viola odorata*). The leaf cools hot flashes and anger. It is an alterative, demulcent, diuretic, and nutritive.

Vitex (*Vitex agnus-castus*). The berry improves the activity of the corpus luteum. It encourages normalization of hormone levels and libido. It is often recommended in treatments for cysts, fibroids, depression, dysmenorrhea, hot flashes, menorrhagia, metrorrhagia, and vaginal dryness. It is phytoprogesteronic.

Wild yam (*Dioscorea opposita, D. villosa*). The rhizome clears chi congestion and can relieve dysmenorrhea. It is an anti-inflammatory, antispasmodic, aphrodisiac, cholagogue, diuretic, kidney tonic, nutritive, and phytoprogesteronic. Avoid therapeutic doses during pregnancy, except under the guidance of your health care provider. The *Dioscorea villosa* species is endangered in the wild; do not use wildcrafted supplies.

Witch hazel (*Hamamelis virginiana*). The bark and leaf contain flavonoids that help heal damaged blood vessels. Witch hazel is often recommended in treatments for dysmenorrhea, leukorrhea, menorrhagia, organ prolapse, and varicose veins. It is anti-inflammatory, astringent, hemostatic, sedative, and tonic.

Yarrow (*Achillea millefolium*). The herb can reduce excessive bleeding during menstruation. However, because it is a diaphoretic, it may intensify hot flashes and night sweats. It is also an anti-inflammatory, antispasmodic, bitter, cholagogue, circulatory stimulant, febrifuge, hemostatic, hypotensive, phytoprogesteronic, and urinary antiseptic.

HOT FLASH STASH TEA

These heat-relieving herbs will help your body keep its cool.

1 quart water

1 teaspoon dandelion root

1 teaspoon elder flower

1 teaspoon violet leaf

½ teaspoon motherwort herb

1 teaspoon red raspberry leaf

Honey (optional)

Bring the water to a boil. Add the dandelion root, cover, and simmer for twenty minutes. Remove from heat and add the remaining herbs. Cover and let steep for ten minutes. Strain. Sweeten with honey, if desired. Store in the refrigerator. Drink 1 quart daily.

HORMONE BALANCING TEA

Instead of taking synthetic or animal-derived hormones to help your body through changing times, use the plant hormones (phytosterols) that Mother Nature provides so richly in her wild garden.

1 quart water

½ teaspoon vitex berries

½ teaspoon wild yam root

½ teaspoon dong quai root

½ teaspoon licorice root

1 teaspoon red clover blossoms

1 teaspoon alfalfa leaf

Bring the water to a boil. Add the vitex, wild yam, dong quai, and licorice. Cover and simmer for twenty minutes. Remove from heat and add the remaining herbs. Cover and let steep ten minutes. Strain. Store in the refrigerator. Drink 1 quart daily.

BONE HEALTH TEA

The health of our bones is bolstered by many practices, including weight-bearing exercises, eating calcium-rich foods, having strong kidneys, and avoiding mineral-depleting foods such as sugar. The mineral-rich herbs in this formula, taken now, will yield healthy bones later.

1 quart water

1 teaspoon nettle leaf

1 teaspoon oatstraw

1 teaspoon alfalfa leaf

1 teaspoon horsetail herb

1 teaspoon red raspberry leaf

Honey (optional)

Bring the water to a boil. Remove from heat, stir in the herbs, cover, and let steep ten minutes. Strain. Sweeten with honey, if desired. Store in the refrigerator. Drink 1 quart daily.

Nutritional Therapy

Although women should be able to derive the nutrition they need from their daily diet, there are cases in which certain nutritional supplements can help ease a woman through "the change."

Vitamin A. If you suffer from vaginal dryness, consider supplementing with vitamin A, which nourishes the body's mucous membranes. Look for beta-carotene, which is the precursor to vitamin A; an overload of vitamin A can be toxic to the body, whereas an overload of beta-carotene is simply flushed out with other waste products. Take 10,000 IU of beta-carotene daily.

Vitamin B complex. Hot flashes increase a woman's need for B vitamins, which are lost in perspiration. The B-complex vitamins can also improve energy levels and reduce nervousness. Take 50 mg daily.

Vitamin C. Vitamin C clears heat, nourishes the adrenal glands, and supports collagen activity so that the skin remains elastic and supple. Look for a vitamin C supplement that also includes bioflavonoids, which have a chemical activity similar to that of estrogen. They can reduce excessive bleeding during menstruation, normalize menstrual cycles, relieve hot flashes, and increase vaginal lubrication. Take 1,000 mg of vitamin C with 500 mg of bioflavonoids.

Calcium and magnesium. These two nutrients are often bundled together into a single supplement. They work together to strengthen the bones, calm the emotions, and promote good sleep. If you're having trouble sleeping or if you have a family history of osteoporosis, I highly recommend that you consider this supplement. Take 1,000 mg of calcium and 500 mg of magnesium daily.

Vitamin E. Vitamin E can reduce hot flashes, restore emotional balance, and prevent vaginal dryness. Take 400–800 IU daily.

Iron. If menstrual bleeding is excessive, an iron supplement can help prevent anemia. Take 18 mg daily. Use only if needed.

Evening primrose oil. Evening primrose oil is rich in essential fatty acids. It can stimulate the production of estrogen and reduce excessive menstrual bleeding. If you can find evening primrose capsules, follow the dosage guidelines given on the package label.

Flaxseed oil. If your skin starts to become very dry during or after menopause, flaxseeds can help. Take 3 tablespoons of freshly ground flaxseeds daily.

Chinese Patent Formulas

There are several Chinese patent formulas that can be used to relieve discomfort and promote good health during menopause. Follow the dosage recommendations given on the package label.

Ba Wei Di Huang Wan. This is the famous Eight-Flavor Rehmannia Pills. It is particularly helpful for women who have deficient kidney yin that causes heat symptoms. It relieves nervous energy, night sweats, hot flashes, hot hands and feet, and insomnia and helps regulate hormonal function and blood pressure.

Da Bu Yin Wan. Also known as Big Tonify Yin Pills, this formula helps relieve the heat effects of menopause, such as night sweats, hot flashes, and migraines.

Er Xian Tang. Women who suffer from kidney yin deficiency, hot flashes, night sweats, hot hands and feet, irritability, fatigue, depression, frequent urination, a burning sensation over the kidneys, and insomnia will find relief with this formula.

Gui Pi Tang. This formula, also known as Restore the Spleen Decoction, can remedy excessive bleeding during the early stages of menopause. It also soothes the nerves.

Tian Wang Bu Xin Wan. Also known as Celestial Emperor Tonify Heart Powder, this formula is helpful for calming emotional disturbances and relieving insomnia.

Zhi Bai Di Huang Wan (Zhi Bai Ba Wei Wan). This formula nourishes yin, tonifies the kidneys, and can help prevent hot flashes, headaches, and irritability.

Zuo Gui Wan. This formula can benefit postmenopausal women who suffer from weak kidneys, lack of libido, coldness, and lack of energy. It is also known as Gathering/Returning to the Left Pills.

Homeopathic Remedies

When the signs of menopause match one of the descriptions below, try the suggested homeopathic remedy. The usual dosage is four pellets, or as many liquid drops as the package label recommends, taken under the tongue four times daily. Rather than swallowing the pellets whole, allow them to dissolve slowly.

Apis Mellifica. The menses are suppressed, although the patient may feel as though they are about to begin. The patient feels apathetic and indifferent; she is fidgety, intolerant of heat and touch, and difficult to please. She may cry or scream suddenly. She suffers from edema and vaginal dryness.

Belladonna. Hot flashes suddenly come and go and are felt most on the face. The woman experiences intense flushing in which heat is given off by the skin. She exhibits red skin, profuse sweating, agitation, and restlessness and suffers from headache or pressure. Her menstrual flow contains bright red blood clots. Her vagina may be dry and too sensitive to touch.

Byronia. The vagina is dry and its walls are thinning. Stools are dry. The patient suffers from headache and irritability.

Calcarea Carbonica. The patient experiences hot flashes that cause her head to sweat. She feels cold easily, is pale, and tends toward flabbiness.

Cantharis. The vagina is raw and irritated and feels as though it is burning.

Cinchona Officinalis. The menses are profuse and painful. The patient is weepy, despondent, and sleepless. After menstruation, she is exhausted. Her skin is sensitive to touch. She may feel cold but perspire profusely. Warmth relieves the symptoms.

Crocus Sativus. Menstrual flow is excessive and filled with blood clots, but it does not cause pain.

Ferrum Metallicum. The patient experiences sudden hot flashes. She is in good health but tires easily.

Graphites. The patient experiences facial flushing. She tends to gain weight and has nosebleeds.

Ignatia. The patient is cultured or refined and also hypersensitive. She feels grief with anger; feeling angry gives her a headache. Her emotions are conflicting, and she bottles them up inside until she explodes. She sighs frequently. She may feel a lump in her throat.

Ipecacuanha. Menstrual flow is bright red. The patient suffers from continuous cramping, weakness, and occasional vomiting.

Kali Carbonicum. Hot flashes are accompanied by backache and a feeling of weakness in the legs.

Lachesis. The patient experiences daytime sweating and flushing. Hot flashes are often worse after going to bed and are accompanied by heart palpitations and headache. The patient is often filled with feelings of irritability, melancholy, gloom, hatred, jealousy, and resentment. She is hypersensitive and suffers from headaches, especially on the top of the head. She may speak rapidly and change subjects frequently. The symptoms are aggravated by heat and improved by cold.

Lycopodium. The skin and vaginal membranes are very dry. The patient has poor self-esteem.

Natrum Muriaticum. The patient is emotionally vulnerable but doesn't express her feelings. She is teary, depressed, and exhausted. She has been disappointed by love and tends to hold on to resentments. She suffers from excessive menstrual flow, headache, and constipation. The vagina may be dry, painful, and irritated. This remedy is also useful for women whose menses have stopped after emotional trauma.

Nux Vomica. The patient experiences hot flashes, night sweats, insomnia, and leg cramps. She is irritable and tends to find fault in others. She is also hypersensitive to noise and light.

Pulsatilla. The patient is moody but not aggressive. She craves approval, affection, and sympathy and fears rejection. Her moods are changeable. She becomes weepy when describing her symptoms. She experiences irregular menses and hot flashes, which may be followed by chills. This remedy is often most helpful for fair women with blue eyes and a gentle nature.

Sabina. The patient experiences intense cramps, weakness, and excessive menstrual flow that contains blood clots.

Sanguinaria Canadensis. The patient's cheeks are red and burning. Her hands and feet are hot.

Secale Cornutum. Menstrual flow is excessive but does not contain any blood clots. The patient suffers from severe cramping.

Sepia. The patient experiences sudden flushes with sweating that leave her exhausted and weak. She experiences feelings of anger, gloom, depression, exhaustion, and irritability. She may be weepy and fidgety, except when talking about herself. She has a heavy feeling in her pelvis, lower back pain, and constipation. Menses are frequent, heavy, and painful. This remedy is often most helpful for women with a sallow complexion who enjoy dance and exercise.

Sulfur. The patient experiences hot flashes over her entire body, including her feet. She has a red face and flushes easily; her perspiration may have an offensive odor. The hot flashes are worse in the evening and after exertion. She is thirsty after night sweats. She may be forgetful, selfish, and untidy and reluctant to work. She may suffer from itchy dermatitis, coarseness of the skin, vaginal itching, and diarrhea. Menstrual flow is heavy, and the patient experiences weight loss and a craving for sweets.

Valeriana. The patient suffers from facial flushing, sweating, and an inability to sleep.

Flower Essences

Flower essences that can help a woman through the challenges of menopause include the following. The usual dosage is 7 drops under the tongue or taken with a glass of water, three or four times daily.

Alpine Lily. This essences helps restore a sense of self in women who feel disconnected from their femininity. Black cohosh is a good complement to this flower essence; it can help open blocked areas in the pelvis and release emotions relating to anger and violence.

Borage. Borage helps gladden the heart and can relieve feelings of despair and depression.

California Wild Rose. This essence can help invigorate and inspire those who feel exhausted and tend to focus on the past rather than the future.

Crab Apple. Crab Apple helps clear feelings of being polluted.

Fairy Lantern. Women who are obsessed with trying to look younger and are resisting menopause will find that this essence eases their emotional passage into wise womanhood.

Fuschia. Fuschia is often recommended in treatments for grief, sorrow, and sexual feelings that cause tension. It can help a woman comprehend repressed memories.

Hibiscus. This essence clears sexual blockages. It can be helpful for those who have lost sexual desire and feel emotionally dry. It is often recommended for women who have suffered sexual trauma.

Mallow. Mallow can relieve fears of aging.

Mimulus. Mimulus can relieve fears of a known origin and oversensitivity to crowds and noise.

Oak. Oak provides strength to those who need it to complete their mission in life.

Pomegranate. Pomegranate helps women channel procreative energy into new realms of creativity. It can clear emotional blockages in the realms of feminine creativity, career, and home life. It can relieve mental stress that leads to sexual dysfunction.

Scarlet Monkeyflower. This essence can help a woman understand the message of hot flashes.

Scleranthus. Scleranthus relieves mood swings and restlessness.

Walnut. Walnut is helpful for the woman who needs stability and has to let go of things that no longer serve her purpose.

Willow. Willow can relieve feelings of bitterness, resentment, and self-pity. It can encourage a woman to make a fresh start in life.

Aromatherapy

Essential oils have a variety of supportive, healing applications for menopause, depending on the particular side effects a woman is experiencing. The oils recommended can be used in massage, in the bath, in inhalations, and as spritzers. (See Chapter 7 for more information.) However, to avoid stimulating hot flashes, take only cool baths, not hot ones.

To stimulate estrogenic activity and ease passage through menopause, use the essential oils of clary sage, sage, anise, fennel, angelica, coriander, cypress, and niaouli.

To relieve or prevent hot flashes, use the essential oils of basil, geranium, grapefruit, and thyme.

To counteract vaginal dryness and thinning vaginal walls, use the essential oils of clary sage and cypress. Clary sage can also help regulate the menses and lift depressed spirits.

19

Women's Health

believe that we are each our own best health care provider. After all, who else can better monitor our physical and emotional health, diagnose symptoms, and gauge the effectiveness of healing therapies? The body is not a simple machine but a loving home for our soul—do we really want someone else tinkering with it?

The current Western system of health care encourages us to relinquish control over our own health, and we are fast coming to regret it. Emergency rooms are full of people with a vast range of mild illness. Patients cry out for miracle drugs. HMOs govern treatment decisions. We have specialists for every ailment under the sun, ingenious treatments designed by some of the best scientists on the planet, and still the population becomes more and more prone to illness.

Gone are the days when we looked after ourselves, knew our own bodies, knew our own medicines, and worked as one with Nature to effect community health.

I believe that making a commitment to self-care is one of the important steps we must take in order to reclaim harmony among ourselves and with the planet. Therefore, the healing techniques and remedies in this chapter focus on self-care as a first solution for sexual health problems. You'll find that the at-home techniques are simple in design and, over time, potent in effect. You may wish to find a holistic health care provider with whom you can consult when more serious illnesses manifest in you or a member of your family.

Herbal Dosages

You'll find many recommendations for herbal therapy in this chapter. Unless stated otherwise, the therapeutic adult dosage for a recommended herb is:

- 1 cup of tea three times daily;
- 1 or 2 capsules three times daily; or
- 1 dropperful of tincture three times daily.

To figure out the appropriate dosage for a child, take the child's weight and divide by 150. The resulting fraction is the fraction of the adult dosage that the child should take. For example, a 50-pound child would take $^{50}/_{150}$, or $\frac{1}{3}$, of the adult dosage.

BASIC GUIDELINES FOR SEXUAL HEALTH

A healthy lifestyle is the most important precept of good self-care; it prevents disease, which relieves you of the responsibility to treat it. So live life fully but wisely. Develop harmonious relationships and seek fulfilling livelihood. Eat healthfully, exercise regularly, get plenty of fresh air, and use herbs and natural therapies on a daily basis to build the health of your body and mind.

Some regular habits are particularly important in maintaining health in the female body:

- Wear loose-fitting, natural-fiber clothing and undergarments. Tight-fitting and synthetic-fiber clothing prevent the skin from breathing, contributing to the buildup of yeast.

- Don't sit around in wet underclothing; change into dry clothing as soon as possible.

- Wipe from front to back after using the toilet. This helps keep the organisms that live in your rectum from moving into your vagina.

- Minimize douching, and never douche with chemically scented or flavored douches. These douches introduce toxins to the vagina, leaving you more susceptible to infection.

- Don't use chemically scented bubble baths, feminine deodorant sprays, or deodorant tampons.

- Use only undyed, unscented toilet paper.

- When you must take antibiotics, add to your diet fermented foods such as plain yogurt and unpasteurized sauerkraut, apple cider vinegar, miso, and tamari. These foods support and replenish the friendly bacteria in the body. Follow antibiotic therapy with a two- to three-month course of probiotics (see page 276).

BARTHOLIN'S GLAND CYSTS

Bartholin's glands, a pair of small glands located between the labia minor and the vaginal wall, produce mucus when a woman is sexually aroused. If the glands become blocked, cysts may develop. The cysts do not usually lead to more serious infection or permanent injury, but they may cause discomfort.

Symptoms

Cysts are indicated by heat and swelling. When you run a finger against the labia minor, you may feel a hard lump in the area where the Bartholin's glands are located.

Treatment

Gonorrhea can trigger the development of cysts in the Bartholin's glands, so check with your gynecologist to find out whether you have contracted the disease.

Support your body's battle against the infection by eating plenty of fruits and vegetables and avoiding white flour and saturated fats, which contribute to congestion. The following natural therapies will also be of assistance. These healing treatments may temporarily increase the discomfort caused by the cyst, but the discomfort will soon pass.

Sitz Baths

Take alternating hot and cold sitz baths. (For information on sitz baths, turn to Chapter 12.) The resulting increase in circulation to the pelvic area can help clear the blockage in the Bartholin's glands.

Calendula-Goldenseal Salve

Apply a salve containing calendula and goldenseal to the area to reduce swelling and speed up healing. Calendula-goldenseal salves are available in most natural food stores and herb shops. You can also make your own, following Cascade Anderson Geller's instructions on page 111.

Clay Poultice

At night, mix cosmetic-quality green clay with enough water to make a paste and apply to the skin over the cysts. This healing poultice draws toxins from the skin as it dries.

Oil Massage

Massage the area with 1 ounce of almond oil to which 10 drops each of chamomile, lavender, and peppermint essential oils have been added. This oil blend helps fight infection and reduce inflammation.

Cleavers Tea

Prepare an infusion of cleavers herb (*Galium aparine*) following the instructions on page 72, and drink 4 cups daily. Cleavers cleanses the lymphatic system, clears heat, and relieves inflammation, all of which make the herb very effective for resolving glandular cysts.

Homeopathic Remedies

When Bartholin's gland cysts are accompanied by the conditions that are described, try the suggested homeopathic remedy. The usual dosage is four pellets, or as many liquid drops as the package label recommends, taken under the tongue four times daily. Rather than swallowing the pellets whole, allow them to dissolve slowly.

Baryta Carbonica. The glands are swollen but not infected.

Belladonna. The cysts are accompanied by vaginal dryness and early, heavy periods.

Mercurius Solubilis. The patient has a strong constitution but feels mentally exhausted from overwork. The patient feels rawness or stinging in the genital area, perhaps accompanied by yellow or greenish vaginal discharge.

CANDIDIASIS

Candida albicans is a one of many yeast fungi that grows on the mucous membranes of most living organisms, including people. *Candida* is usually present on the surface of the skin and in the intestinal tract, vagina, and rectum, living in harmony with many other microbial species. The presence of these other flora and the highly acidic vaginal environment—which ranges in pH from 3.5 to 4.5—normally keep *Candida* growth in the vagina under control. When vaginal pH becomes more alkaline, when excess sugar is available to feed the yeast, when the immune system is weakened, or when the species of bacteria that keep *Candida* growth in check are removed, *Candida* proliferates wildly, and vaginal candidiasis—otherwise known as a yeast infection—results.

There are many known factors that cause these changes to the vaginal environment, and probably many more that have yet to be discovered. What we do know is this: Menstruation, pregnancy, birth control pills, some antibiotics, hormone supplements, and diabetes all lead to an increase in vaginal alkalinity. Excess sugar and simple carbohydrates in the diet offer yeast a veritable feast. By stressing the body's cleansing and immune systems, common toxins such as environmental pollutants, fluoride, chlorine, and mercury dental fillings can all encourage the growth of yeast. And antibiotics—particularly broad-spectrum antibiotics—destroy the "friendly" bacteria in the vagina, allowing *Candida* to spread unchecked.

Seventy-five percent of all women have a yeast infection at some time in their lives; about half of these women have the infection more than once.

Symptoms

Symptoms of vaginal candidiasis include vaginal discharge, vaginal itching, vaginal odor, rectal itching, a craving for sweets, depression, mood swings, endometriosis, frequent urination, lack of sexual desire, lethargy, and even premenstrual syndrome.

Treatment

Natural therapy is just as effective, if not more so, than standard medical care for vaginal candidiasis. It's based on three precepts:

1. Restore the balance of vaginal flora.

Symptoms of Non-Vaginal Candidiasis

Candidiasis is by no means limited to the vaginal area. Yeast overgrowth can occur almost anywhere on or in the body. Symptoms of other types of candidiasis can include acne, alcoholism, allergies, asthma, athlete's feet, bad breath, bloating, bronchitis, burning and tingling muscles, chronic constipation, chronic cough, chronic fatigue, diaper rash, diarrhea, extreme sensitivity to smells, frequent infections, frequent sore throats, gas, headaches, impotence, jock itch, joint swelling, lack of sexual desire, lethargy, nail fungus, nasal congestion, oral thrush, redness, ringworm, schizophrenia, small white patches on the skin, feeling spaced-out, and seeing spots in front of the eyes. The tongue is likely to be coated white.

2. Normalize vaginal pH.

3. Support the immune system.

When you begin a yeast-control program, it's not unusual to feel worse at first. The proteins made available by dead yeast can stimulate a histamine reaction, resulting in further irritation of the vaginal tissues and feelings of anxiety and malaise. This is a temporary side effect; taking powdered vitamin C in 1,000 mg doses two or three times daily will help clear the symptoms.

It is vital that you stick with the treatment program. *Candida* is resilient. If you stop the treatment too soon, you sabotage the cure, and the infection will soon return.

Refrain from Sexual Contact

The yeast can be spread by oral, vaginal, and anal sex, so refrain from sexual contact until the infection has cleared. Men carry genital *Candida* underneath the foreskin and in the prostate; if you pass *Candida* to a male partner, he may later pass it back to you, allowing the yeast to circumvent and thus survive the treatment protocol you've undertaken. Researchers do not really agree on *Candida* transmission, but it is more likely to occur if either partner is immuno-compromised.

Probiotics

Yeast, bacteria, and other microbial organisms maintain a finely poised balance in the body. Antibiotics destroy "friendly" bacteria, allowing opportunistic *Candida* to expand. Probiotics replenish and support bacteria, bringing balance back to the flora of the body.

The bacterium *Lactobacillus acidophilus,* more commonly known as acidophilus, is among the most effective probiotics for treating yeast infections. Acidophilus and *Candida* have similar binding sites in the intestinal tract. The more acidophilus present, the less room there is for *Candida*. Acidophilus also produces lactic acid, which helps normalize the acidity of the vaginal environment, and competes with *Candida* for food sources.

Another useful bacterium is *Bacillus laterosporus,* which seems to destroy yeasts and support friendly bacteria.

Both *Lactobacillus acidophilus* and *Bacillus laterosporus* can be taken as supplements, in either powdered or pill form. Most natural food stores carry these probiotics.

After a course of antibiotic therapy, begin a course of probiotic therapy. Take one or two capsules of *Lactobacillus acidophilus* or *Bacillus laterosporus* three times daily (not with meals) for three to four months.

While you are taking antibiotics, incorporate fermented foods, such as plain yogurt and unpasteurized sauerkraut, apple cider vinegar, miso, and tamari, into your diet. Fermented foods are a good source of probiotics. Eat at least one serving a day.

Suppositories

Vaginal suppositories are very effective for treating yeast infections; they introduce the cure directly to the infected area. A garlic clover suppository is a potent antiyeast treatment. At bedtime, peel the skin from a single clove and insert the raw clove into the vagina. Do not to cut the clove, as the potent juices can be irritating to the delicate tissues of the vagina. In the morning, remove the clove. You shouldn't have any trouble removing it, but if you're overly concerned, place the clove in a square of cheesecloth, gather the corners of the cloth together, and tie it off with dental floss, leaving a string of floss hanging out far enough to aid retrieval.

Boric acid is another effective antiyeast suppository. Insert a "0" capsule filled with boric acid high into the vagina five to seven nights in a row. (Do not ingest boric acid, as it is mildly toxic.)

Probiotic suppositories help resupply the vagina with friendly bacteria. Try using two "00" capsules of acidophilus or, preferably, a broad-spectrum probiotic formula containing acidophilus and *Bifidobacterium bifidum* (sometimes called *bifidus*) or *Lactobacillus bulgaricus*. Insert the capsules high into the vagina five to seven nights in a row.

Plain yogurt can also be used as a vaginal suppository to introduce acidophilus directly to the vagina. At bedtime, insert a small amount into the vagina; the applicator that comes with spermicidal cream or jelly makes this an easy task. Wear a cotton menstrual pad to prevent the yogurt from dripping over the bedsheets. Repeat for five to seven nights.

> If you are pregnant, do not insert anything into the vagina, including suppositories and douches, without consulting your health care provider.

Douches

Douches, like suppositories, introduce the cure directly to the point of infection. For an effective antiyeast douche, mix 1 quart of water with one of the following:

- ¼ tablespoon of apple cider vinegar
- 1 teaspoon acidophilus powder
- 1 teaspoon salt and 1 teaspoon 3 percent hydrogen peroxide

Douche just twice daily; getting overzealous with this treatment can wash away friendly vaginal flora. Follow up with a plain yogurt suppository.

Antifungal Teas

After bowel movements or urination, wipe the perineal area and then squirt onto it some antifungal herbal teas, such as calendula, echinacea, garlic, myrrh, rosemary, thyme, or yarrow tea.

These teas should be stored in the refrigerator, where they'll keep for up to a week. However, you certainly don't want to squirt cold tea on your sensitive parts. Instead, every morning pour a day's supply of tea into a container, cover, and keep in the bathroom. What isn't used by the end of the day should be discarded.

Diet

For every book that discusses how to treat *Candida,* there's a different dietary theory. To my mind, there's no need to dip into the sophisticated underpinnings of nutritional science to understand what sort of diet supports or counteracts a yeast infection. Instead, follow these six simple, common-sense guidelines.

1. **Avoid simple sugars.** For yeast, sugar is food, and simple sugars make that food readily available. So don't eat sweets; if you must use a sweetener, try using stevia, an herb that has twenty times the sweetening power of sugar without the simple sugars. Don't drink fruit juices, sodas, or alcohol; they're packed with sugar. Simple carbohydrates are another source of simple sugars. Avoid anything made with white flour or gluten-rich grains such as wheat, oats, rye, and barley. Also avoid high-carbohydrate vegetables such as peas, potatoes, winter squashes, and lima beans.

2. **Avoid common allergens.** Whether or not you have a bona fide allergy, common allergens stress the immune system and prevent it from focusing its attention on the *Candida* infection. This is another reason to avoid foods that are rich in wheat and gluten, both common allergens. Also avoid peanuts, pistachios, and cashews. (Substitute them with almonds, hazelnuts, pine nuts, and sunflower and pumpkin seeds, which are not common allergens.)

3. **Acidify your system.** For a *Candida* infection to exist, the vaginal environment must be more alkaline than is normal. The solution is to acidify the body. A good method for this is to start each day by drinking a pint of warm water to which the juice of a fresh lemon has been added.

4. **Eat high-fiber foods.** Backed-up bowels create an alkaline environment in which excess *Candida* can shelter. Fiber encourages healthy bowel movements. High-fiber foods include vegetables, fruits, nuts, and seeds. Most whole grains are rich in fiber, but because they are also rich in carbohydrates, they should be avoided.

5. **Eat foods that warm the system.** In Oriental medicine, a yeast overgrowth is considered a cold, damp condition that obstructs the flow of chi. The remedy is to increase warmth and the circulation of chi. Warming culinary herbs fit the bill. Try seasoning your food with black pepper, cayenne, cinnamon, cloves, curry powder, garlic, ginger, oregano, and turmeric, all of which help dry damp conditions and inhibit yeasts.

6. **Support friendly flora.** Rather than killing *Candida,* simply help the "opposition" outnumber it! Fermented foods, such as plain yogurt, unpasteurized sauerkraut, unpasteurized apple cider vinegar, and miso, help defeat *Candida* by supporting and replenishing friendly bacteria in the body. Chlorophyll-rich foods such as barley grass and wheat grass juices also support healthy intestinal flora and help cool the heat of this damp condition. Also consider seaweeds, which contain beneficial yeasts that compete with *Candida.*

Biotin

Biotin, a member of the vitamin B complex, helps prevent *Candida* from developing. Take 300 mcg daily. Avoid vitamin formulas that use yeast as a base.

Herbal Therapy

Several herbs can be used to inhibit *Candida* growth.

Aloe vera (*Aloe vera, A. barbadensis*). Squeeze the juice from the leaves and apply to the irritated tissue. It is an antifungal, anti-inflammatory, antiseptic, demulcent, and rejuvenative. Avoid internal use during pregnancy and in cases of intestinal inflammation.

Asafoetida (*Ferula foetida, F. assa-foetida, F. rubricaulis*). The resin is warming to the digestive tract and counteracts *Candida* overgrowth. It is an antiseptic, a carminative, and a digestive tonic. In rare cases, it may cause diarrhea. Avoid therapeutic doses during pregnancy and in cases of ulcers.

Black walnut (*Juglans nigra*). The hull contains juglone, an antifungal compound. It is an alterative, antifungal, anti-inflammatory, antiseptic, antiparasitic, and astringent.

Calendula (*Calendula officinalis*). The flower is a time-tested remedy against chronic infection. It is an alterative, anti-inflammatory, antifungal, astringent, and vulnerary.

Cayenne (*Capsicum annuum*). The fruit dries cold, damp conditions. It is an antifungal, alterative, anti-inflammatory, antioxidant, antiseptic, circulatory stimulant, and tonic. Avoid contact with eyes and mucous membranes. Avoid therapeutic doses during pregnancy and while nursing.

Chaparral (*Larrea tridentata*). The leaf inhibits the growth of molds, bacteria, and pathogens. It also dries dampness in the body. It is an alterative, antifungal, antioxidant, antiseptic, and immunostimulant. Avoid in cases of liver or kidney disease, cirrhosis, or hepatitis and during pregnancy. Discontinue use if nausea, fatigue, fever, or jaundice occur. Do not use for more than a month at a time. Consult with your health care provider before use.

Cubeb (*Piper cubeba*). The berry helps eliminate bladder mucus and clears cold and dampness. It is an antiseptic, carminative, stomach tonic, and yang tonic. Avoid in cases of acute digestive and kidney irritation.

Echinacea (*Echinacea purpurea, E. angustifolia*). The root stimulates the immune system and inhibits fungal growth. It also dries dampness. It is an alterative, antifungal, anti-inflammatory, antiseptic, carminative, digestive tonic, and vulnerary.

Evening primrose (*Oenothera biennis*). The oil of the seeds stimulates the T cells of the immune system.

Garlic (*Allium sativum*). The clove cleanses mucous membranes and helps clear yeast infections. It can be used as a suppository and incorporated in liberal amounts into the diet. It is an alterative, antifungal, antioxidant, antiseptic, carminative, immunostimulant, and yang tonic. Some people are allergic to garlic. Excessive use can cause emotional irritability and irritation of the stomach and kidneys. Avoid therapeutic doses during pregnancy, and avoid during the first three months of nursing, as it can cause breast milk to become unpalatable for infants. Avoid use the week before having surgery.

Goldenseal (*Hydrastis canadensis*). The root clears infection and increases blood supply to the spleen. It is an alterative, antifungal, anti-inflammatory, antiseptic, bitter tonic, and cholagogue. Goldenseal is very bitter, and most people find it easiest to ingest in capsule form. The tea can be used as a douche. Goldenseal salves and powders can be applied topically. This herb is endangered in the wild; do not use wildcrafted supplies. Avoid during pregnancy.

Marsh mallow (*Althaea officinalis*). The root soothes and moistens irritated mucous membranes and stimulates white blood cell production. Use as a tea or a douche. It is an alterative, demulcent, immunostimulant, nutritive, rejuvenative, and vulnerary.

Nettle (*Urtica dioica, U. urens*). The herb increases the oxygen available to mucous membranes, which helps make them stronger and less susceptible to infection. It also dries dampness and helps lessen the effect of food sensitivities. It is an adrenal tonic, alterative, astringent, cholagogue, circulatory stimulant, kidney tonic, mucolytic, and nutritive. Contact with the fresh plant will irritate the skin. Use only dried herb. Wear gloves when collecting.

Oregano (*Origanum vulgare*). The herb inhibits the growth of *Candida*. It is an antifungal, anti-inflammatory, antiseptic, carminative, cholagogue, and digestive tonic. Oregano-infused oil is often available in natural food stores and herb shops and can be applied topically. Avoid therapeutic doses of this herb during pregnancy.

Oregon grape (*Mahonia aquifolium*). The root contains antiseptic properties that are especially beneficial to the skin and intestinal tract. It is an alterative, anti-inflammatory, antiseptic, astringent, bitter tonic, cholagogue, digestive tonic, immunostimulant, and liver tonic. Avoid during pregnancy, and do not exceed the recommended dosage.

Pau d'arco (*Tabebuia impetiginosa*). The bark contains antifungal compounds, strengthens a weakened immune system, and dries dampness. It is an alterative, antifungal, anti-inflammatory, antioxidant, antiseptic, and immunostimulant.

Prickly ash (*Zanthoxylum americanum, Z. clava-herculis*). The bark improves circulation to mucous membranes and inhibits yeast overgrowth. It is an alterative, antiseptic, astringent, carminative, circulatory stimulant, and digestive tonic. Avoid during pregnancy and in cases of stomach inflammation.

Spilanthes (*Spilanthes acmella*). The herb counteracts yeast infections and thrush. It is antifungal and antiseptic. Avoid during pregnancy.

Turmeric (*Curcuma longa, C. aromatica*). The rhizome helps heal ulcerated intestinal mucus and stabilizes microflora, thus inhibiting yeast overgrowth. It is an alterative, antifungal, anti-inflammatory, antioxidant, antiseptic, astringent, cholagogue, circulatory stimulant, digestive tonic, and vulnerary.

Usnea (*Usnea barbata*). This lichen is often recommended in treatments for deep-seated infections of the body. It is an antifungal, antiseptic, and immunostimulant.

Yarrow (*Achillea millefolium*). The herb opens pores and aids in the elimination of wastes, helping flush toxins from the body. It is an anti-inflammatory, antifungal, antiseptic, astringent, bitter tonic, carminative, cholagogue, circulatory stimulant, digestive tonic, and urinary antiseptic. Avoid during pregnancy.

Homeopathic Remedies

When a yeast infection is accompanied by the conditions that are described, try the suggested homeopathic remedy. The usual dosage is four pellets, or as many liquid drops as the package label recommends, taken under the tongue four times daily. Rather than swallowing the pellets whole, allow them to dissolve slowly.

Borax. The infection is diagnosed as thrush.

Calcarea Carbonica. Vaginal itching occurs just before menses. The infection is accompanied by a milky discharge. The patient experiences headache, anxiety, and depression. The symptoms improve in the morning and worsen before and after menses, after exertion, between 2 and 3 A.M., when the weather is cold, damp, and windy.

Candida. Using homeopathic *Candida* can stimulate an immune response in fighting *Candida* yeast. It is especially effective against intestinal and vaginal yeast overgrowth.

Ipecacuanha. The infection is accompanied by diarrhea and profuse mucous secretions. The patient experiences nausea. The symptoms worsen in heat and humidity.

Sepia. The infection is accompanied by a foul-smelling, whitish discharge and vaginal itching, soreness, and burning. The patient is irritable and tearful. Symptoms improve after sleep, eating, exercising, and application of heat to the vulva region. Symptoms worsen in the cold, when the patient is fatigued, during exposure to smoke, during intercourse, and in the early morning and the evening.

Sulfur. The infection is accompanied by a yellow or whitish discharge and vaginal itching, soreness, and burning. The patient experiences pain in the vagina during intercourse, constipation or diarrhea, and anal itching. Symptoms improve with fresh air and dry warmth. Symptoms worsen after spending excessive time standing, in cold and damp conditions, with consumption of alcohol, and in the morning and the night.

Therapeutic Baths

Therapeutic baths are beneficial for both men and women. They are especially well-suited for pregnant women, who should not use douches or suppositories.

Fill the tub with warm water, then add the following:

- 1 cup of unpasteurized apple cider vinegar (to support and replenish friendly bacteria)

- 1 pound of salt (to inhibit yeast)

- 7 drops of allspice, chamomile, cinnamon, cloves, eucalyptus, geranium, lavender, patchouli, rosemary, or tea tree essential oil (to inhibit yeast)

When bathing, use coconut-based soaps. Coconut contains caprylic acid, which has anti-*Candida* properties. Avoid soaps and lubricants that contain glycerin, which is sweet and can feed yeasts.

CERVICAL DYSPLASIA

Cervical dysplasia is an abnormal precancerous cellular growth on the cervix. Though its causes are unknown, cervical dysplasia has been linked to having intercourse at an early age, having had numerous sexual partners, birth control pills, hormonal therapy, smoking, and sexually transmitted diseases, including venereal warts. If caught in its early stages, cervical dysplasia is benign.

Practices that may lessen your risk for developing cervical dysplasia include using barrier methods of contraception (such as condoms and diaphragms), washing before and after intercourse, and maintaining a strong immune system.

Having cervical dysplasia is not the same thing as having cancer. In fact, most cases of cervical dysplasia resolve themselves, returning to normal without treatment. However, once a Pap smear has shown that you have cervical dysplasia, you will require regular Pap smear testing for the next year to monitor the condition. One should have regular followups with a health care provider.

Symptoms

Cervical dysplasia most often yields no outward symptoms, although in some cases it may cause blood-stained discharge or bleeding between periods, with defecation, or after intercourse. In late stages, the condition may cause a foul-smelling discharge. The problem is usually detected by a Pap smear.

Treatment

Natural therapies for treating cervical dysplasia focus on supporting the liver and immune system, preventing cancerous growths, relieving irritation of mucous membranes, and reducing inflammation. Overall, they encourage the dissolution of cervical growths.

The most important treatment for cervical dysplasia is getting healthy. If you're on hormone replacement therapy, talk to your doctor about stopping. Give up addictions. Enforce a healthy diet. Eliminate sources of stress. And consult with a holistic health care provider to create a personalized health care program that supports vibrant health.

Nutritional Therapy

The following nutrients can have a positive effect on cervical dysplasia. Try to incorporate natural sources of these nutrients into your diet; you may also wish to use supplements.

Antioxidants. Antioxidants prevent free-radical damage in the body, which is believed to contribute to cancerous growths. They also strengthen mucous membranes and help the body resist infections. Antioxidants are best absorbed through natural sources of the nutrients beta-carotene, vitamin C, vitamin E, selenium, and superoxide dismutase. Good sources of each are listed in Chapter 5.

Folic acid. In some cases, an irregular Pap smear results from a folic acid deficiency. This is most often the case for women on the Pill, because the synthetic estrogens tend to have a combative effect on folic acid levels. Take 400 mcg daily. Also add plenty of leafy greens, a great source of folic acid, to your diet.

Vitamin B$_6$. Vitamin B$_6$, also known as pyridoxine, supports healthy cellular growth and may encourage normal cells to replace dysplastic cells on the cervix. Take 50 mg daily. For a list of natural sources of B$_6$, see Chapter 5.

Vitamin A. Vitamin A can prevent cells from becoming malignant. The best source of vitamin A is beta-carotene, which is a precursor to vitamin A. Take 25,000–50,000 IU of beta-carotene daily. Better yet, incorporate natural sources of beta-carotene into your diet.

Herbal Therapy

Herbs that can be used to treat cervical dysplasia include:

Burdock (*Arctium lappa*). The root supports proper functioning in the organs of elimination and relieves lymphatic congestion. It is an alterative, antifungal, antiseptic, anti-inflammatory, antitumor, choleretic, demulcent, diuretic, laxative, nutritive, and rejuvenative.

Celandine (*Chelidonium majus*). The root and leaves contain berberine, an alkaloid that fights infection. They have alterative, anodyne, anti-inflammatory, and cholagogue properties. Use only in small doses; 2 or 3 drops of tincture three times daily is adequate. Consult with your health care provider before use, and avoid during pregnancy.

Chaparral (*Larrea tridentata*). The leaf inhibits the growth of some cancer cells. It is an alterative, antifungal, antioxidant, antiseptic, antitumor, and immunostimulant. Avoid in cases of liver or kidney disease, cirrhosis, or hepatitis and during pregnancy. Discontinue use if nausea, fatigue, fever, or jaundice occur. Do not use for more than a month at a time. Consult with your health care provider before use.

Dandelion (*Taraxacum officinale*). The root improves liver function, which relieves stagnation in the reproductive organs. It is an antifungal, antitumor, cholagogue, and liver tonic.

Echinacea (*Echinacea purpurea, E. angustifolia*). The root stimulates T-cell production and macrophage activity in the immune system. It also dilates peripheral blood vessels, thus increasing circulation to the genitourinary area and helping to flush toxins from the area. It is an alterative, antifungal, anti-inflammatory, antiseptic, antitumor, and depurative.

Goldenseal (*Hydrastis canadensis*). The root inhibits a wide range of pathogens. It is alterative, anti-inflammatory, antiseptic, cholagogue, deobstruent, and hemostatic. Goldenseal is very bitter, and most people find it easiest to ingest in capsule form. The tea can be used as a douche. This herb is endangered in the wild; do not use wildcrafted supplies. Avoid during pregnancy.

Licorice (*Glycyrrhiza glabra, G. uralensis*). The root helps the body produce interferon, its own anticancer treatment. It also inhibits the production of prostaglandin E_2, which contributes to inflammation, and soothes irritated mucous membranes. It is an anti-inflammatory, antiseptic, antitumor, chi tonic, demulcent, nutritive, and rejuvenative. Avoid during pregnancy and in cases of edema, high blood pressure, or diabetes. Do not use in combination with digoxin drugs. Excessive use can cause sodium retention and potassium depletion.

Lomatium (*Lomatium dissectum*). The root is an anti-inflammatory, antiseptic, and immunostimulant. In rare cases, lomatium root may cause skin irritation. This herb is endangered in the wild; do not use wildcrafted supplies.

Pau d'arco (*Tabebuia impetiginosa*). The bark inhibits cancerous growths and improves liver function. It is an alterative, antifungal, anti-inflammatory, antioxidant, antiseptic, antitumor, and immunostimulant.

Red clover (*Trifolium pratense*). The blossom is an excellent lymphatic cleanser. It is alterative, anti-inflammatory, and antitumor.

Red raspberry (*Rubus idaeus*). The leaf tonifies the uterus and the cervix. It is an alterative, antiseptic, hemostatic, hormonal regulator, and yin tonic.

Suppositories

Purchase capsules that contain vitamin A in liquid form. Every night for one week, saturate a pure cotton tampon with 25,000 IU of vitamin A and insert it as high as possible into the vagina. Remove the tampon in the morning.

After one week, make an herbal vaginal bolus from the Radical Resistance Yoni Suppository formula. Every night for one week, insert it as high as possible into the vagina. Wear a cotton menstrual pad to avoid any leakage on your bedsheets.

When the week is up, begin with the vitamin A treatment again. Alternate weekly between the vitamin and herbal applications for at least three cycles. Take a break during menses.

RADICAL RESISTANCE YONI SUPPOSITORY

Designed to be a vaginal suppository to help deter infection and yeasts.

1 part yellow dock root

1 part chaparral leaf

1 part echinacea root

1 part calendula blossoms

1 part pau d'arco bark

½ part witch hazel bark

½ part black walnut hull

1 drop cedar leaf essential oil or infused oil
(usually sold as *thuja oil*)

1 drop cypress essential oil

Coconut oil

Combine the herbs with enough coconut oil to make a thick paste. Roll into a suppository shape the size of your pinkie, and store in a glass jar in the refrigerator. Insert before bed. You may wish to wear a cotton menstrual pad to prevent the oil from dripping on the bedsheets.

OVARIAN CYSTS

There are two types of functional (as opposed to neoplastic) ovarian cysts. A follicular ovarian cyst may develop when a follicle has grown—as one or more does every month as part of the menstrual cycle—but does not rupture and release its egg. A luteal ovarian cyst may develop from the corpus luteum if it does not deteriorate as it should after ovulation.

Cysts are by definition filled with fluid. They're quite common, and most are benign and resolve on their own. In some cases, however, ovarian cysts produce large amounts of sex hormones, are painful, or cause irregular menses. Sometimes they rupture, which can be very painful and cause bleeding. In the rare cases where ovarian cysts become extremely painful or dangerous to a woman's health, they should be removed.

Although it is not common, cysts can also be caused by endometriosis or cancer, or they may be dermoid cysts, which are small tumors that contain skin and skin derivatives. In these cases, removal of the cyst by a health care professional is recommended.

Reoccurrence of cysts can be a symptom of hormonal imbalance. If you find yourself getting cysts regularly, stop taking birth control pills and discontinue hormone replacement therapy. Intense exercise can also bring on cysts by banging around the ovaries, which don't have much cushioning to support them.

Symptoms

A cyst is usually first discovered during a routine pelvic exam. If cysts are large or numerous, they can cause lower abdominal swelling, pain in the lower pelvic area, pain during intercourse, and irregular menses. If you experience any of these symptoms, bring them to the attention of your gynecologist.

Treatment

Natural medicine can be quite effective for treating smaller cysts, but larger cysts may require surgery. However, even if you must go the surgery route, consider the dietary and lifestyle changes suggested here; they will help prevent reoccurrence.

The protocol for treating ovarian cysts focuses on regulating hormones, decreasing outside sources of estrogen, improving liver function, promoting prostaglandin production to reduce inflammation, improving lymphatic drainage, increasing circulation to the womb, and removing toxins from the body.

Herbal Therapy

Several herbs can be helpful in preventing and treating ovarian cysts.

Angelica (*Angelica archangelica, A. atropurpurea*). The root normalizes menstrual bleeding and inhibits blood platelet aggregation. It is an anti-inflammatory, astringent, diuretic, emmenagogue, tonic, and uterine stimulant. Avoid during pregnancy and in cases of heavy bleeding or diabetes. In rare cases, the root causes photosensitivity.

Black cohosh (*Actaea racemosa*). The root soothes irritation and congestion of the cervix, uterus, and vagina. It is often recommended to relieve menstrual pain. It is an alterative, anti-inflammatory, antiseptic, antispasmodic, astringent, circulatory stimulant, emmenagogue, and vasodilator. Avoid during pregnancy, except in the final stages, and then only under the guidance of your health care provider. Avoid while nursing and in cases of high blood pressure or pressure in the inner eye. Consult with your health care provider before use. This herb is endangered in the wild; do not use wildcrafted supplies.

Blessed thistle (*Cnicus benedictus*). The herb strengthens the spleen and the liver. It is an alterative, antihemorrhagic, and emmenagogue.

Blue cohosh (*Caulophyllum thalictroides*). The root can be used to relieve pain caused by ovarian cysts and *Mittelschmerz* (ovulation pain). It is an anti-inflammatory, antispasmodic, diuretic, emmenagogue, oxytocic, and uterine tonic. Avoid during pregnancy, except in the final stages, and then only under the guidance of your health care provider. Make sure the root is dried, not fresh. This herb is endangered in the wild; do not use wildcrafted supplies.

Bupleurum (*Bupleurum chinense, B. falcatum*). The root stabilizes menses and relieves liver stagnation. It is an alterative, analgesic, anti-inflammatory, chi tonic, choleretic, and tonic. Avoid in cases of fever, headache, or high blood pressure.

Celandine (*Chelidonium majus*). The herb helps detoxify the liver, supporting its ability to break down excess hormones. It is an alterative, anti-inflammatory, cholagogue, and diuretic. Use only in small doses; 2 or 3 drops of tincture three times daily is adequate. Consult with your health care provider before use, and avoid during pregnancy.

Chaparral (*Larrea tridentata*). The leaf helps reduce the size of growths associated with elevated estrogen levels. It is an alterative, antifungal, antioxidant, antiseptic, antitumor, antiparasitic, and immunostimulant. Avoid in cases of liver or kidney disease, cirrhosis, or hepatitis and during pregnancy. Discontinue use if nausea, fatigue, fever, or jaundice occur. Do not use for more than a month at a time. Consult with your health care provider before use.

Chickweed (*Stellaria media*). The herb helps dissolve cysts in the body; it can be used to treat not only ovarian cysts but also breast cysts and fibroids. It is an alterative, anti-inflammatory, astringent, discutient, and vulnerary.

Codonopsis (*Codonopsis pilosula*). The root relieves stagnation in the pelvic area. It is an adaptogen, a chi tonic, and a nutritive.

Cramp bark (*Viburnum opulus*). The bark relieves uterine pain. It is an analgesic, anti-inflammatory, antispasmodic, astringent, diuretic, and uterine sedative.

Dandelion (*Taraxacum officinale*). The root is a cholagogue and helps the liver break down excess estrogen.

Dong quai (*Angelica sinensis*). The root relieves blood stagnation in the pelvic area. It is an alterative, anticoagulant, blood tonic, emmenagogue, and uterine tonic. Avoid during pregnancy, except under the guidance of your health care provider. Do not use in cases of diarrhea, heavy menstrual flow, poor digestion, or bloating. Do not use in conjunction with blood-thinning medications such as ibuprofen.

False unicorn (*Chamaelirium luteum*). The root is both an antiseptic and a uterine tonic. It can be helpful in treating uterine cysts as well as amenorrhea, dysmenorrhea, endometriosis, infertility, leukorrhea, and uterine prolapse. The bitter taste of this herb can cause vomiting. Excessive amounts may cause kidney and stomach irritation, blurred vision, and hot flashes. Do not use without employing birth control during sex unless pregnancy is desired. Discontinue use during pregnancy. False unicorn is endangered in the wild; do not use wildcrafted supplies.

Figwort (*Scrophularia nodosa*). The herb and root help decongest the lymphatic system. They are often recommended in treatments for polycystic ovarian disease and ovarian cysts. They are alterative, anodyne, antifungal, antiseptic, anti-inflammatory, demulcent, depurative, and vulnerary.

Fraxinus (*Fraxinus americana*). The bark is a circulatory stimulant and helps reduce uterine inflammation.

Ginger (*Zingiber officinale*). The root improves circulation to the reproductive system and reduces blood platelet aggregation. It is an analgesic, anti-inflammatory, antioxidant, antiseptic, and anticoagulant. Avoid large doses in cases of acne and eczema. Discontinue use if heartburn results.

Goldenseal (*Hydrastis canadensis*). The root is a tonic to mucous membranes of the genitourinary tract. It is an alterative, anti-inflammatory, astringent, cholagogue, and deobstruent. Goldenseal is very bitter, and most people find it easiest to ingest in capsule form. The tea can be used as a douche. This herb is endangered in the wild; do not use wildcrafted supplies. Avoid during pregnancy.

Lady's mantle (*Alchemilla xanthochlora*). The herb promotes blood coagulation and tissue healing. It is helpful for reducing heavy bleeding caused by uterine cysts. It is an anti-inflammatory, astringent, diuretic, emmenagogue, hemostatic, liver decongestant, and vulnerary.

Licorice (*Glycyrrhiza glabra, G. uralensis*). The root soothes irritated mucous membranes and inhibits prostaglandin production. It is anti-inflammatory. Avoid during pregnancy and in cases of edema, high blood pressure, or diabetes. Do not use in combination with digoxin drugs. Excessive use can cause sodium retention and potassium depletion.

Motherwort (*Leonurus cardiaca*). The herb inhibits blood platelet aggregation. It is often recommended for treating both breast and ovarian cysts. It is an astringent, circulatory stimulant, diuretic, emmenagogue, rejuvenative, and vasodilator. Avoid in cases of heavy menstrual bleeding and during pregnancy, except during the final stages, and then only under the supervision of your health care provider.

Oregon grape (*Mahonia aquifolium*). The root (including the bark) improves liver function and helps dilate blood vessels. It is an anti-inflammatory, antiseptic, alterative, astringent, cholagogue, diuretic, and immunostimulant. Avoid during pregnancy, and do not exceed the recommended dosage.

Partridge berry (*Mitchella repens*). The herb has a long tradition of use as a uterine normalizer. It is an alterative, astringent, emmenagogue, uterine stimulant, and uterine tonic. Dosages in excess of what is recommended can irritate the mucous membranes. This herb is endangered in the wild; do not use wildcrafted supplies.

Peony (*Paeonia lactiflora*). The root nourishes muscles, including those of the uterus, and improves blood flow to the reproductive organs. It is an alterative, anti-inflammatory, antiseptic, antispasmodic, astringent, blood tonic, emmenagogue, hepatotonic, immunostimulant, and vasodilator. Avoid during pregnancy and in cases of diarrhea.

Pipsissewa (*Chimaphila umbellata*). The herb improves all uterine disorders, including cysts. It is an alterative, anti-inflammatory, astringent, diuretic, and urinary antiseptic.

Pokeweed (*Phytolacca americana*). The root increases T-cell activity in the immune system. It is an alterative, anti-inflammatory, immunostimulant, and lymphatic decongestant. In large amounts, pokeweed root can be toxic. Take only 2 or 3 drops of the tincture daily; after one week, increase the dosage to 5 drops (2 drops in the morning, 3 drops at night). Drink copious amounts of water while you are taking pokeweed root. Consult with your health care provider before use.

Prickly ash (*Zanthoxylum americanum, Z. clava-herculis*). The bark cleanses the body, especially the lymphatic system. It is an alterative, anodyne, antiseptic, antispasmodic, astringent, emmenagogue and circulatory stimulant. Avoid during pregnancy and in cases of stomach inflammation.

Red clover (*Trifolium pratense*). The blossom is an excellent lymphatic cleanser and can be helpful for clearing breast and ovarian cysts. It is alterative, anti-inflammatory, and antitumor.

Red raspberry (*Rubus idaeus*). The leaf is a universal remedy for all women's health concerns. It is an alterative, antiseptic, antispasmodic, astringent, hemostatic, hormonal regulator, nutritive, and uterine tonic.

Redroot (*Ceanothus americanus*). The root encourages the elimination of catabolic waste and breaks up congestion in the body. It is often recommended in treatments for cysts, dysmenorrhea, and lymphatic congestion. It is antispasmodic and astringent.

Sarsaparilla (*Smilax* spp.). The root is a blood and lymphatic cleanser. It helps purify the genitourinary tract by binding with toxins and carrying them from the body. It is an alterative, antispasmodic, diuretic, and rejuvenative.

Saw palmetto (*Serenoa repens*). The berry reduces ovarian enlargement and pain. It is a diuretic, nutritive, rejuvenative, and urinary antiseptic.

Trillium (*Trillium* spp.). The root is an antispasmodic pain reliever and is often recommended in treatments for dysmenorrhea. It also can stanch uterine hemorrhage. It is an alterative, antiseptic, antispasmodic, astringent, emmenagogue, hemostatic, and uterine tonic. Avoid during pregnancy, except under the guidance of your health care provider. This herb is endangered in the wild; do not use wildcrafted supplies.

Turmeric (*Curcuma longa, C. aromatica*). The root inhibits yeast overgrowth and prevents blood platelet aggregation. It is an alterative, anticoagulant, antifungal, anti-inflammatory, antioxidant, cholagogue, circulatory stimulant, emmenagogue, hepatotonic, and vulnerary.

Vervain (*Verbena hastata, V. officinalis*). The herb stimulates uterine activity and improves the body's assimilation of nutrients. It is an anticoagulant, anti-inflammatory, antitumor, astringent, cholagogue, diuretic, emmenagogue, hepatostimulant, vasoconstrictor, and vulnerary. Avoid during pregnancy.

Violet (*Viola odorata*). The leaf is often used in traditional Oriental medicine to treat cysts and abscesses. It also helps break up congestion in the lymphatic system. It is an alterative, antifungal, antiseptic, demulcent, and diuretic. You can incorporate violets, flowers and all, into your diet; try tossing them into fresh salads. You can also use the leaves as a compress.

Vitex (*Vitex agnus-castus*). The berry inhibits excessive cellular growth in the ovaries. It is an emmenagogue, phytoprogesteronic, and vulnerary.

Wild yam (*Dioscorea opposita, D. villosa*). The root can reduce inflammation, move congested chi, and relieve ovarian pain. It also helps normalize hormone production. It is an anti-inflammatory, antispasmodic, cholagogue, diuretic, nutritive, and uterine sedative. Avoid therapeutic doses during pregnancy, except under the guidance of your health care provider. The *Dioscorea villosa* species is endangered in the wild; do not use wildcrafted supplies.

Yarrow (*Achillea millefolium*). The herb increases circulation to the reproductive system. It is an anti-inflammatory, antiseptic, antispasmodic, astringent, cholagogue, circulatory stimulant, diuretic, hemostatic, and urinary antiseptic. Avoid during pregnancy, except under the guidance of your health care provider.

Yoni Suppository

Use a Radical Resistance Yoni Suppository (see page 286) for five nights in a row. Every morning, douche with a tea made from yellow dock root and myrrh resin. Take a two-day break, then repeat. Continue this cycle for a month.

Nutritional Therapy

Any of the nutritional supplements recommended for cervical dysplasia will also be helpful for resolving ovarian cysts. See page 283 for more information.

Castor Oil Compress

The application of castor oil is thought to stimulate prostaglandin and immune system activity. Soak a flannel cloth in castor oil and apply to the lower abdominal area, over the liver and ovaries. Cover with a sheet of plastic and a hot water bottle, and relax for ninety minutes. Apply the compress once daily for three days. Take a four-day break, then repeat the cycle.

Aromatherapy Massage

The essential oils of clary sage, lavender, neroli, rose, and thuja (cedar leaf) can help disperse congestion. Make a massage oil from one of these essential oils, or a combination thereof, following the instructions in Chapter 7, and use it to massage over the abdominal area. You can also add 5 drops of essential oil to the bath.

ENDOMETRIOSIS

The endometrium is the mucous membrane that lines the uterus and is shed during menstruation. Endometriosis occurs when tissue similar to endometrial tissue starts growing outside the uterus, such as on the ovaries, the fallopian tubes, the ligaments outside the uterus, the abdomen, the bladder, and the intestines. In extreme cases, endometrial tissue has been found in the nasal passages, lungs, arms, legs, and brain. These endometrial growths sometimes respond, like the endometrium itself, to the body's hormonal cycle: They build up, break down, and bleed. Intense pain and cramping can result. If endometriosis progresses, the renegade endometrial tissue can strangle the fallopian tubes and cause infertility or increase the likelihood of ectopic pregnancy.

The exact cause of endometriosis is unknown. Symptoms of endometriosis range greatly. Researchers believe there may be a genetic link or altered immune system function at the roots. More research is needed. Dioxin, a toxin found in herbicides, pesticides, and industrial waste, has proven to be a trigger. Women who bleed heavily, experience strong cramps, have short cycles, and had early menarche are more likely candidates for endometriosis. IUDs and tampons may be factors because they cause irritation and sometimes scarring in the uterine area. (In fact, tampons are themselves a carrier of dioxin.) And endometriosis is often accompanied by other conditions, such as candidiasis, lupus, eczema, asthma, and a range of immune system disorders, although the connections between the diseases has not yet been discovered.

For more information about the causes, symptoms, and treatments of endometriosis, contact the Endometriosis Association (see Resources).

Symptoms

Classic symptoms of endometriosis include chronic pelvic pain, severe menstrual cramps, pain during intercourse, fatigue, inflammatory bowel syndrome, and allergies. However, symptoms vary greatly, and diagnosis is difficult. The only way to confirm endometriosis is with laparoscopy, a surgical procedure in which a small viewing tube is inserted into the abdomen, usually through a horizontal incision above the navel.

If you do have a laparoscopy, use homeopathic *Arnica* to reduce swelling and homeopathic *Bellis* to help the tissue heal. Use 30C potencies of both, and take 4 drops or four pellets under the tongue four times daily for several months, or as directed by a homeopath.

Treatment

In treating endometriosis, it's important to focus on five goals:

1. **Improve the health of the liver.** The liver breaks down hormones and filters out toxins that contribute to the disease.

2. **Build up the health of the blood.** Healthy blood supports good health, good energy, and good circulation.

3. **Dispel stagnation.** Stagnation in the liver interferes with the breakdown of excess hormones, and stagnation in the pelvic area contributes to the development of blockages and growths.

4. **Dry mucous membranes.** Endometriosis is considered to be a condition of excess moisture and lymphatic congestion. Drying out the mucous membranes helps reduce this congestion.

5. **Relieve pain.** Endometriosis can be extremely painful, and the pharmaceutical painkillers that are often recommended for it can stress or even harm the liver. Natural methods for relieving pain generally often won't eliminate it altogether, but they can reduce both the severity and duration of pain.

Though endometriosis can be difficult to cure completely, symptoms and pain can be greatly improved. Plan on spending eight months to a year on improving the condition. If treatment doesn't show immediate results, don't become discouraged. Pain may remain unresolved for the first couple of months as old clots and stagnation are released from the body.

High levels of estrogen stimulate the endometrium and outlying endometrial tissues to grow. Pregnancy produces high levels of progesterone, which overpowers estrogen. Therefore, some health care providers might suggest pregnancy as a treatment for endometriosis. This solution is of questionable value. First, it's temporary; when the pregnancy is over, the symptoms often return. And second, pain relief seems like a silly reason to have a baby, unless you really want one.

Sitz Baths

Alternating hot and cold sitz baths is a helpful hydrotherapy technique for increasing circulation to and clearing congestion in the pelvic area. See Chapter 12 for instructions.

Herbal Therapy

Herbal therapy for endometriosis is gaining recognition in the medical community for its effectiveness. For best results, continue therapy for at least six months.

Alfalfa (*Medicago sativa*). The leaf aids in cellular detoxification. It is an anti-inflammatory, diuretic, and nutritive.

Asparagus (*Asparagus officinalis, A. cochinchinensis*). The root supports and moistens yin, which, in turn, supports the endocrine system. It is a demulcent, diuretic, female tonic, nutritive, and sedative.

Black cohosh (*Actaea racemosa*). The root dries mucous membranes and helps regulate menses. It also improves circulation and relieves congestion in the cervix, uterus, and vagina. It is often recommended for dysmenorrhea. It is an alterative, anti-inflammatory, antispasmodic, astringent, diuretic, emmenagogue, and muscle relaxant. Avoid during pregnancy, except in the final stages, and then only under the guidance of your health care provider. Avoid while nursing and in cases of high blood pressure or pressure in the inner eye. Consult with your health care provider before use. This herb is endangered in the wild; do not use wildcrafted supplies.

Blue cohosh (*Caulophyllum thalictroides*). The root relieves endometrial pain and helps regulate menses. It also dries mucous membranes. It is an anti-inflammatory, antispasmodic diuretic, emmenagogue, and uterine tonic. Avoid during pregnancy, except in the final stages, and then only under the guidance of your health care provider. Make sure the root is dried, not fresh. This herb is endangered in the wild; do not use wildcrafted supplies.

Bupleurum (*Bupleurum chinense, B. falcatum*). The root clears stagnation from the liver and blood. It helps normalize menses and can relieve pain. It is an alterative, anti-inflammatory, and muscle relaxant. Avoid in cases of fever, headache, or high blood pressure.

Burdock (*Arctium lappa*). The root cleanses glands and normalizes their function. It also improves the function of the organs of elimination, thereby reducing the load on the liver, and removes dampness. It is an alterative, anti-inflammatory, cholagogue, diuretic, laxative, and nutritive.

Chamomile (*Matricaria recutita*). The blossom helps detoxify liver. It is often recommended in treatments for amenorrhea and dysmenorrhea. It is an analgesic, anodyne, anti-inflammatory, antispasmodic, emmenagogue, and mild sedative.

Cramp bark (*Viburnum opulus*). The bark relaxes muscles, relieving pain. It is an alterative, analgesic, anti-inflammatory, antispasmodic, diuretic, nervine, sedative, and uterine sedative.

Dandelion (*Taraxacum officinale*). The root clears congestion from the liver. It is a cholagogue, diuretic, and liver tonic.

Dong quai (*Angelica sinensis*). The root clears stagnation from the blood and improves circulation. It also relieves congestion in pelvic tissue, helps regulate menses, and relaxes smooth muscles. It is an alterative, anticoagulant, antispasmodic, blood tonic, and uterine tonic. Avoid during pregnancy, except under the guidance of your health care provider. Do not use in cases of diarrhea, heavy menstrual flow, poor digestion, or bloating. Do not use in conjunction with blood-thinning medications such as ibuprofen.

Ginger (*Zingiber officinale*). The root improves circulation and helps relieve inflammation. It is often recommended for amenorrhea and dysmenorrhea. It is an analgesic, anticoagulant, anti-inflammatory, and antispasmodic. Avoid large doses in cases of acne and eczema. Discontinue use if heartburn results.

Hibiscus (*Hibiscus sabdariffa*). The flower is antiestrogenic, suppressing estrogen-induced growths in the uterus. It also helps regulate menses. It is an alterative, anti-inflammatory, antispasmodic, astringent, emmenagogue, and hemostatic.

Ho shou wu (*Polygonum multiflorum*). The root discourages blood clotting and helps reduce benign growths. It is an alterative, analgesic, antispasmodic, anti-inflammatory, and hepatotonic.

Jamaican dogwood (*Piscidia piscipula*). The bark is excellent for endometriosis affecting the fallopian tubes and pain that causes nausea. It is a potent pain-relieving agent, calming ovarian and uterine discomfort. It is also an anti-inflammatory and a sedative.

Lady's mantle (*Alchemilla xanthochlora*). The herb helps prevent excess menstrual bleeding and clears congestion from the liver. It promotes blood coagulation and healing of tissue. It is often recommended for dysmenorrhea and menorrhagia. It is an anti-inflammatory, astringent, diuretic, emmenagogue, and hemostatic.

Licorice (*Glycyrrhiza glabra, G. uralensis*). The root inhibits the production of the prostaglandins that contribute to irritation of the mucous membranes. It is anti-inflammatory, antispasmodic, demulcent, and phytoestrogenic. Avoid during pregnancy and in cases of edema, high blood pressure, or diabetes. Do not use in combination with digoxin drugs. Excessive use can cause sodium retention and potassium depletion.

Motherwort (*Leonurus cardiaca*). The herb relaxes vaginal muscles, thereby improving blood flow to the pelvic region and contributing to the breakdown and removal of endometrial tissue. It is often recommended for amenorrhea and dysmenorrhea. It is an antispasmodic, astringent, circulatory stimulant, emmenagogue, nervine, sedative, and uterine tonic. Do not use for excessive bleeding. Avoid in cases of heavy menstrual bleeding and during pregnancy, except during the final stages, and then only under the supervision of your health care provider.

Myrrh (*Commiphora myrrha*). The resin clears stagnation from the blood and dries out mucous membranes. It is often recommended for amenorrhea and dysmenorrhea. It is an alterative, analgesic, antispasmodic, and emmenagogue. Avoid during pregnancy, and do not use for more than one month at a time.

Oregon grape (*Mahonia aquifolium*). The root strengthens the liver and helps curb excessive menstrual bleeding. It is an alterative, anti-inflammatory, astringent, cholagogue, and diuretic. Avoid during pregnancy, and do not exceed the recommended dosage.

Partridge berry (*Mitchella repens*). The herb relieves pelvic congestion. It is an astringent and a uterine tonic. Dosages in excess of what is recommended can irritate the mucous membranes. This herb is endangered in the wild; do not use wildcrafted supplies.

Peony (*Paeonia lactiflora*). The root relieves cramps and relaxes uterine muscles. It also improves blood flow to the uterus. It is an alterative, anti-inflammatory, antispasmodic, emmenagogue, hepatotonic, and uterine astringent. Avoid during pregnancy and in cases of diarrhea.

Prickly ash (*Zanthoxylum americanum, Z. clava-herculis*). The bark is warming to the abdominal region, thereby helping to clear congestion from the pelvic area. It is an alterative, anodyne, analgesic, antispasmodic, astringent, circulatory stimulant, emmenagogue, and glandular stimulant. Avoid during pregnancy and in cases of stomach inflammation.

Red clover (*Trifolium pratense*). The blossom reduces blood clots. It's a wonderful tonic for general health. It is an alterative, anodyne, anticoagulant, anti-inflammatory, antispasmodic, diuretic, nutritive, and phytoestrogenic.

Red raspberry (*Rubus idaeus*). The leaf helps prevent premenstrual spotting, decreases uterine swelling, and relieves muscle cramps. It is an alterative, antispasmodic, anodyne, astringent, demulcent, hemostatic, and uterine tonic.

Rehmannia (*Rehmannia glutinosa*). The root strengthens and purifies the liver and relieves abdominal pain. It is an alterative, anti-inflammatory, blood tonic, diuretic, hemostatic, and uterine tonic. Avoid in cases of loose stools, poor appetite, bloating, or a coated tongue.

Turmeric (*Curcuma longa, C. aromatica*). Compounds in the root may compete with estrogen for receptor sites, reducing the production of hormones in the body. It can reduce blood clots and uterine tumors and is often recommended for amenorrhea and dysmenorrhea. It is an alterative, anticoagulant, anti-inflammatory, astringent, cholagogue, circulatory stimulant, emmenagogue, and hepatotonic.

Valerian (*Valeriana officinalis*). The root encourages smooth muscles to relax, relieving pain. It is an anodyne, antispasmodic, astringent, nervine, and sedative.

Vitex (*Vitex agnus-castus*). The berry reduces estrogen production and thus reduces endometrial growth. It helps normalize menstrual cycles and regulate the pituitary gland. It is an antispasmodic, emmenagogue, and phytoprogesteronic.

White willow (*Salix alba*). The bark sedates the pelvis, repressing the perception of pain. It inhibits prostaglandin production, thereby reducing inflammation. It is an alterative, analgesic, anodyne, anti-inflammatory, antispasmodic, and astringent.

Wild yam (*Dioscorea opposita, D. villosa*). The root reduces inflammation, clears congested chi, and calms painful cramps, particularly in the fallopian tubes. It contains phytosterols, which help normalize the body's production of hormones. It is an anti-inflammatory, antispasmodic, cholagogue, diuretic, and nervine. Avoid therapeutic doses during pregnancy, except under the guidance of your health care provider. The *Dioscorea villosa* species is endangered in the wild; do not use wildcrafted supplies.

Yarrow (*Achillea millefolium*). The herb can curb the excess menstrual bleeding sometimes associated with endometriosis. It is an anti-inflammatory, antispasmodic, astringent, cholagogue, diuretic, emmenagogue, hemostatic, and uterine sedative. Avoid during pregnancy.

Yoni Suppository

Use a Radical Resistance Yoni Suppository (see page 286) for ten nights in a row. Take two days off, then repeat. Continue this cycle for a month.

To Wan

The Chinese patent formula To Wan, also known as the "Regulate Menses Pill," disperses blood stagnation and relieves cramping. In my experience, and that of my fellow herbalists, To Wan has been effective in resolving many cases of endometriosis.

Nutritional Therapy

Food is always the first choice in providing nutrients for the body. Turn to Chapter 5 to identify natural sources of these nutrients. But as you work on improving your diet, you may also wish to use supplements.

Vitamin B₆. Vitamin B_6 encourages progesterone production and supports the liver's ability to break down estrogen. Take 25–300 mg daily.

Choline and inositol. These two members of the vitamin B complex help the liver break down fats and fat-soluble hormones such as estrogen. Take 25–500 mg of each daily.

Vitamin C with bioflavonoids. Vitamin C, combined with bioflavonoids, supports the oxygenation of tissues, which reduces blockages and promotes tissue elasticity and capillary strength. Take 1,000 mg of vitamin C with 500 mg of bioflavonoids daily.

Vitamin E. Vitamin E can improve the body's use of oxygen and prevent the formation of scar tissue, thereby reducing the development of blockages. Take 100–1,200 IU daily.

Magnesium. Magnesium helps nerves relax, allowing chi to flow freely, and also encourages muscles to relax, relieving pain. Take 500–750 mg daily.

Methionine. This amino acid, like choline and inositol, aids in the breakdown of fats and fat-soluble hormones. Take 500 mg daily. You won't find methionine listed in Chapter 5; good natural sources include apples, Brazil nuts, Brussels sprouts, cabbage, cauliflower, chicken, chives, corn, cottage cheese, eggs, fish, garlic, lentils, milk, nuts, pineapple, rice, ricotta cheese, sesame seeds, soy foods, sunflower seeds, watercress, whole grains, and yogurt.

Castor Oil Compress

Castor oil compresses improve circulation to the pelvic area, stimulate immune system activity, are very helpful for pain relief, and soften scar tissue. See page 292 for instructions on making and applying the compress.

Homeopathic Remedies

When endometriosis is accompanied by the conditions that are described, try the suggested homeopathic remedy. The usual dosage is four pellets, or as many liquid drops as the package label recommends, taken under the tongue four times daily. Rather than swallowing the pellets whole, allow them to dissolve slowly.

Apis Mellifica. The pain feels similar to bee stings and is worse on the right side. The abdomen and uterus feel tender. The patient lacks thirst and produces scant urine.

Arsenicum Album. The ovarian area burns. The patient experiences early, heavy menses with throbbing pain. She feels restless and thirsty. Movement and cold worsen symptoms and cause fatigue.

Aurum Muriaticum Natronatum. The endometriosis is chronic. The uterus is enlarged, and the vagina and cervix are ulcerated.

Belladonna. The pain comes on and disappears suddenly. Sensations of burning, clutching, and stitching occur. The patient feels tired but is unable to sleep. She may experience incontinence.

Cantharis. The ovaries are inflamed. The patient may have had gonorrhea.

Chamomilla. The patient is irritable and oversensitive to the pain, which shoots down the thighs.

Cimicifuga Racemosa. The pain occurs just before the menses. The menses are irregular, accompanied by backache, and produce dark, profuse blood.

Colocynthis. The patient experiences intense emotions, especially vexation. Doubling over and the application of hard pressure lessens the pain.

Dioscorea. The pain is sharp and shoots out in multiple directions. The pain is worse when the patient is lying down or doubled over; it lessens when the patient is moving, stretched out, or bending backward.

Gelsemium. The uterus feels like it is being squeezed. The patient experiences dysmenorrhea and light menses. The pain affects the hips and back.

Helonias Dioica. The menses are frequent and profuse. The patient feels swelling and burning in the endometrial region.

Lachesis. The menses are light and painful. Soreness extends from the pelvic region to the chest. The ovaries are inflamed. The pain decreases during menstruation.

Lycopodium. Sharp pain extends across the body in the pelvic area. The patient discharges blood from the genitals during bowel movements.

Magnesium Phosphate. The pain comes on suddenly and increases with cold, touch, and at night. Warmth and the application of pressure lessen pain.

Mercurius Corrosivus. The patient experiences pain similar to labor pain in the vagina and abdomen. There is a yellowish discharge from the vagina. The menses arrive early.

Mercurius Vivus. The patient experiences abdominal pain, stinging pain in the ovaries, and heavy menses. There is a greenish bloody discharge from the vagina.

Nux Vomica. The pain is worse in the early morning and when cold or pressure is applied. The pain lessens during menstruation, when heat is applied, and when pressure is applied to the head.

Pulsatilla. The menses are light. The patient has diarrhea before the onset of menstruation. There are cutting pains in the uterus, which is sensitive to touch. Intercourse is painful.

Sepia. Menses are either excessively light or profuse and late or early. The patient experiences a sharp clutching or bearing-down pain.

Silicea. The patient experiences bleeding between cycles and feels cold. There is an acrid, milky, leukorrhea-like discharge during urination.

Viburnum. The pain is more sudden and more severe before menstruation. The pain lessens when pressure is applied.

Flower Essences

There are a couple of flower essences that can support the treatment of endometriosis. The usual dosage is 7 drops under the tongue or taken with a glass of water three or four times daily.

Blackberry. This essence stimulates the liver, boosts blood circulation, and improves hormonal function.

Star Tulip. Star Tulip helps people who seem to have a protective wall around their emotions open up.

Aromatherapy

Try the following essential oils in massage oil, the bath, or inhalations. For instructions on preparing these treatments, turn to Chapter 7.

- Angelica—disperses stagnation and is phytoestrogenic.

- Chamomile—relieves pain and inflammation.

- Cypress—disperses stagnation.

- Geranium—disperses stagnation.

- Hyssop—disperses stagnation.

- Lavender—relieves inflammation and calms the nerves.

- Oregano—disperses stagnation.

- Rosemary—improves circulation to the pelvic area.

FIBROCYSTIC BREAST CONDITIONS

According the tenth edition of *Merriam Webster's Collegiate Dictionary,* the term *fibrocystic* is "characterized by the presence or development of fibrous tissue and cysts." *Fibrocystic breast disease,* a term sometimes still heard in the medical community to describe having lumps in the breast, is a misnomer. Every woman has had cysts or fibrous tissue in her breasts at one time or another; a fibrocystic condition, then, is normal, not a disease.

Some lumps in the breast are simple cysts, or fluid-filled sacs. Others are fibroadenomas, or benign tumors of glandular origin. Still others are simply dense areas of otherwise normal breast tissue. Only 10 to 15 percent of breast lumps are cancerous.

Most noncancerous breast lumps do not require medical treatment. If cysts are large, a surgeon can remove the fluid from them. If a lump is large enough to interfere with your ability to properly examine the tissue around it, your health care provider may recommend that you have it surgically removed.

Symptoms

Monthly breast exams will help you become familiar with the normal lumps of your breasts. These may grow or decrease in size through the evolution of the menstrual cycle. If you find a new lump in your breast, don't panic. Unless you have a family history of breast cancer—in which case you should bring the lump to the immediate attention of your health care provider—you may want to keep an eye on the lump for a couple of menstrual cycles. If it disappears or grows smaller during this time, it's probably not a cancerous growth. If it stays the same size or grows, have it evaluated by your health care provider. Nipple discharge, especially bloody, should be evaluated by a health care provider.

To prevent or reduce the size of noncancerous lumps in the breasts, consider the treatment suggestions that follow.

Treatment

The breasts have a high concentration of lymphatic tissue and lymph nodes. If lymph glands or lymph flow in the breasts is obstructed, inflammation and cysts can develop. Therefore, supporting the health of the breasts involves, in part, supporting proper lymphatic circulation. That's good news for our immune system, because the lymph system, which transports the liquid lymph throughout the body, is a vital component of our immune function. Lymph is filled with white blood cells called lymphocytes; some of these lymphocytes evolve into lymphoblasts, which are capable of recognizing and eliminating antigens.

It's also important to support the liver and the colon. The liver breaks down excess hormones in the body. If liver function is impaired, the resulting hormonal overload can result in the development of cysts in the breasts as well as many other maladies. The colon is the organ of elimination. If colon function is impaired, waste matter builds up in the body, imbuing it with toxins.

Wear Natural-Fiber Clothing

Most women are conscious these days of the importance of wearing natural-fiber clothing to allow skin to breathe. Yet most bras are made with synthetic fibers, and we encase our breasts with polyester foam fill and metal wires. These synthetic materials prevent sweat—a waste product—from flowing freely, trapping toxins in the breast region. Stop the madness! Wear bras that are made of cotton or another natural fiber (preferably organic). And go braless when possible.

Exercise

Exercise boosts circulation in the lymph system and supports the elimination of metabolic wastes, helping to prevent cysts from developing. Good exercises for improving lymphatic drainage include jumping on a trampoline and walking while allowing the arms to swing freely.

Yoga postures that help alleviate sore cystic breasts include Laid-Back Camel, Corner Hang, and Twisted Angle. These postures can be learned in a yoga class or from books on yoga.

Avoid Antiperspirants

Commercial antiperspirants are designed to keep you from sweating. Many contain aluminum, which, when it comes in contact with the skin, causes an allergic-type reaction. The pores of the skin swell and close, preventing perspiration from escaping.

Now let's think about this. Perspiration is one of the means by which we excrete metabolic wastes. If we can't excrete metabolic wastes, they must be stored somewhere in the body. So when we apply antiperspirant to our armpits, the metabolic wastes in that area must find a storage location. What roomy, fleshy area is located just around the corner? That's right—our breasts.

Years ago, I had a wise older woman friend who told me she would never use antiperspirant because she thought that they contributed to breast cancer. In my sixteen-year-old naïveté, I thought she was being ridiculous. A few weeks later, while at boarding school, I accidentally knocked a bottle of commercial antiperspirant behind my dresser, and it smashed on the floor. But then the bell rang, and I had to run off to class. Being a sloppy kid, it was a few days before I got around to moving the dresser to clean up the mess behind it. I was amazed to see that the deodorant had hardened into a plasticlike sheet. Gross! I never bought another commercial antiperspirant after that; I use instead only natural, aluminum-free deodorants.

Diet

If you have breast cysts, avoid coffee, tea, cola drinks, and chocolate. They contain caffeine, and most health care practitioners agree that caffeine in any form contributes to the development of breast cysts and pain. These products also contain methylxanthines, compounds that impair the enzymatic activity of cells, contributing to poor digestion and the development of blockages in the body. Even decaffeinated coffee contains methylxanthines.

Avoid hydrogenated oils, such as those found in fried foods and margarine, because they congest the liver. Minimize your intake of dairy products, which cause mucous congestion and often contain the residues of synthetic hormones that were used in raising the dairy animals. The one exception to this rule is plain yogurt; eat at least one serving every day to promote the growth of friendly microorganisms in the colon. Just be sure that the yogurt contains live bacteria cultures and was made from the milk of animals raised by organic methods and without hormone treatments.

To support healthy elimination, drink plenty of water. Juice made from an equal mix of carrots, beets, and celery can improve the functions of all the organs of elimination and provide the body with a great range of minerals. Try drinking a cup of it several times a week.

Include plenty of seaweeds in your diet as they help drain and disperse congestion and also support the endocrine system. If seaweed doesn't suit your palate, take a kelp supplement.

You should see results in two to six months.

Herbal Therapy

There are many herbs that can help reduce the size and occurrence of non-cancerous breast lumps.

Agrimony (*Agrimonia eupatoria*). The herb inhibits blood platelet aggregation, which can be a factor in the development of cysts. It is an anti-inflammatory, astringent, diuretic, emmenagogue, and tonic. Avoid during pregnancy and in cases of constipation.

Astragalus (*Astragalus membranaceus*). The root stimulates immune system response and inhibits the development of free radicals. it is an adaptogen, antiviral, blood tonic, chi tonic, circulatory stimulant, immunostimulant, and vasodilator.

Black cohosh (*Actaea racemosa*). The root helps reduce pain in the breasts. It is an alterative, anti-inflammatory, antiseptic, antispasmodic, astringent, circulatory stimulant, emmenagogue, and vasodilator. Avoid during pregnancy, except in the final stages, and then only under the guidance of your health care provider. Avoid while nursing and in cases of high blood pressure or pressure in the inner eye. Consult with your health care provider before use. This herb is endangered in the wild; do not use wildcrafted supplies.

Blessed thistle (*Cnicus benedictus*). The herb strengthens the spleen and the liver. It is an alterative, emmenagogue, and hemostatic.

Burdock (*Arctium lappa*). The root supports proper functioning in the organs of elimination. It also relieves lymphatic congestion. It is an alterative, antifungal, antiseptic, anti-inflammatory, antitumor, choleretic, demulcent, diuretic, laxative, nutritive, and rejuvenative.

Calendula (*Calendula officinalis*). The flower improves liver and lymphatic function. It reduces glandular swelling and improves peripheral circulation. It is an alterative, anti-inflammatory, astringent, and vulnerary.

Cleavers (*Galium aparine*). The herb is a lymphatic cleanser. It clears heat and relieves inflammation and pain in the breasts. It is an alterative, anti-inflammatory, antitumor, astringent, and vulnerary.

Dandelion (*Taraxacum officinale*). The root improves liver function and supports the elimination of toxins. It also relieves stagnation in the reproductive organs. It is an antifungal, antitumor, cholagogue, and liver tonic.

Dong quai (*Angelica sinensis*). The root improves circulation and clears stagnation in the liver. It is an alterative, anticoagulant, and blood tonic. Avoid during pregnancy, except under the guidance of your health care provider. Do not use in cases of diarrhea, heavy menstrual flow, poor digestion, or bloating. Do not use in conjunction with blood-thinning medications such as ibuprofen.

Echinacea (*Echinacea purpurea, E. angustifolia*). The root stimulates T-cell production and macrophage activity in the immune system. It also improves peripheral blood circulation. It is an alterative, antifungal, anti-inflammatory, antiseptic, antitumor, and depurative.

False unicorn (*Chamaelirium luteum*). The root normalizes estrogen production and helps reduce both the occurrence and size of breast cysts. It is often recommended as a reproductive tonic. The bitter taste of this herb can cause vomiting. Excessive amounts may cause kidney and stomach irritation, blurred vision, and hot flashes. Do not use without employing birth control during sex unless pregnancy is desired. Discontinue use during pregnancy. False unicorn is endangered in the wild; do not use wildcrafted supplies.

Fringe tree (*Chionanthus virginicus*). The bark improves liver function, clears circulatory obstructions, and reduces inflammation. It is an alterative and cholagogue.

Ginger (*Zingiber officinale*). The root improves circulation, helps clear stagnation, and encourages lymphatic cleansing. It is an anti-inflammatory, antispasmodic, antioxidant, and anticoagulant. Avoid large doses in cases of acne and eczema. Discontinue use if heartburn results.

Goldenseal (*Hydrastis canadensis*). The root improves liver function. It is an alterative, anti-inflammatory, antiseptic, astringent, cholagogue, and vasoconstrictor. Goldenseal is very bitter, and most people find it easiest to ingest in capsule form. This herb is endangered in the wild; do not use wildcrafted supplies. Avoid during pregnancy.

Hawthorn (*Crataegus* spp.). The leaf, flower, and berry help break down fatty deposits in the body, including those that form lumps in the breasts. They are astringents, circulatory stimulants, and vasodilators.

Lady's mantle (*Alchemilla xanthochlora*). The herb is a hormonal balancer. It reduces inflammation, clears heat, and relieves congestion in the liver. It is an astringent.

Licorice (*Glycyrrhiza glabra, G. uralensis*). The root stimulates the immune system and inhibits the production of prostaglandin E_2, which contributes to inflammation. It also soothes irritated mucous membranes. It is an anti-inflammatory, antiseptic, antitumor, chi tonic, demulcent, nutritive, and rejuvenative. Avoid during pregnancy and in cases of edema, high blood pressure, or diabetes. Do not use in combination with digoxin drugs. Excessive use can cause sodium retention and potassium depletion.

Nettle (*Urtica dioica, U. urens*). The leaf benefits all systems of the body. It is an alterative, astringent, cholagogue, circulatory stimulant, galactagogue, nutritive, and rubefacient. Contact with the fresh plant will irritate the skin. Use only dried herb. Wear gloves when collecting.

Pau d'arco (*Tabebuia impetiginosa*). The bark increases red blood cell production, helps the body resist autoimmune diseases, and improves liver function. It also can reduce both the size and occurrence of tumors. It is an alterative, antifungal, anti-inflammatory, antioxidant, antiseptic, antitumor, and immunostimulant.

Pokeweed (*Phytolacca americana*). The root improves lymphatic function and increases T-cell activity in the immune system. It is an alterative, anti-inflammatory, immunostimulant, and lymphatic decongestant. In large amounts, pokeweed root can be toxic. Take only 2 or 3 drops of the tincture daily; after one week, increase the dosage to 5 drops (2 drops in the morning, 3 drops at night). Drink copious amounts of water while you are taking pokeweed root. Consult with your health care provider before use.

Red clover (*Trifolium pratense*). The flower is an excellent lymphatic cleanser. It is alterative, anti-inflammatory, and antitumor.

Red raspberry (*Rubus idaeus*). The leaf helps normalize hormone production. It is an alterative, antiseptic, astringent, hemostatic, hormonal regulator, nutritive, and yin tonic.

Sarsaparilla (*Smilax* spp.). The root is a blood and lymphatic cleanser. It contains compounds that bind with toxins and carry them from the body. It is an alterative and a rejuvenative.

Vervain (*Verbena hastata, V. officinalis*). The herb improves the body's assimilation of nutrients and helps reduce the size and occurrence of breast and ovarian cysts. It is an anticoagulant, anti-inflammatory, antitumor, astringent, cholagogue, diuretic, emmenagogue, hepatostimulant, vasoconstrictor, and vulnerary. Avoid during pregnancy.

Violet (*Viola odorata*). The leaf has long been used as treatment for cysts, breast cancer, lymphatic congestion, and mastitis. Eat as a salad herb and use topically as a poultice. It is an alterative, antifungal, antiseptic, demulcent, and diuretic.

Wild yam (*Dioscorea opposita, D. villosa*). The root is a hormonal balancer. It reduces inflammation and clears congested chi. It is an anti-inflammatory, cholagogue, diuretic, and nutritive. Avoid therapeutic doses during pregnancy, except under the guidance of your health care provider. The *Dioscorea villosa* species is endangered in the wild; do not use wildcrafted supplies.

Yellow dock (*Rumex crispus*). The root improves liver, kidney, and lymphatic function. It is an alterative, astringent, blood tonic, and cholagogue.

Nutritional Therapy

Food should always be first source of nutrients for the body. You may also wish to use supplements as you work on improving your diet.

Antioxidants. Antioxidants support the body's immune system. Antioxidants are best absorbed through natural sources of the nutrients beta-carotene, vitamin C, vitamin E, selenium, and superoxide dismutase. Good sources of each are provided in Chapter 5.

Essential fatty acids. EFAs can reduce pain and inflammation. Evening primrose oil, borage seed oil, and black currant seed oil are good sources of EFAs; take 1 tablespoon daily. Purslane, sesame seeds, sunflower seeds, and walnuts are also good sources of EFAs; incorporate these foods into your diet, amounting to 3 tablespoons daily.

Potassium. Potassium encourages the body to get rid of excess fluid. Eat plenty of potassium-rich foods, such as apricots, avocados, bananas, beans, beets and beet greens, blackstrap molasses, brown rice, cantaloupe, carrots, currants, dates, figs, fish, grapes, green, leafy vegetables, lentils, oranges, papaya, peaches, potatoes, pumpkin seeds, raisins, seafood, spinach, sunflower seeds, tomatoes, watermelon, and wheat germ. You might also consider supplementing with 99–300 mg of potassium daily.

Vitamin B complex. The B vitamins support the immune system. Take 50 mg daily, or incorporate into the diet natural sources, such as alfalfa, beans, brown rice, Brussels sprouts, eggs, green, leafy vegetables, nuts, and peas.

Vitamin E. Vitamin E can help reduce the size and number of breast cysts. Take 400 IU daily. Look for a vitamin E supplement that also contains selenium; women prone to breast cysts have been found to have low levels of selenium in their blood.

Homeopathic Remedies

When fibrocystic breast conditions are accompanied by the conditions that are described, try the suggested homeopathic remedy. The usual dosage is four pellets, or as many liquid drops as the package label recommends, taken under the tongue four times daily. Rather than swallowing the pellets whole, allow them to dissolve slowly.

Belladonna. The patient has a strong constitution. She is filled with energy but may lack creative outlets for it.

Byronia. The breasts are sore and swollen during the menses.

Conium. The breasts are tender and swollen just before menstruation. The patient experiences aching muscles and disturbing dreams.

Lachesis. The patient is absentminded and has swollen, aching breasts.

Phytolacca. The breasts are sore and lumpy. There are enlarged lymph nodes under the arms.

Pulsatilla. The breasts are swollen and tender.

Silicea. The lumps in the breast are hard.

Aromatherapy Massage

Massage the breasts daily to improve circulation and lymphatic drainage. For added benefit, use a massage oil infused with essential oils that support cleansing of the circulatory and lymphatic systems, such as cypress, geranium, juniper, lavender, rose, rose geranium, and/or rosemary. (See Chapter 7 for instructions on making a massage oil.) Also try adding 7–10 drops of any of these essential oils to the bath. Be sure to soak your breasts in the tub while bathing.

LEUKORRHEA

Leukorrhea is a whitish vaginal discharge containing mucus and pus that results from inflammation or congestion of the mucous membrane. Having a slight discharge before the menses and a thicker discharge around the time of ovulation is normal. A change in that cycle or a consistent abnormal discharge signals a possible infection.

Causes of Leukorrhea

The causes of leukorrhea are many. Candidiasis can cause excessive vaginal discharge; if the discharge is accompanied by itchiness and burning, suspect a *Candida* infection, and turn to page 274. If the discharge is greenish and foul smelling, Trichomoniasis (*T. vaginalis*) is the most likely culprit; see page 399 for more details. If the discharge is thin and grayish, suspect bacterial vaginosis (caused by the bacterium *Hemophilus*). If the discharge contains blood, you may have chlamydia, and you should see your health care provider for a proper diagnosis.

In all other cases, if leukorrhea is not accompanied by other symptoms, you may wish to try the treatments suggested below. If treatment does not clear up the symptoms within two to three weeks, visit your gynecologist for a proper diagnosis.

Treatment

Treatments for leukorrhea focus on supporting the immune system and reducing inflammation and irritation of mucous membranes.

Diet

Dairy products and wheat contribute to the production of excess mucus, so they should be minimized in the diet. The one exception to this rule is plain yogurt, which contains live bacteria cultures that support friendly vaginal microorganisms and combat yeast overgrowth. Eat at least one serving of plain, organic yogurt daily. Vegans can use almond or sesame yogurt.

Herbal Therapy

The following herbs can be very effective in clearing up leukorrhea.

Burdock (*Arctium lappa*). The root is alterative, antibacterial, and anti-fungal. It improves the function of all the organs of elimination.

Dandelion (*Taraxacum officinale*). The root is an antifungal, cholagogue, and diuretic. It supports the body's cleansing systems.

Echinacea (*Echinacea purpurea, E. angustifolia*). The root strengthens the immune system and stimulates white blood cell production. It is alterative, antibiotic, antifungal, antiseptic, and antiviral.

Garlic (*Allium sativum*). The bulb counteracts a wide range of infectious conditions. It is an alterative, antibiotic, antifungal, antioxidant, antiprotozoan, and immunostimulant. Some people are allergic to garlic. Excessive use can cause emotional irritability and irritation of the stomach and kidneys. Avoid therapeutic doses during pregnancy, and avoid during the first three months of nursing, as it can cause breast milk to become unpalatable for infants. Avoid use the week before having surgery.

Myrrh (*Commiphora myrrha*). The resin helps normalize mucous membrane activity. It is an alterative, antifungal, antiseptic, decongestant, and emmenagogue. Avoid during pregnancy, and do not use for more than one month at a time.

Yellow dock (*Rumex crispus*). The root improves kidney, liver, lymph system, and colon function, thus aiding all of the body's natural cleansing processes. It is an alterative, antiseptic, and astringent.

Disinfectant Douche

The Disinfectant Douche is both germicidal and astringent. It can clear infection and dry mucous membranes, helping eliminate the leukorrheal discharge. Douche just twice daily; getting overzealous with this treatment can wash away friendly vaginal flora. Follow up with a plain yogurt suppository.

DISINFECTANT DOUCHE

This douche inhibits unfriendly microorganisms.

1 part bayberry root

2 parts calendula flower

⅕ part goldenseal root

1 part lady's mantle herb

1 part white oak bark

1 quart plus 2 cups water

Combine all the herbs. Bring the water to a boil. Add 4 heaping teaspoons of the mixed herbs. Remove from heat, cover, and let steep for one hour. Strain the liquid from the herbs, and compost the spent herbs. Pour the infused liquid into a douche bag. Add 2 cups of water. Douche.

Therapeutic Bath

Add to the bath 7–10 drops of the essential oil of eucalyptus, lavender, tea tree, or a combination thereof. These oils are both germicidal and astringent and can help clear up infection and congestion in mucous membranes.

PAINFUL INTERCOURSE

Pain during intercourse can manifest as a deep aching pain, a sudden sharp twinge, a burning sensation, itchiness, or simple discomfort. The possible causes are many and can include allergies (to soap, bath bubbles, latex, contraceptive gel, and so on), candidiasis, constipation, endometriosis, herpes, pelvic inflammatory disease, scar tissue, urinary tract infection, vaginal dryness, and venereal warts. Seek the advice of a gynecologist to determine the cause and the appropriate treatment.

PELVIC INFLAMMATORY DISEASE

Pelvic inflammatory disease (PID) has become one of the most common gynecological infections contracted by young women. It is a leading cause of infertility. It is usually caused by an infection, such as gonorrhea, chlamydia, or *E. coli,* that travels up from the vagina and infects the ovaries, uterine lining, or fallopian tubes. If untreated, PID can cause scarring of the reproductive organs, which in turn can lead to infertility or, if conception is achieved, ectopic pregnancy.

Symptoms

About one-third of the population suffering from PID experiences no symptoms. When symptoms are experienced, they range from mild to severe and can include vaginal bleeding, vaginal discharge, abdominal pain, fever, chills, nausea, painful intercourse, and pelvic tenderness.

Treatment

Allopathic medicine, which tends to make use of antibiotics, is generally best suited for treating PID. Natural medicine may be used to support the effect of the allopathic treatment and to strengthen the body.

If you've been diagnosed with PID, note that your sexual partner should receive the same treatment that you are undergoing, even if he or she exhibits no symptoms of an infection. Most cases of PID are caused by sexually transmitted diseases, and it won't help to cure you of the disease only to have you catch it again from your partner.

Herbal Therapy

The following herbs are potent activators of the body's immune and cleansing systems.

Calendula (*Calendula officinalis*). The flower is a time-tested remedy against deep-seated infections of the body. It improves liver and lymphatic function as well as peripheral circulation. It is an alterative, anti-inflammatory, antifungal, astringent, and vulnerary.

Cleavers (*Galium aparine*). The herb clears heat and reduces inflammation. It is an alterative, anti-inflammatory, mild antiseptic, and diuretic.

Echinacea (*Echinacea purpurea, E. angustifolia*). The root stimulates immune response, including T-cell production and macrophage activity. It also dilates peripheral blood vessels, thus increasing circulation to the genitourinary tract. It is an alterative, antibiotic, antifungal, anti-inflammatory, antiviral, immunostimulant, and vulnerary.

Garlic (*Allium sativum*). The bulb neutralizes a wide range of pathogens. It is an alterative, antibiotic, antifungal, and immunostimulant. Some people are allergic to garlic. Excessive use can cause emotional irritability and irritation of the stomach and kidneys. Avoid therapeutic doses during pregnancy, and avoid during the first three months of nursing, as it can cause breast milk to become unpalatable for infants. Avoid use the week before having surgery.

Goldenseal (*Hydrastis canadensis*). The root is effective against a wide range of pathogens. It is an anti-inflammatory, astringent, cholagogue, deobstruent, hemostatic, oxytocic, and vasoconstrictor. Goldenseal is very bitter, and most people find it easiest to ingest in capsule form. The tea can be used as a douche. This herb is endangered in the wild; do not use wildcrafted supplies. Avoid during pregnancy.

Myrrh (*Commiphora myrrha*). The resin normalizes mucous membrane activity and stimulates white blood cell production. It is an alterative, anti-inflammatory, antifungal, antiseptic, astringent, and vulnerary. Avoid during pregnancy, and do not use for more than one month at a time.

Parsley (*Petroselinum crispum*). The leaf is rich in chlorophyll, which builds the blood and helps the body resist infection. It is antioxidant, antiseptic, and diuretic. Avoid therapeutic doses during pregnancy and in cases of kidney inflammation.

Pokeweed (*Phytolacca americana*). The root increases T-cell activity in the immune system. It is an alterative, anti-inflammatory, immunostimulant, and lymphatic decongestant. In large amounts, pokeweed root can be toxic. Take only 2 or 3 drops of the tincture daily; after one week, increase the dosage to 5 drops (2 drops in the morning, 3 drops at night). Drink copious amounts of water while you are taking pokeweed root. Consult with your health care provider before use.

Thyme (*Thymus vulgaris*). The herb expels mucus and relieves congestion throughout the body. It is an antibiotic, antifungal, antiseptic, diaphoretic, emmenagogue, and vulnerary.

Nutritional Therapy

A healthy diet is imperative to overcoming a deep-seated infection of the body. Vitamin C and antioxidants may be of particular help.

Antioxidants. Antioxidants help prevent cellular damage to the body and speed the healing process. Antioxidants are best absorbed through natural sources of the nutrients beta-carotene, vitamin C, vitamin E, selenium, and superoxide dismutase. Good sources of each are listed in Chapter 5.

Vitamin C. Large doses of vitamin C help the body resist infection and stimulate white blood cell production. Take 1,000 mg three or four times daily. Also incorporate into the diet natural sources of vitamin C; see Chapter 5 for information.

Poultices and Compresses

Poultices and compresses placed over an affected area can help draw out infection and relieve both congestion and pain. Apply these healing poultices or compresses at a time when you can lie low, relax, and really focus on the healing process.

Castor oil compress. A castor oil compress improves circulation to the pelvic area, thus helping clear congestion, and softens scar tissue. See page 292 for instructions on making and applying the compress. Apply the compress for three days in a row, then take four days off. Repeat this pattern for as long as necessary.

Chamomile tea poultice. A chamomile tea poultice applied over the abdominal area can relieve pain, reduce inflammation, and provide a mild antiseptic action. The herb's gentle healing compounds are absorbed through the skin and pass into the bloodstream at the site of infection. To make the poultice, bring a quart of water to a boil. Remove from heat, stir in four heaping teaspoons of chamomile flowers or four chamomile tea bags, cover, and let steep for twenty minutes. Then remove the tea bags or strain out the blossoms. Soak a clean cloth in the hot tea, wring out, and apply to the pelvic area. Cover with a dry towel to help hold in the heat. When the cloth cools, resoak it in the hot tea and reapply. When it cools again, resoak and reapply one more time, so that you've made three applications total. Repeat once daily for as long as necessary.

Clay poultice. Clay poultices can help draw toxins from the body. Use only dry, cosmetic-quality clay. In a glass bowl, mix together about ½ cup of clay powder with enough water to make a paste. Apply over the liver area.

Leave on until it dries thoroughly, then rinse off. Repeat once daily for as long as necessary.

Aromatherapy

Daily sitz baths (see Chapter 12) increase circulation to the pelvic area, clearing congestion and stimulating immune system activity. For germicidal action, add to the water the essential oil of geranium, lavender, rosemary, or a combination thereof.

Massaging the abdominal area with a massage oil that includes some of the aforementioned essential oils will also be helpful in banishing the infection.

URINARY TRACT INFECTIONS

Urinary tract infections can affect the bladder (cystitis), the urethra (urethritis), or the kidneys (nephritis). They are usually caused by the bacterium *E. coli* traveling from the colon to the bladder and urethra. Although urinary tract infections can be treated effectively with natural medicine, some cases are caused by a sexually transmitted disease, so it's wise to visit your health care provider for a diagnosis of the cause.

Symptoms

If you need to urinate frequently and feel a burning sensation when you do so, even if you don't produce much urine, you probably have cystitis. If vaginal discharge or lumps around the genitals and anus are also present, suspect urethritis. If back pain, fever, chills, or a bloody discharge are also present, suspect kidney infection, and contact your health care provider immediately.

Treatment

The holistic approach to treating urinary tract infections focuses on supporting the urinary system, reducing inflammation, and stimulating the immune system.

Diet

To soothe irritation in the urinary tract, include in your diet plenty of cooling foods, such as asparagus, barley, carrots, celery, corn, cucumbers, grapes, green, leafy vegetables, lotus root, millet, mung beans, parsley, pomegranates, squash, strawberries, vegetable juices, water chestnuts, and watermelon (eat the seeds too).

Also include foods that strengthen the kidneys and bladder, including adzuki beans, black beans, black sesame seeds, black quinoa, kidney beans, and sea vegetables.

Avoid foods that irritate the urinary system, such as alcohol, artificial sweeteners, cheese, fried foods, juices, coffee, sodas, spicy food, tomatoes, and vinegar.

To keep the urinary system well flushed, drink at least eight tall glasses of water every day.

Unsweetened cranberry juice is an excellent remedy for urinary tract infections because it contains hippuric acid, which inhibits the adhesion of bacteria to the walls of the urinary tract. Blueberries, which are in the same family as cranberries, also contain compounds that help prevent bacteria from adhering to the walls of the urinary tract.

Herbal Therapy

Useful herbs for treating urinary tract infections include the following.

Buchu (*Agathosma betulina*). The leaf soothes and strengthens the urinary system. It is an antiseptic, diuretic, kidney tonic, and urinary antiseptic. Avoid during pregnancy and while nursing.

Cleavers (*Galium aparine*). The herb clears heat and reduces inflammation. It can help relieve the urge to urinate constantly. It is an alterative, anti-inflammatory, mild antiseptic, and diuretic.

Cornsilk (*Zea mays*). The stigma regenerates and soothes irritated tissue. It can help relieve the urge to urinate constantly. It is an alterative, antiseptic, diuretic, demulcent, and tonic.

Couchgrass (*Elymus repens*). The rhizome has a high mucilage content and can soothe renal (kidney) tissue. It is antiseptic, demulcent, diuretic, and tonic.

Flax (*Linum usitatissimum*). The seeds help relieve the symptoms of cystitis, particularly the burning sensation associated with urination. They are anti-inflammatory, demulcent, and nutritive. Try grinding the seeds in a blender and incorporating 3 tablespoons daily into salads, salad dressings, and other dishes.

Goldenrod (*Solidago* spp.) The herb cleanses the kidneys. It is an anti-inflammatory, antioxidant, mild antiseptic, astringent, diuretic, and tonic. Do not use in cases of hot inflammation, such as fever or high blood pressure.

Hibiscus (*Hibiscus sabdariffa*). The flower relieves the symptoms of cystitis. It is an alterative, mild antiseptic, anti-inflammatory, antispasmodic, demulcent, and diuretic.

Horsetail (*Equisetum arvense*). The herb soothes irritated tissue. It is an alterative, anti-inflammatory, genitourinary antiseptic and astringent, diuretic, and nutritive. Use horsetail that has been collected in spring.

Juniper (*Juniperus communis*). The berry stimulates the flow of urine. It is an anti-inflammatory, antiseptic, antiviral, diuretic, and urinary antiseptic. Avoid during pregnancy, during acute renal inflammation, and in cases of blood in the urine. Do not use for longer than one month at a stretch.

Marsh mallow (*Althaea officinalis*). The root nourishes kidney yin and can soothe an irritated bladder. It is an alterative, demulcent, diuretic, nutritive, and rejuvenative.

Nettle (*Urtica dioica, U. urens*). The herb dries the dampness associated with some cases of urinary tract infections. It is an alterative, circulatory stimulant, diuretic, kidney tonic, and nutritive. Contact with the fresh plant will irritate the skin. Use only dried herb. Wear gloves when collecting.

Oregon grape (*Mahonia aquifolium*). The root is a urinary antiseptic and is especially helpful in cases of chronic infections. It is an alterative, anti-inflammatory, antiseptic, diuretic, and tonic. Avoid during pregnancy, and do not exceed the recommended dosage.

Pipsissewa (*Chimaphila umbellata*). The herb is an anti-inflammatory, urinary antiseptic, astringent, diuretic, and tonic. It may give urine a greenish color.

Plantain (*Plantago major*). The leaf clears heat and soothes irritated tissue. It is an alterative, anti-inflammatory, antiseptic, antispasmodic, demulcent, diuretic, and refrigerant.

Usnea (*Usnea barbata*). The lichen counteracts bacterial infections. It is an antibiotic, antifungal, and immunostimulant.

Uva ursi (*Arctostaphylos uva-ursi*). The leaf contains arbutin, which the body converts to hydroquinone, which helps alkalinize the urine. It is an antiseptic, astringent, bladder tonic, diuretic, and vulnerary. Avoid during pregnancy.

Nutritional Therapy

Supplementation with vitamin C and vitamin E, in combination with the dietary measures suggested above, may bolster the body's defenses against urinary tract infections. Natural sources of these vitamins are listed in Chapter 5.

Vitamin C. Vitamin C helps prevent bacterial infection. Take 1,000 mg three or four times daily.

Vitamin E. Vitamin E can help prevent scarring of bladder tissues. Take 400 IU daily.

Homeopathic Remedies

When bladder infection is accompanied by the conditions that are described, try the suggested homeopathic remedy. The usual dosage is four pellets, or as many liquid drops as the package label recommends, taken under the tongue four times daily. Rather than swallowing the pellets whole, allow them to dissolve slowly.

Apis Mellifica. Urination causes a burning, stinging sensation, and the vaginal area is itchy and swollen. The patient is nervous and unable to urinate fully; the last few drops of urine are particularly painful.

Berberis Vulgaris. The bladder infection starts to settle in the kidneys or lower back area. Motion aggravates the symptoms, and there may be a reddish color to the urine.

Cantharis. The patient feels a severe burning in the vaginal area and a constant urge to urinate, yet when she urinates, only a few drops pass. She may feel agitated, and there may be blood in the urine.

Equisetum. The patient experiences a feeling of fullness in the bladder, even after urinating.

Mercurius Corrosivus. The burning is less intense but ever-present, as is the urge to urinate. The patient may experience bladder spasms and painful urination. Symptoms tend to worsen when temperatures fluctuate.

Sarsaparilla. Urination is painful and causes stress.

Sepia. The patient is pregnant, and experiences bladder pressure rather than pain.

Staphysagria. The symptoms are caused by "honeymoon cystitis" (more sex than you're accustomed to having). The patient may feel an ever-present burning sensation. This remedy is also helpful for a bladder infection induced by emotional stress.

Pipsissewa Sitz Bath

A sitz bath in an infusion of pipsissewa will help disinfect the pelvic area. Bring a quart of water to a boil, add a large handful of pipsissewa herb, cover, and let steep twenty minutes. Then strain and pour into the sitz bath. Add more water if necessary.

For extra antiseptic action, add 16 ounces of baking soda (a whole box) or 1 cup of apple cider vinegar to the water.

Aromatherapy

Gentle abdominal massage can increase circulation to the area, transmit caring touch, and, when combined with antiseptic essential oils, help the body resist or fight off infection. Use a massage oil infused with the essential oil of eucalyptus, lavender, lemon, or niaouli. These antiseptic oils can also be added to the bath. See Chapter 7 for advice on these techniques.

UTERINE FIBROIDS

Uterine fibroids, also called leiomyomas, are benign tumors that grow outside, inside, or in the walls of the uterus, sometimes distorting its shape. They range in size from that of a pea to that of a full-term fetus, and they are more common in women who have not had children. They tend to grow slowly, and their growth seems to be stimulated by estrogen. (Because they are dependent on estrogen, fibroids usually decrease in size after menopause.)

Symptoms

Most cases of fibroids are free of symptoms. However, if fibroids are of sufficient size or number, they may cause heavy or prolonged periods, painful periods, bleeding between cycles, anemia, the urge to urinate frequently, pain during intercourse, backache, constipation, and abdominal enlargement.

Treatment

You may be able to reduce the size of fibroids with some of the natural therapies suggested below. However, in cases where fibroids are causing serious pain, surgery may be necessary.

Natural therapy for treating fibroids focuses on supporting three important systems:

- The liver, which breaks down excess estrogen in the body

- The kidneys, which relieve stagnation, thereby preventing the formation of masses in the body

- The blood, which prevent blockages

If you have fibroids, avoid birth control pills and hormone replacement therapy, both of which provide the body with synthetic estrogen.

Diet

First things first. If you're overweight and fibroids are giving you trouble, lose the extra pounds. Overweight women tend to secrete proportionately higher levels of estrogen, which stimulates fibroid growth.

Avoid meat, egg, and dairy products that derive from animals treated with hormones. Incorporate fermented soy products, like miso, into your diet, because soy helps regulate estrogen levels in the body.

Eat violet leaves and chickweed in salads as much as possible, taking in their healing, cleansing, soothing energy.

Herbal Therapy

Herbs that help reduce the size of uterine fibroids include the following.

Angelica (*Angelica archangelica, A. atropurpurea*). The root regulates menstrual bleeding and inhibits blood platelet aggregation. It is an anti-inflammatory, astringent, diuretic, emmenagogue, tonic, and uterine stimulant. Avoid during pregnancy and in cases of heavy bleeding or diabetes. In rare cases, the root causes photosensitivity.

Astragalus (*Astragalus membranaceus*). The root stimulates the immune system and inhibits the formation of free radicals. It is an adaptogen, antiviral, blood tonic, chi tonic, circulatory stimulant, immunostimulant, and vasodilator.

Black cohosh (*Actaea racemosa*). The root helps relieve the pain of fibroids. It soothes irritation and relieves congestion in the cervix, uterus, and vagina. It is an alterative, anti-inflammatory, antiseptic, antispasmodic, astringent, circulatory stimulant, emmenagogue, and vasodilator. Avoid during pregnancy, except in the final stages, and then only under the guidance of your health care provider. Avoid while nursing and in cases of high blood pressure or pressure in the inner eye. Consult with your health care provider before use. This herb is endangered in the wild; do not use wildcrafted supplies.

Blessed thistle (*Cnicus benedictus*). The herb strengthens the spleen and the liver. It is an alterative, antihemorrhagic, and emmenagogue.

Blue cohosh (*Caulophyllum thalictroides*). The root reduces pain and spasms in the uterus. It is an anti-inflammatory, antispasmodic, diuretic, emmenagogue, oxytocic, and uterine tonic. Avoid during pregnancy, except in the final stages, and then only under the guidance of your health care provider. Make sure the root is dried, not fresh. This herb is endangered in the wild; do not use wildcrafted supplies.

Burdock (*Arctium lappa*). The root improves the functions of the organs of elimination, such as the liver, the lymph nodes, and the kidneys. It is an alterative, antifungal, antiseptic, anti-inflammatory, antitumor, choleretic, demulcent, diuretic, laxative, nutritive, and rejuvenative.

Calendula (*Calendula officinalis*). The flower improves liver and lymphatic function as well as peripheral circulation. It is an alterative, anti-inflammatory, astringent, and vulnerary.

Celandine (*Chelidonium majus*). The herb detoxifies the liver. It is an alterative, anodyne, anti-inflammatory, and cholagogue. Use only in small doses; 2 or 3 drops of tincture three times daily is adequate. Consult with your health care provider before use, and avoid during pregnancy.

Chamomile (*Matricaria recutita*). The flower can relieve pain in the uterus. It is an antispasmodic, anti-inflammatory, and emmenagogue.

Chaparral (*Larrea tridentata*). The herb helps reduce the size of uterine fibroids occurring with elevated estrogen levels. It is an alterative, antifungal, antioxidant, antiseptic, antitumor, and immunostimulant. Avoid in cases of liver or kidney disease, cirrhosis, or hepatitis and during pregnancy. Discontinue use if nausea, fatigue, fever, or jaundice occur. Do not use for more than a month at a time. Consult with your health care provider before use.

Cleavers (*Galium aparine*). The herb is a lymphatic cleanser. It clears heat and reduces inflammation. It is an alterative, antitumor, astringent, and vulnerary.

Collinsonia (*Collinsonia canadensis*). The root can shrink small fibroids that congest the uterus, causing chronic irritation. It relieves congestion in the pelvic area and helps remove masses from the reproductive organs. It is a diuretic and an emmenagogue.

Cotton root (*Gossypium hirsutum, G. herbaceum*). The bark constricts blood vessels and is recommended for uterine fibroids accompanied by hemorrhage. It is an antitumor, emmenagogue, nutritive, and uterine tonic. Avoid during pregnancy. Large doses may cause nausea and vomiting. Avoid in cases of urogenital irritation.

Cramp bark (*Viburnum opulus*). The bark relaxes muscles, thereby relieving pain. It also improves dysmenorrhea. It is an anti-inflammatory, antispasmodic, astringent, nutritive, and uterine sedative.

Dandelion (*Taraxacum officinale*). The root and leaf improve liver function and aid in the elimination of toxins. They reduce stagnation in the reproductive organs. They are antifungals, antitumors, cholagogues, and liver tonics.

Dan shen (*Salvia miltiorrhiza*). The root invigorates the blood and breaks up congestion. It can relieve pain in the uterus.

False unicorn (*Chamaelirium luteum*). The root strengthens the genitourinary tract and helps balance estrogen levels. It is an antiseptic and a uterine tonic. The bitter taste of this herb can cause vomiting. Excessive amounts may cause kidney and stomach irritation, blurred vision, and hot flashes. Do not use without employing birth control during sex unless pregnancy is desired. Discontinue use during pregnancy. False unicorn is endangered in the wild; do not use wildcrafted supplies.

Fraxinus (*Fraxinus americana*). The bark reduces the size of fibroids, particularly when they are in the earlier stages of development. It is a circulatory stimulant.

Fringe tree (*Chionanthus virginicus*). The bark removes obstructions, including fibroids, and clears heat from the liver. It also reduces inflammation. It is an alterative, cholagogue, and hepatic.

Ginger (*Zingiber officinale*). The root improves circulation and helps clear stagnant material from the pelvic region. It encourages lymphatic cleansing and reduces blood platelet aggregation. It is an analgesic, anti-inflammatory, antioxidant, antiseptic, antispasmodic, and anticoagulant. Avoid large doses in cases of acne and eczema. Discontinue use if heartburn results.

Goldenseal (*Hydrastis canadensis*). The root reduces pelvic congestion, improves liver function, and reduces bleeding. It is an anti-inflammatory, astringent, cholagogue, deobstruent, hemostatic, oxytocic, and vasoconstrictor. Goldenseal is very bitter, and most people find it easiest to ingest in capsule form. The tea can be used as a douche. This herb is endangered in the wild; do not use wildcrafted supplies. Avoid during pregnancy.

Hawthorn (*Crataegus* spp.) The berry, flower, and leaf improve circulation and help break down fatty deposits in the body. They are astringents, circulatory stimulants, and vasodilators.

Lady's mantle (*Alchemilla xanthochlora*). The herb normalizes hormone production, reduces heavy bleeding, promotes blood coagulation, and encourages tissue healing. It is an anti-inflammatory, astringent, diuretic, emmenagogue, hemostatic, liver decongestant, uterine tonic, and vulnerary.

Motherwort (*Leonurus cardiaca*). The herb inhibits blood platelet aggregation and helps normalize hormone production. It is an astringent, circulatory stimulant, diuretic, emmenagogue, rejuvenative, uterine tonic, and vasodilator. Avoid in cases of heavy menstrual bleeding and during pregnancy, except during the final stages, and then only under the supervision of your health care provider.

Oregon grape (*Mahonia aquifolium*). The root improves liver function and circulation. It is an alterative, anti-inflammatory, antiseptic, astringent, cholagogue, diuretic, and immunostimulant. Avoid during pregnancy, and do not exceed the recommended dosage.

Partridge berry (*Mitchella repens*). The herb helps relieve pelvic congestion. It is an alterative, astringent, emmenagogue, uterine stimulant, and uterine tonic. Dosages in excess of what's recommended can irritate the mucous membranes. This herb is endangered in the wild; do not use wildcrafted supplies.

Pipsissewa (*Chimaphila umbellata*). The herb improves liver and kidney function, cleansing the body and helping to eliminate fluids. It is an alterative, anti-inflammatory, astringent, diuretic, and urinary antiseptic.

Pokeweed (*Phytolacca americana*). The root increases T-cell activity in the immune system. It is an alterative, anti-inflammatory, immunostimulant, and lymphatic decongestant. In large amounts, pokeweed root can be toxic. Take only 2 or 3 drops of the tincture daily; after one week, increase the dosage to 5 drops (2 drops in the morning, 3 drops at night). Drink copious amounts of water while you are taking pokeweed root. Consult with your health care provider before use.

Prickly ash (*Zanthoxylum americanum, Z. clava-herculis*). The bark improves circulation throughout the body. It is an alterative, anodyne, antiseptic, antispasmodic, astringent, emmenagogue and circulatory stimulant. Avoid during pregnancy and in cases of stomach inflammation.

Red clover (*Trifolium pratense*). The herb and flower are excellent lymphatic cleansers. They are alterative, anti-inflammatory, and antitumor.

Red raspberry (*Rubus idaeus*). The leaf tonifies the uterus and the cervix. It prevents hemorrhage and helps balance hormones. It is an alterative, antiseptic, astringent, hemostatic, hormonal regulator, nutritive, and yin tonic.

Redroot (*Ceanothus americanus*). The root encourages the elimination of catabolic waste and breaks up congestion in the body. It is often recommended for treating cysts, dysmenorrhea, and lymphatic congestion. It is antispasmodic and astringent.

Sarsaparilla (*Smilax* spp.). The root contains compounds that help purify the genitourinary tract by binding with toxins and carrying them out of the body. It is an alterative, antispasmodic, diuretic, and rejuvenative.

Saw palmetto (*Serenoa repens*). The berry reduces ovarian enlargement and pain, which can contribute to impaired circulation and drainage in the uterus. It is a diuretic, nutritive, rejuvenative, reproductive tonic, and urinary antiseptic.

Trillium (*Trillium* spp.). The root helps control excessive bleeding associated with fibroids. It is an alterative, antihemorrhagic, antiseptic, antispasmodic, astringent, emmenagogue, and uterine tonic. Avoid during pregnancy, except under the guidance of your health care provider. This herb is endangered in the wild; do not use wildcrafted supplies.

Turmeric (*Curcuma longa, C. aromatica*). The root prevents blood platelet aggregation. It is an alterative, anticoagulant, antifungal, anti-inflammatory, antioxidant, cholagogue, circulatory stimulant, emmenagogue, hepatotonic, and vulnerary.

Vervain (*Verbena hastata, V. officinalis*). The herb stimulates uterine activity and improves the body's assimilation of nutrients. It is an anticoagulant, anti-inflammatory, antitumor, astringent, cholagogue, diuretic, emmenagogue, hepatostimulant, vasoconstrictor, and vulnerary. Avoid during pregnancy.

Vitex (*Vitex agnus-castus*). The berry helps normalize the production of hormones and inhibits excessive cellular growth in the reproductive organs. It is an antispasmodic, emmenagogue, phytoprogesteronic, and vulnerary.

Wild yam (*Dioscorea opposita, D. villosa*). The root reduces inflammation, clears congested chi, and helps normalize hormones. It is an anti-inflammatory, antispasmodic, cholagogue, diuretic, nutritive, and uterine sedative. Avoid therapeutic doses during pregnancy, except under the guidance of your health care provider. The *Dioscorea villosa* species is endangered in the wild; do not use wildcrafted supplies.

Yarrow (*Achillea millefolium*). The herb increases circulation to the pelvic region and promotes liver detoxification. It is an anti-inflammatory, antiseptic, antispasmodic, astringent, cholagogue, circulatory stimulant, diuretic, hemostatic, and urinary antiseptic.

Chinese Patent Medicines

The Chinese patent medicine To Jing Wan helps regulate the menstrual cycle and break up stagnation in the blood. Tang Kwei Gin can help shrink fibroids.

Nutritional Therapy

Several supplements can contribute to the healing of fibroids.

Vitamin B complex. Elevated estrogen levels can result from a B vitamin deficiency. Choline and inositol, both part of the vitamin B complex, help the liver break down fats and fat-soluble hormones such as estrogen. Take 50–300 mg of vitamin B complex daily.

Vitamin E. Vitamin E helps regulate bleeding and normalizes estrogen levels. Take 400 IU daily.

Iron. If fibroids cause heavy menstrual bleeding, use an herbal liquid iron supplement, available at most natural food stores. Follow the dosage guidelines given on the product label.

Methionine. This amino acid aids in the breakdown of fats and fat-soluble hormones. Take 500 mg daily.

Sitz Baths

Alternate hot and cold sitz baths, as directed in Chapter 12. This treatment increases circulation to the pelvic region, moving blockages and allowing reabsorption.

Castor Oil Packs

To improve circulation to the pelvic area and soften scar tissue, apply castor oil packs to the abdominal region three times a week. See page 292 for instructions.

Pelvic Exercise

Practice exercises that move energy in the pelvis, such as the Cat Stretch (see page 33) and Kegels (see page 30).

Aromatherapy

Massage over the abdominal area with oil infused with a blockage-dispelling essential oil, such as jasmine, lotus, rose, rose geranium, or a combination thereof. (See Chapter 7 for instructions on making an aromatherapy massage oil.) These oils can also be used in an aromatherapy diffuser.

Acupuncture

Acupuncture treatments can be very effective for moving blockages, such as fibroids, in the body. Begin treatment as soon as the fibroids are discovered, because they are easier to eliminate when they are still small and have not yet tightly adhered to surrounding organs. To find an acupuncturist in your area, contact the American Association of Oriental Medicine; see Resources.

UTERINE PROLAPSE

Prolapse means an organ has "slipped down" from its normal position. Prolapse of the uterus can be caused by childbirth, constipation, obesity, and the normal forces of gravity. In most cases it is not a serious health condition and may resolve itself. If it doesn't, surgical repair is always an option. Ask your health care provider for advice on the method of treatment that is best suited for your condition.

Symptoms

Signs of uterine prolapse include a heavy feeling in the lower abdomen, painful intercourse, backache, incontinence, frequent or difficult urination, constipation, urinary tract infections, and vaginal discharge.

Treatment

Try natural remedies for six months to a year before resorting to surgery. You might end up not needing it, and you'll certainly improve your health in the meantime.

The holistic approach to treating uterine prolapse focuses on resting the body, strengthening the genitourinary system, and stimulating the body's healing response.

Rest

The most important treatment for uterine prolapse is simply rest. Give your body a chance to heal itself. Make sure you get plenty of sleep, avoid heavy lifting, and don't stand on your feet for long periods at a time.

Bodywork and Exercise

Bodywork and exercise directed toward strengthening the pelvic area can help the uterus find its way back home. Locate a bodyworker who knows how to do uterine massage and visit him or her for weekly sessions. Practice pelvic-strengthening exercises such as those described in Chapter 3, and do lots of Kegels. Try inversion yoga postures such as the shoulder stand or head stand, or spend thirty minutes or so every day lying on a slant board (available at many sports shops and by mail-order from Bodyslant; see Resources).

One note of caution: Do not undertake these exercises if you have just given birth, because bleeding could still occur. Also, headstands should not be done unless one is adept at doing them. Avoid inversion poses during the menses.

Herbal Therapy

Herbs that can help the body lift the uterus back to its proper position include the following.

Black cohosh (*Actaea racemosa*). The root stimulates the flow of chi in the body, which can provide the body with the strength to lift prolapsed internal organs. It relieves congestion in the cervix, uterus, and vagina. It is an alterative, anti-inflammatory, astringent, circulatory stimulant, emmenagogue, and vasodilator. Avoid during pregnancy, except in the final stages, and then only under the guidance of your health care provider. Avoid while nursing and in cases of high blood pressure or pressure in the inner eye. Consult with your health care provider before use. This herb is endangered in the wild; do not use wildcrafted supplies.

Dong quai (*Angelica sinensis*). The root nourishes vaginal tissues and clears stagnation of blood in the pelvic area. It is an alterative, anticoagulant, blood tonic, emmenagogue, and uterine tonic. Avoid during pregnancy, except under the guidance of your health care provider. Do not use in cases of diarrhea, heavy menstrual flow, poor digestion, or bloating. Do not use in conjunction with blood-thinning medications such as ibuprofen.

False unicorn (*Chamaelirium luteum*). The root strengthens the genitourinary tract. It is an antiseptic and a uterine tonic. The bitter taste of this herb can cause vomiting. Excessive amounts may cause kidney and stomach irritation, blurred vision, and hot flashes. Do not use without employing birth control during sex unless pregnancy is desired. Discontinue use during pregnancy. False unicorn is endangered in the wild; do not use wildcrafted supplies.

Horsetail (*Equisetum arvense*). The herb encourages the healing of bones, tissue, and cartilage. It has a high silica content, which helps strengthen the body's connective tissues. It is an anti-inflammatory, astringent, hemostatic, nutritive, and vulnerary. Use horsetail that has been collected in spring.

Lady's mantle (*Alchemilla xanthochlora*). The herb promotes tissue healing. It is an anti-inflammatory, astringent, diuretic, emmenagogue, hemostatic, liver decongestant, and vulnerary.

Red raspberry (*Rubus idaeus*). The leaf tonifies the uterus. It is an astringent, hormonal regulator, kidney tonic, nutritive, uterine tonic, and yin tonic.

If prolapse occurs after menopause, lack of estrogen may be a factor. In this case, herbs with phytoestrogenic activity, such as hops, sage, and wild yam, can be helpful. See Chapter 18 for more information.

Vaginal Suppository
The astringent herbal bolus made from the Tissue-Tonifying Yoni Suppository formula supports the body's healing response and prevents infection.

TISSUE-TONIFYING YONI SUPPOSITORY

Supports the body's healing response and prevents infection.

5 parts powdered witch hazel bark

1 part powdered goldenseal root

Coconut oil

Combine the herbs with enough coconut oil to make a thick paste. Roll into a suppository shape the size of your pinkie, and store in a glass jar in the refrigerator. Insert it as high as possible before going to bed. You may wish to wear a cotton menstrual pad to prevent the oil from dripping over the bedsheets.

Homeopathic Sepia

Homeopathic *Sepia* tightens tissues and may benefit women with uterine prolapse. The usual dosage is four pellets, or as many liquid drops as the package label recommends, taken under the tongue four times daily. Rather than swallowing the pellets whole, allow them to dissolve slowly.

Aromatherapy

Abdominal massage can strengthen the muscles, helping the body pull the uterus back where it belongs. Use a massage oil combined with an antiseptic essential oil, such as lemon and rosemary. (See Chapter 7 for instructions for making an aromatherapy massage oil.) These oils can also be included in the bath.

Sitz Baths

To improve circulation to and move blockages in the pelvic region, take a cold sitz bath every day for thirty seconds.

VAGINAL DRYNESS

Vaginal lubrication is often a woman's initial response to sexual excitement. Small drops of mucuslike secretions appear throughout the vaginal folds; as the excitement continues, the drops of moisture fuse to form a lubricating coat.

Lack of vaginal lubrication is not always a sign of lack of excitement. It may, instead, be a symptom of a deeper health problem.

Causes

According to Oriental medicine, a deficiency in vaginal lubrication is often an indication of kidney yin or liver deficiency. Menopause and hysterectomies often affect vaginal lubrication; the drop in estrogen production can leave the mucous membranes high and dry. Other factors that can contribute to vaginal dryness include yeast overgrowth, diabetes, overdouching, sexually transmitted disease, stress, overwork, and excessive exercise. Alcohol and marijuana can cause vaginal dryness, as can some common prescription drugs, such as antihistamine-filled allergy medications and birth control pills.

Treatment

Natural therapy for treating vaginal dryness focuses on nourishing mucous membranes, strengthening vaginal tissue, and normalizing estrogen production. Most important, visualize your river flowing!

Diet

Drink copious amounts of fluids. Barley water is highly nourishing and emollient; cook 2 cups of lightly pearled barley in 10 cups of water for two hours, then strain and sweeten to taste. To strengthen mucous membranes, eat plenty of foods that are rich in beta-carotene, including dark green, leafy vegetables, winter squash, sweet potatoes, and spirulina. To nourish the kidneys, which govern yin moisture in the body, incorporate black sesame seeds and black soybeans into your diet.

Sitz Bath

Take a sitz bath using emollient herbs such as comfrey leaf and marsh mallow root, which will soothe and protect the skin. Bring a quart of water to a boil, add a large handful of the herb of choice, cover, and let steep twenty minutes. Then strain and pour into the sitz bath. Add more water if necessary.

Herbal Therapy

The following herbs all help promote vaginal lubrication:

Black cohosh (*Actaea racemosa*). The root soothes vaginal irritation. It is an alterative, anti-inflammatory, circulatory stimulant, and muscle relaxant. Avoid during pregnancy, except in the final stages, and then only under the guidance of your health care provider. Avoid while nursing and in cases of high blood pressure or pressure in the inner eye. Consult with your health care provider before use. This herb is endangered in the wild; do not use wildcrafted supplies.

Fennel (*Foeniculum vulgare*). The seed contains phytoestrogens and soothes irritated mucous membranes. It is a smooth muscle relaxant.

Longan (*Euphoria longan*). The berry is moistening and helps build the blood. It is a restorative.

Vitex (*Vitex agnus-castus*). The berry is phytoprogesteronic.

Herbal Suppository

Use this suppository at night to encourage moisture in the vaginal mucous membranes.

YONI MOISTENING SUPPOSITORY

Encourages moisture in the vaginal mucous membranes.

1 ounce cocoa butter

1 tablespoon powdered dong quai

1 tablespoon powdered licorice root

1 tablespoon powdered marsh mallow root
or slippery elm bark

1 tablespoon powdered wild yam

2 tablespoons vitamin E oil

2 drops essential oil of rose (optional)

Melt the cocoa butter, then add the powdered herbs and vitamin E oil. Scent with 2 drops of rose essential oil, if desired. Roll into a suppository shape the size of your pinkie, and store in a glass jar in the refrigerator. Insert before bedtime.

Nutritional Therapy

Several supplements may be of assistance in relieving vaginal dryness.

Essential fatty acids. EFAs soothe irritated tissue and have an anti-inflammatory effect. Hempseed and flaxseed oils are excellent sources of EFAs; take 3 tablespoons daily.

Vitamin A. Vitamin A helps strengthen and soothe mucous membranes. It is best taken in the form of beta-carotene; try 25,000–50,000 IU of beta-carotene daily.

Vitamin C. Vitamin C supports collagen production, thereby improving tissue tone. Take 1,000 mg twice daily.

Vitamin E. Vitamin E helps moisten tissues and soothes inflammation.

Take 400 IU daily. You can also apply the oil from a vitamin E capsule directly to vaginal tissues.

Zinc. Zinc helps strengthen the vaginal lining. Take 15 mg daily.

Acidophilus

Yeast overgrowth is often a contributing factor in vaginal dryness. An acidophilus capsule inserted into the vagina inhibits yeast overgrowth and can help produce lubrication. Make sure you are not using an enteric-coated capsule, which will not dissolve in the vagina. You can use acidophilus in this manner on a continuing basis for as long as you need to.

Lubricants

If you can't produce your own lubricant, import it! The ideal lubricant should not become sticky, should liquefy at body temperature, and should stay slick for long periods of time. In preparation for intercourse, you can always use a water-based lubricant or a glycerin suppository. Coconut oil is also an excellent lubricant, but it cannot be used with barrier methods of contraception because it degrades the quality of the barrier. Check out the Resources for sources of yummy natural lubricants.

VAGINISMUS

Vaginismus is the occurrence of vaginal muscle spasms that close the vagina so tightly that intercourse is difficult or impossible. The cause of this condition has yet to be discovered, although psychological factors are certainly a factor. It can be helpful to work with a therapist.

The best approach to overcoming vaginismus is to proceed slowly, backing off whenever psychological stress or muscle spasms set in. Try looking at your genitals in a mirror after a relaxing bath. With a lubricated finger, try to insert a finger into the vagina while lightly bearing down. Enter a littler bit at a time. When you can do this effectively on your own, try it with a partner you trust. Practice Kegels.

When you feel you're ready for intercourse, use lubrication, and make sure that foreplay is both extensive and fun. If the tension of the situation—will it happen, or won't it?—starts to affect you, back off, and save the actual penetration for another time. There are plenty of ways to make love, after all! When you are ready for penetration, use plenty of lubrication.

VAGINITIS

Vaginitis is the general term for a nonspecific vaginal infection. Most cases of vaginitis are caused by overgrowth of a bacteria that is normally present in the body; the bacterium *Hemophilus,* for example, is a common culprit. Hormonal changes, birth control pills, excessive douching, tears in or irritations to vaginal tissue, stress, and synthetic-fiber clothing may all be contributing factors.

Symptoms

Symptoms of vaginitis are varied and range from mild to severe. The most common are abnormal discharge, burning or itching in the vulva, burning or stinging upon urination, and the need to urinate frequently.

Treatment

Treatment for vaginitis entails stimulating the body's immune response and nourishing the mucous membranes.

Herbal Therapy

Herbs that can counteract a bacterial vaginal infection include the following.

Astragalus (*Astragalus membranaceus*). The root stimulates the body's immune response. It is an adaptogen, antiseptic, circulatory stimulant, and vasodilator.

Echinacea (*Echinacea purpurea, E. angustifolia*). The root stimulates the body's immune response. It is an alterative, antibiotic, antifungal, anti-inflammatory, antiviral, immunostimulant, and vulnerary.

Garlic (*Allium sativum*). The bulb neutralizes a wide range of pathogens. It is an alterative, antibiotic, antifungal, antiprotozoan, and immunostimulant. Some people are allergic to garlic. Excessive use can cause emotional irritability and irritation of the stomach and kidneys. Avoid therapeutic doses during pregnancy, and avoid during the first three months of nursing, as it can cause breast milk to become unpalatable for infants. Avoid use the week before having surgery.

Goldenseal (*Hydrastis canadensis*). The root helps dry up excessive discharge from mucous membranes, and it is an effective antibiotic against a wide range of pathogens. It is also alterative and anti-inflammatory. Goldenseal is very bitter, and most people find it easiest to ingest in capsule form. The tea can be used as a douche. This herb is endangered in the wild; do not use wildcrafted supplies. Avoid during pregnancy.

Isatis (*Isatis tinctoria*). The root is a strong antimicrobial, anti-inflammatory agent.

Myrrh (*Commiphora myrrha*). The resin normalizes mucous membrane activity and stimulates white blood cell production. It is an alterative, anti-inflammatory, antifungal, antiseptic, astringent, and vulnerary. Avoid during pregnancy, and do not use for more than one month at a time.

Oregon grape (*Mahonia aquifolium*). The root has antibacterial activity against a wide range of pathogens. It is an alterative, anti-inflammatory, antibiotic, febrifuge, and immunostimulant. Avoid during pregnancy, and do not exceed the recommended dosage.

Suppositories

Suppositories of garlic, yogurt, or boric acid can all help conquer a bacterial infection. See page 277 for more information.

Antiseptic Bath

A warm bath increases circulation to and moves blockages from the pelvic region. To help clear infection, add 1 cup of apple cider vinegar and 7 drops of tea tree or lavender essential oil to the bathwater.

20

Men's Health

On average, men don't live as long as women. They also are more likely to have type A personalities, which foster stress and anxiety. And from boyhood to manhood, men are usually encouraged to be strong, both physically and emotionally. As a result, they tend to pay less attention to their health, ignoring signs and symptoms and avoiding medical care at all costs.

Men can greatly benefit from a healthy lifestyle. It prolongs life, reduces the physical effects of stress, and promotes overall good health. It also builds sexual energy and ability. When a man develops a health problem, a healthy lifestyle will both support and speed up his body's recovery process. Most important, a healthy lifestyle is a vital component of self-care. If medical care is a pesticide that keeps the human body free of "bugs," self-care is the river that waters and fertilizes the landscape of the body in harmony with the rhythms of nature. Furthermore, self-care allows a man independence, so that he himself can gauge the state of his health and decide whether a problem can be addressed at home or needs the expertise of a health care professional.

The healing techniques and remedies in this chapter focus on self-care as a first solution for sexual health problems. Men may also wish to consult with a health care provider whom they feel comfortable communicating and working with. Men over the age of forty, especially those with a family history of cancer, should consider having a yearly physical, including a rectal exam.

Herbal Dosages

You'll find many recommendations for herbal therapy in this chapter. Unless stated otherwise, the therapeutic adult dosage for a recommended herb is:

- 1 cup of tea three times daily;
- 1 or 2 capsules three times daily; or
- 1 dropperful of tincture three times daily.

To figure out an appropriate dosage for a child, take the child's weight and divide by 150. The resulting fraction is the fraction of the adult dosage that the child should take. For example, a 50-pound child would take $^{50}/_{150}$, or $\frac{1}{3}$, of the adult dosage.

TESTICULAR SELF-EXAM

Self-examinations, including testicular exams, are an integral part of self-care. Weekly testicular exams, begun at about age fifteen, take only about three minutes and can catch testicular cancer in its early stages, when it is still treatable, as well as many other reproductive dysfunctions. If you discover any irregularities, bring them to the attention of your health care provider.

1. Hold the scrotum in the palms of your hands. Gently roll each testicle between the thumb and forefingers of a hand, checking for lumps.

2. Probe the epididymis, a comma-shaped cord behind the testicles, for lumps. This is a site where many noncancerous reproductive problems occur.

3. Examine the vas deferens, which is right under the skin that runs up from the epididymis. It should feel firm and smooth and should move under the pressure of your fingers.

CIRCUMCISION AND FORESKIN HEALTH

I'm going to make an argument here that many people would disagree with: Circumcision is an unnecessary, painful amputation that leaves the penis more vulnerable to disease than if left intact. We've been trained to think of a circumcised penis as "normal," when, in fact, it is quite abnormal. English-speaking countries began popularizing circumcision in the general population in the late 1800s in the hope that it would deter masturbation. (Didn't work, did it?) Today, the United States is the only country that still performs circumcision for reasons other than religious doctrine or medical necessity; about 80 percent of the planet's men are not circumcised.

Most of us would agree that the practice of removing the clitoris from a young girl qualifies as mutilation. What, then, is removal of the foreskin of an infant boy? The foreskin is a sensitive anatomical extension of the penis. It is rich in nerve endings and blood vessels, contains glands that produce antibacterial and antiviral proteins that help prevent infection, and protects a layer of emollient smegma that moisturizes the glans or head of the penis, keeping it supple, warm, and free of bacteria.

The glans is designed to be an internal organ, protected by the foreskin, which emerges upon erection. Think of the foreskin as a protective hood, much like the eyelids. Its removal exposes the glans to friction (especially from rubbing against clothes) and takes away its moisturizing protection. The end result is that the penis becomes tougher and less sensitive.

Circumcision will not, as common myth would tell you, prevent cancer of the penis. This rare disease affects only 1 in 100,000 males, and it is most prevalent in elderly men. Should women cut off their breasts to prevent breast cancer?

Circumcision is a fifteen-minute operation; although it's usually quite safe, infection, scarring, and damage to the penis are all risks. And it's painful. Most babies scream during the procedure, and some even go into shock. A study done at Washington University School of Medicine showed that most infant boys would not nurse right after being circumcised, and those who did would not look into their mother's eyes.

It's my vehement position that no one should have his or her genitals mutilated without his or her own informed consent. Should a male really want to be circumcised, he should be able to make that decision for himself when he reaches the age of eighteen.

Save the foreskins!

Cleaning under the Foreskin

Never retract the foreskin of an infant to clean underneath it. Retracting the foreskin before it is ready can cause pain and bleeding and can contribute to infection and scarring. Furthermore, washing underneath the foreskin removes friendly flora that protect the penis against infection.

The foreskin will gradually separate from the glans during childhood. The exact age of separation differs from child to child, but it usually happens at the age of four. Once their foreskin has separated from the glans on its own, little boys can be taught to pull it back gently to clean the glans, wiping away any accumulated discharge.

Phimosis

Phimosis is a condition in which the orifice at the top of the foreskin is constricted, so that the foreskin cannot be retracted back over the glans. This is a normal condition in infants, but in rare cases it persists into adulthood. Gentle stretching of the foreskin, as well as topical creams available upon prescription from a physician, can encourage flexibility of the foreskin and, eventually, retractability.

The constriction of phimosis may be relieved by supplementation with vitamin C (500–1,000 mg three times daily) and zinc (25–50 mg daily), which improve skin elasticity. (Consult with your health care provider to determine proper dosages for children.)

Irritations and Infections of the Foreskin

If an uncircumcised infant, boy, or man develops irritation around the foreskin area, the following remedies should clear it up in about five days.

Topical Herb Applications

Three times daily, rinse the area with warm water, then apply one of the following:

- A few drops of calendula-infused oil, which has soothing, infection-fighting, and anti-inflammatory properties. It is available at most natural food stores and herb shops.

- 10 drops each of calendula tincture and echinacea tincture diluted in ⅓ cup of warm water. This remedy is a bit stronger than calendula-infused oil and can be used to treat a more stubborn irritation. It is drying rather than lubricating.

- A dusting of powdered goldenseal root and/or slippery elm bark. Goldenseal fights infection and slippery elm soothes the inflammation.

- 1 tablespoon of cornstarch and 2 drops of lavender essential oil mixed in ¼ cup of warm water and 2 drops of lavender essential oil. After one to two minutes, wipe this mixture off with a soft cloth. Lavender essential oil is antiseptic, antifungal, and anti-inflammatory.

Antiseptic Bath

Add ½ cup of apple cider vinegar and 5 drops of lavender essential oil to a full bath. If you're using a baby-sized bath, use only 3 drops of the essential oil.

Support for the Immune System

If an infection persists, take one dropperful each of echinacea, calendula, and marsh mallow root tinctures three times daily. You can mix the tinctures in a bit of juice or water to make them more palatable. (To calculate a child's dosage, see "Herbal Dosages" on page 336.)

CRYPTORCHIDISM

As a male fetus develops, the testes are formed in the abdominal area. Some time before birth, they drop from the body into the scrotum. Cryptorchidism is a condition in which the testes fail to descend into the scrotum. About 10 percent of newborn male infants are cryptorchid; although most cases will resolve within a few weeks, in rare cases the testes remain undescended. Increased hormone levels at puberty, then, usually encourage descent in cryptorchid boys. There is some evidence indicating that parental exposure to xenoestrogens and pesticides may be a contributing factor to cryptorchidism.

Treatment: Encouraging the Descent

Cryptorchidism can impair sperm production and cause sterility if the testicles do not descend by puberty. For this reason, it is a good idea to try to resolve the problem during a boy's childhood. Physicians may suggest hormonal therapy or surgery. The following techniques are more natural alternatives that you may wish to try first, before resorting to surgery.

Physical Manipulation

A urologist or trained health care provider can encourage the testes to drop through gentle manipulation, as long as there is no structural condition contributing to the obstruction. Consult with your health care provider to discuss this option.

Moxa

An acupuncturist may use moxa, which entails burning the herb mugwort (*Artemisia vulgaris*) and bringing the heat and aromatic smoke close to the area. The moxa treatment increases circulation in the area, which can help move blockages.

Herbal Therapy

An herbalist would recommend herbs that stimulate hormonal production, such as fennel and saw palmetto. An adult dosage of these herbs is one dropperful of tincture three times daily. (To calculate a child's dosage, see "Herbal Dosages" on page 336.)

Fennel (*Foeniculum vulgare*). The seed contains phytosterols, which provide the body with raw material for creating its own hormones.

Saw palmetto (*Serenoa repens*). The berry is anabolic, meaning that it aids in the development of muscle tissue, thereby preventing atrophy of the genitals. It also contains phytosterols. It is a nutritive, stimulant, and tonic for the genitourinary system.

DELAYED EJACULATION

It is common for men to begin to experience delayed ejaculation as they age. However, it's also likely to be a symptom of drug or alcohol abuse, stress, anger, or lack of trust in a partner. Check in with yourself, and if you find that your lifestyle is contributing to this deficiency in your sexual chi, do what it takes to resolve the problem before other, more negative symptoms begin appearing.

For some older men, delayed ejaculation or the inability to ejaculate may be a permanent condition. This is not detrimental to health, so long as underlying health problems have been ruled out by a health care professional. In fact, making love without ejaculating can help build sexual chi.

EPIDIDYMITIS

The epididymis is a system of long, tangled ducts connected to the testes. It holds sperm until maturation and then feeds it to the vas deferens. Inflammation in the epididymis is called epididymitis, and it can be very painful. The cause of the inflammation cannot always be determined, although chlamydia and gonorrhea may be contributing factors. (Therefore, if you have epididymitis, it's a good idea to get checked for STDs.)

Symptoms

Epididymitis manifests as pain in the scrotum. There is often a lump on the back of the testicles that is hot and tender to the touch. There may be a discharge from the penis or difficulty in urinating.

Treatment

Antibiotics are usually prescribed, but consider the following natural therapies:

Elevation

Elevating an inflamed area helps reduce the swelling. Whenever you're able to take a few minutes to relax, lie down with a pillow under your bottom to elevate the scrotum. You could also try sleeping in this position.

Cold Packs and Sitz Baths

Twice daily, alternate ice compresses on the testicles with hot sitz baths. This treatment can help clear the blockage. (For information on preparing a sitz bath, see Chapter 12.)

Herbal Therapy

Herbal therapy for epididymitis focuses on stimulating the body's immune system and eliminating pathogens.

Echinacea (*Echinacea purpurea, E. angustifolia*). The root stimulates the immune system. It is also an alterative, antifungal, and antiseptic.

Goldenseal (*Hydrastis canadensis*). The root is effective against a wide range of pathogens and is especially effective for inflammation of the mucous membranes. It is an alterative and an antibiotic. Goldenseal is very bitter, and most people find it easiest to ingest in capsule form. This herb is endangered in the wild; do not use wildcrafted supplies.

Usnea (*Usnea barbata*). The lichen stimulates the immune system and is effective against a wide range of pathogens. It is also an antibiotic and an antifungal.

ERECTILE DYSFUNCTION

Erection occurs when blood rushes in from the penile arteries, engorging the erectile tissue. Valves in the veins close down, limiting blood flow back to the body. The engorged penis expands to accommodate the extra blood, which amounts to sixteen times the amount of blood it normally contains.

The penile arteries are tiny; their lumens, or cavities, are just slightly larger than the head of a pin. When blood flow to the penis is impeded—as may happen when circulation through the penile arteries is limited by blockages or muscle constriction due to tension—achieving and maintaining erection becomes difficult.

Identifying the Cause

Although aging is sometimes accompanied by the onset of erectile dysfunction, it is not itself the cause. Rather, as the raging hormonal tides of young adulthood subside to normal rhythms, erection becomes less a "default" state and more the result of healthy sexual impulses. A man, then, must be in good health, both physically and mentally, to achieve and maintain an erection.

It is estimated that about 80 percent of cases of erectile dysfunction are caused by physical dysfunction, with the other 20 percent resulting from psychological concerns. Distinguishing between a physical and a psychological dysfunction is not always easy, but two general guidelines should be considered:

- If the dysfunction gained hold slowly but progressively over time, with a gradual decrease in erectile ability, it is probably physical in nature. If it appeared suddenly, with no gradual buildup of symptoms, it is probably psychological in nature.

- If the inability to achieve or maintain erection occurs in all situations, including masturbation, it is probably a physical problem. If it occurs only with a particular partner or in certain situations, it is probably a psychological problem.

Direct a sharp eye at what's going on in your life or what was happening at the time the dysfunction began. Make a list of the situations in which erection is possible and impossible. If you can uncover a trigger or pattern, you're close to discovering the cause, and with it, the cure.

If you suspect that the dysfunction is physical in nature, visit your health care provider as soon as possible for a full examination. There are many diseases and health conditions that can contribute to erectile dysfunction, including atherosclerosis, diabetes, endocrine disorders, heart disease, high cholesterol, kidney disease, Leriche's disease, liver disease, Lou Gehrig's disease, multiple sclerosis, Parkinson's disease, penile dysfunctions, prostate disease, sickle-cell anemia, and vascular disease. Exposure to toxic substances, including radiation treatments for cancer, can also impair erectile function.

Treatment

It makes sense to try natural remedies, rather than drug therapy, as a first recourse. Natural therapies encourage your body to heal itself, and they generally have a wide-ranging healing effect, supporting many of the body's systems, rather than just those related to erection.

Seek Alternatives to Pharmaceuticals

Many medications, including antidepressants, antihistamines, antipsychotics, and tranquilizers, can adversely affect libido. Medications designed to reduce high blood pressure can be especially problematic, because erection depends upon the mechanics of raising blood pressure.

If you're taking any of the aforementioned medications, ask your health care provider if there are alternatives that do not have erectile dysfunction as a side effect. However, do not stop taking medication without first consulting with your health care provider. If you must continue to take these drugs, incorporate natural, health-supporting therapies such as massage, herbal supplements, nutritional supplements, and relaxation techniques to improve your overall health and, with luck, counteract the side effects of your medication.

Take a Break

A prohibition on intercourse and ejaculation for four to six weeks can do wonders for building sexual energy and pulling your head, heart, and health together. Sex therapists suggest sensate therapy: getting naked, touching, caressing, exploring, and communicating, all the while avoiding intercourse and ejaculation. If arousal and erection does occur, avoid ejaculation, focusing instead on building sexual chi, much like adding money to your savings account.

Spend more time on sensate therapy than you would having sex. Becoming more sexually active, rather than less, helps improve erectile function by boosting circulation to the genitals. It also helps couples revive feelings of sensuality and togetherness.

Support Testosterone Levels

Testosterone plays a large role in generating libido. It also facilitates erection, although the connection is not fully understood.

Stress and lack of exercise can diminish testosterone levels. Exercise itself is a good remedy for stress, so be sure to get plenty of it. However, be aware that very intense exercise decreases testosterone levels.

Elevated estrogen levels can interfere with testosterone activity, contributing to erectile dysfunction. Products from animals that have been treated with hormones to encourage growth and early maturation often contain estrogens; eating them can elevate your estrogen levels. Eat products only from animals that were raised without the "benefit" of hormones.

Testosterone levels are highest between 6 and 8 A.M.; if you're having trouble with erectile dysfunction, try to time lovemaking sessions so that they occur in the early morning.

Stop Smoking

Smokers are twice as likely as nonsmokers to develop erection problems. Smoking reduces lung capacity, sexual endurance, libido, and the intensity of orgasms. Nicotine, just one of many noxious cigarette ingredients, constricts the arteries and veins that supply blood to the penis and diminishes testosterone levels. It seems capable of causing erectile dysfunction all on its own.

Stop Drinking

Men with erection difficulties should, at the very least, abstain from alcohol on the days they desire to make love. Alcohol is a depressant and can, at high levels, prevent arousal and erection. Drinking beer, in particular, contributes to elevated levels of prolactin, which can decrease testosterone levels.

Massage

There are many simple types of massage that can stimulate hormone production, strengthen sexual chi, boost circulation to the penis, and help a man achieve and maintain an erection.

The meridians that support sexual potency run through the big toe. Try massaging the whole foot, focusing on the big toe, to encourage erectile ability.

In a Taoist exercise, the man sits in a hot bath and stimulates himself manually to the point of erection. When erect, he grasps the testicles and gently pulls down on them one hundred to two hundred times. A traditional Japanese technique is similar; men are advised to firmly but gently squeeze the testicles daily, once for every year of age.

Kegel exercises, of course, are also excellent therapy for erectile dysfunction, because they encourage blood flow in the genitals. See page 30 for instructions on how to perform Kegels. While you're there, check out The Deer, which follows.

Foreplay can itself consist of therapeutic massage. To stimulate circulation, a man's partner can stroke the penis from the base to the tip, massaging the frenulum and glans and squeezing and massaging the penis's shaft. Form a ring with the forefinger and thumb around the area of the penis just below the frenulum; squeeze gently but firmly to prevent blood from flowing out of the penis. This can encourage erection and greatly build a man's confidence. Take care not to squeeze too tightly or for more than a couple of minutes.

Nutritional Therapy

Cut out saturated fats, hydrogenated and partially hydrogenated oils, sugar, and cold foods and beverages. Cold and cooked fatty foods can impair circulation, and sugar actually robs the body of nutrients, such as calcium and the B-complex vitamins, causing nutritional deficiencies and fatigue. Focus on eating foods that are rich in the following nutrients, or try supplementation.

Arginine. The amino acid arginine is a precursor to nitric oxide, a compound that is responsible for vasodilation and, thus, plays a role in blood flow to the genitals. Creams that deliver arginine transdermally (through the skin) are now available; consult with your health care provider for advice on whether this treatment is right for you. Arginine is also available, often in combination with other erection-enhancing compounds, in tablets or powders, which can be found at natural food stores and vitamin shops.

Protein. To improve erectile ability, be sure to eat adequate protein. Protein helps normalize physiological chemicals; without it, our body deteriorates. Avocados, nuts, and seeds are excellent sources of protein.

Zinc. Through indirect action, zinc stimulates testosterone production. Take 25–50 mg daily, or eat a handful of raw sunflower and pumpkin seeds every day.

Herbal Therapy

Any of the herbs suggested in Chapter 6 would be appropriate for a man suffering from erectile dysfunction. Turn to the "Herbal Compendium" on page 73 for more information.

ORCHITIS

Orchitis is inflammation of a testis. It can arise spontaneously, but it can also be a side effect of mumps, gonnorrhea, syphilis, or other infections. If you experience orchitis, see your health care provider for an examination to rule out these other causes.

Symptoms

Orchitis is usually accompanied by pain, swelling, and a heavy feeling in the testicles.

Treatment

Treatment for orchitis focuses on reducing the inflammation and clearing the infection from the testes.

Ice

Two or three times a day, lie down with a pillow under your buttocks and apply an ice compress to the testicles. The elevation and ice will work together to reduce inflammation.

Herbal Therapy

Herbs that help reduce inflammation and move stagnation in cases of orchitis include the following.

Chamomile (*Matricaria recutita*). The flower helps detoxify liver, reduce inflammation, and move stagnation. It is an analgesic, anodyne, anti-inflammatory, antispasmodic, and mild sedative.

Cleavers (*Galium aparine*). The herb clears heat and reduces inflammation. It is an alterative, anti-inflammatory, antitumor, astringent, lymphatic cleanser, and vulnerary.

Cramp bark (*Viburnum opulus*). The bark relieves pain. It is an analgesic, anti-inflammatory, antispasmodic, astringent, and diuretic.

Dong quai (*Angelica sinensis*). The root clears stagnation from the blood, relieves congestion in pelvic tissue, and relaxes smooth muscles. It is an alterative, anticoagulant, antispasmodic, and blood tonic. Do not use in cases of diarrhea or poor digestion. Do not use in conjunction with blood-thinning medications such as ibuprofen.

Echinacea (*Echinacea purpurea, E. angustifolia*). The root stimulates the body's immune response. It is an alterative, antibiotic, antifungal, anti-inflammatory, antiviral, immunostimulant, and vulnerary.

PEYRONIE'S DISEASE

Also known as the "bent penis" syndrome, Peyronie's disease is a condition in which erection produces what's called a fibrous chordee, or downward bowing of the penis. In some cases, the bend is so severe that intercourse is not feasible. It is often the result of scarring or the development of fibrous plaque in the penis.

For proper diagnosis, visit your health care provider. The penis may look normal when flaccid, so it's helpful to bring a photograph of what the penis looks like when erect (assuming that you might have a difficult time achieving erection in the doctor's office).

Treatment

Surgery is sometimes recommended for Peyronie's disease, but it may cause further damage. Natural therapies don't risk additional harm, so it makes sense to try them first.

First clean up the diet, eliminating hydrogenated oils, fried foods, excess red meat, and dairy products. These foods can contribute to arteriosclerosis, causing circulatory blockage and impairing blood flow throughout the body.

Some men suffering from Peyronie's disease have had positive results with vitamin E, which reduces scarring. Take 400 IU twice daily, or eat a handful of almonds, sunflower seeds, or pumpkin seeds daily. Vitamin E supplementation is most effective when undertaken within two years of the onset of the condition.

You might also try massaging the penis with castor oil, which can help break up scar tissue.

PRIAPISM

Priapism is a persistent abnormal erection. Though an erection that doesn't give up might sound like a man's (or woman's) dream come true, it can result in permanent impotence if not treated within a few hours.

Priapism is named for Priapus, the Greek and Roman god of male generative power, who is often depicted with a huge erect penis. It occurs when blood in the engorged penis is unable to drain back into the body; the blockage is usually caused by high blood pressure medications, some antidepressants, some aphrodisiacs, blood disorders, anesthesia, or damage to the penis, brain, or spinal cord.

Symptoms

Priapism is characterized by a persistent erection accompanied by pain and tenderness. The erection often occurs without sexual desire.

Treatment

Get thee to a doctor! Apply an ice pack to the genitals until you receive medical attention; this will encourage the blood vessels to constrict. Your health care provider will probably give you medication—a shot or pill—to deflate the erection.

PROSTATE HEALTH

The prostate gland is composed of both muscular and glandular tissue. It's shaped much like a chestnut and surrounds the neck of the bladder and the urethra, which is the beginning of the urinary tract. The prostate secretes a milky fluid that makes up about 30 percent of the volume of semen; the fluid is alkaline, which makes the vaginal environment less acidic and, thus, less hostile to sperm.

Common Disorders of the Prostate

It is estimated that half of the men in the United States over the age of fifty will have prostate difficulty at some time. That staggering statistic may be, in part, a result of the placid Western lifestyle. In cultures where a high-fiber diet and exercise are the norm, prostate problems are considered rare.

Benign Prostatic Hyperplasia

Benign prostatic hyperplasia (BPH), also known as prostatism or prostatic adenoma, is nonmalignant enlargement of the prostate. It is characterized by the swelling of prostatic tissue, sometimes accompanied by the development of small nodes. The enlargement is thought to be triggered by increased production of the androgen dihydrotestosterone (DHT), a common phenomenon in men over the age of forty-five.

An enlarged prostate can constrict the urethra, resulting in the need to urinate frequently, the inability to empty the bladder completely, painful urination, and occasional dribbling of urine. It's generally not a serious health problem, although advanced cases can manifest as bladder infections, kidney problems, and sexual dysfunction. It does cause discomfort, however, and the disruption of sleep caused by having to get up three or four times a night to urinate can lead to general malaise.

There are many pharmaceutical treatments for this common disorder. Surgery is also sometimes recommended. However, natural therapies are often very effective at reducing the symptoms of BPH; given the risks associated with surgery and the sometimes annoying side effects of pharmaceuticals, they are a wise choice for initial treatment.

Prostatitis

Prostatitis is inflammation of the prostate, usually due to a bacterial infection. It can cause fever, discharge, back pain upon defecating, and blood in the urine. It often afflicts men who abstained from sex for a long period of time and then overindulged.

When you exhibit symptoms of prostatitis, it is important to rule out several more serious infections that may be triggering the inflammation. Chlamydia and other venereal parasites are common causes. Sometimes prostatitis is not bacterial but a symptom of an autoimmune disorder or a glandular dysfunction. Consult with your health care provider for guidance.

Prostatitis usually responds readily to natural therapy. Cease sexual activity until the irritation has disappeared. Avoid caffeine, alcohol, and spicy foods, which can contribute to prostate irritation. Follow the guidelines for prostate health given below. Echinacea, pipsissewa, and zinc will be especially helpful in fighting off infection and supporting the prostate. If natural therapies do not clear the infection within ten days, seek the advice of your health care provider.

Prostate Cancer

In its early stages, prostate cancer exhibits symptoms similar to those of BPH: the need to urinate frequently, inability to empty the bladder completely, painful urination, and occasional dribbling of urine. In a more advanced stage, prostate cancer may also manifest as blood in the urine, fatigue, bone pain, and weight loss.

Most prostate cancers form in the side of the gland that faces the rectum. Prostate cancer appears to be most prevalent in men whose diets are high in animal fat, such as is found in meat, eggs, and dairy products.

Though surgery and chemotherapy are the usual treatments for prostate cancer, you may also wish to explore raw food therapy and herbal medicine under the guidance of your health care provider. Saw palmetto and pygeum may be of particular benefit.

The Prostate Exam

Any time you suspect you have a problem with your prostate, consult with your health care provider for a proper diagnosis. Early symptoms of prostate cancer can be similar to those of BPH, and a check-up with a competent urologist is needed to distinguish between the two. This will mean a rectal exam; for those of you who dread the procedure, remember that it is easier if you relax. The urologist will be able to determine the condition of the prostate from the way it feels.

Improving the Health of the Prostate

Natural therapies for supporting the health of the prostate focus on strengthening the prostate, improving the function of the liver and kidneys, cleansing the urinary and bowel systems, counteracting or reducing levels of DHT, and relieving inflammation.

Nutritional Therapy

Avoid heated fats, including red meat. A high-fat diet leads to elevated cholesterol levels, which can impair prostate function and contribute to BPH. Also minimize coffee, alcohol, salt, and dairy products, which irritate the prostate gland. Focus on incorporating the following nutrients and supplements into your diet.

Acidophilus. An acidophilus supplement will help discourage unfriendly microorganisms from invading the prostate region. Try taking one or two capsules three times daily.

Amino acids. The amino acids alanine, glutamine, and glycine can help shrink an enlarged prostate gland. They can often be purchased in combination with beneficial herbs for reducing enlargement.

Bee pollen. Small amounts of bee pollen or flower pollen (which differs from bee pollen only in that it is collected directly from the flowers and saves the bees lots of work) can be helpful in treating prostatitis. It has anti-inflammatory properties and is antiandrogenic, meaning it helps to counteract some of the effects of excess DHT. Take 1 teaspoon or two 500 mg tablets twice daily. If you have a pollen allergy, start with just a couple of grains a day, increasing by one grain a day until you reach the recommended dosage.

Estrogenic foods. Foods that have estrogen-like activity are considered beneficial, because they help reduce elevated testosterone levels. These include apples, barley, brown rice, carrots, cherries, soy products, olives, and yams.

Flaxseed and pumpkin seed. To soothe inflammation of the prostate, take 3 tablespoons of freshly ground flaxseed or pumpkin seed daily. Also take 50 mg of vitamin B_6 to help reduce the prostate's size.

High-fiber foods. A thin tissue separates the prostate from the rectum. Because a blockage in one system tends to back up nearby systems, avoiding constipation supports not only the colon but also the prostate. A diet that is rich in high-fiber foods such as raw fruits and vegetables, nuts, and seeds promotes normal elimination.

Natural diuretics. It is also important to keep the urinary system fully functional. When watermelon is in season, chew up the seeds—which are diuretic—to help clean out the urinary tract. Drink plenty of pure water to make the urine less acidic and irritating. Diluted pure cranberry and wheat grass juice are also beneficial drinks; cranberry juice is antiseptic and wheat grass helps the body make better use of oxygen.

Seaweeds. Seaweeds such as kelp and kombu have a softening and draining effect on hardened masses in the body; they can help relieve cases of BPH and prostatitis.

Vitamin E and selenium. As antioxidants that support cellular health, vitamin E and selenium also support prostate health. Take a 400 IU vitamin E–selenium formula daily. Also consider incorporating natural sources of vitamin E and selenium into your diet; see Chapter 5 for information.

Zinc. The prostate gland contains more zinc than any other part of the body, and having plenty of zinc in the diet supports the health of the prostate. Good sources of zinc include almonds, beans, eggs, nutritional yeast, oatmeal, oysters, pumpkin seeds, sunflower seeds, and tahini. Also consider supplementing with 50 mg of chelated zinc daily.

Herbal Therapy

Herbs that support and improve the health of the prostate include the following.

Buchu (*Agathosma betulina*). The leaf soothes and strengthens the urinary system. It is a diuretic, kidney tonic, and urinary antiseptic.

Cleavers (*Galium aparine*). The herb soothes prostate inflammation. It is particularly helpful in cases where one feels the urge to urinate but is unable to do so. It clears heat and improves lymphatic function. It is an alterative, anti-inflammatory, antitumor, soothing diuretic, and vulnerary.

Cornsilk (*Zea mays*). The stigma helps relieve inflammation of the prostate and irritation or infection in the urinary tract. It relieves the urge to urinate frequently by soothing irritated tissues. It is an alterative, demulcent, diuretic, and tonic.

Couchgrass (*Elymus repens*). The rhizome is particularly helpful in treating prostatitis. Its mucilaginous nature helps it cool irritated mucous membranes. It is an antiseptic, demulcent, diuretic, and tonic.

Cubeb (*Piper cubeba*). The berry is used to treat infections of the genitourinary tract and can help relieve cases of prostatitis. It is an antiseptic and a diuretic. Avoid in cases of acute digestive and kidney irritation.

Echinacea (*Echinacea purpurea, E. angustifolia*). The root remedies infections of the urinary tract. It is an alterative, antifungal, anti-inflammatory, antiseptic, and vulnerary.

Fringe tree (*Chionanthus virginicus*). The root clears heat and reduces inflammation. It is an alterative, cholagogue, diuretic, and hepatic.

Goldenrod (*Solidago* spp.). The herb reduces inflammation, sedates urinary passages, promotes urination, prevents infection, and strengthens the bladder. It is an anti-inflammatory, antiseptic, astringent, diuretic, hepatic, and tonic. Do not use in cases of hot inflammation, such as fever or high blood pressure.

Gravel root (*Eupatorium purpureum*). The root helps break up accumulations, such as stones in the urinary system. It clears heat, reduces inflammation, and soothes irritated mucous membranes of the urinary tract. It is often recommended for prostatitis. It is astringent, diuretic, and tonic.

Horsetail (*Equisetum arvense*). The herb reduces benign prostatic enlargement. It is an alterative, antiseptic, anti-inflammatory, astringent, diuretic, and vulnerary. Use horsetail that has been collected in spring.

Hydrangea (*Hydrangea arborescens*). The root soothes irritated mucous membranes and sedates the urinary tract. It is a diuretic and a tonic.

Marsh mallow (*Althaea officinalis*). The root soothes inflammation; it is useful for treating prostatitis in particular. It is an alterative, demulcent, diuretic, immunostimulant, rejuvenative, vulnerary, and yin tonic.

Nettle (*Urtica dioica, U. urens*). The leaf and root improve the metabolism of the prostate gland and reduce benign prostatic hyperplasia. They contain sterols, including beta sitosterol, stigmasterol, and campesterol, that decrease DHT activity. Treats bladder infection, cystitis, kidney inflammation, and stones. They are alteratives, cholagogues, circulatory stimulants, diuretics, kidney tonics, and nutritives. Contact with the fresh plant will irritate the skin. Use only dried herb. Wear gloves when collecting.

Oregon grape (*Mahonia aquifolium*). The root is an alterative, anti-inflammatory, antiseptic, astringent, cholagogue, diuretic, glandular tonic, immunostimulant, and tonic. Do not exceed the recommended dosage.

Parsley (*Petroselinum crispum*). The leaf and root help relieve pain during urination and help men to empty the bladder completely. They are antioxidant, antiseptic, diuretic, and nutritive. Avoid therapeutic doses in cases of kidney inflammation.

Pipsissewa (*Chimaphila umbellata*). The herb contains hydroquinone, which has genitourinary antiseptic properties. It is an alterative, anti-inflammatory, urinary antiseptic, astringent, diuretic, and urinary sedative.

Pygeum (*Pygeum africanum*). The bark has a decongesting action that blocks cholesterol buildup in the prostate gland. It is also anti-inflammatory. It is often recommended for treating erectile dysfunction, prostate cancer, prostatic hyperplasia, chronic prostate inflammation, and urinary disorders. This herb is endangered in the wild; do not use wildcrafted supplies.

Saint John's wort (*Hypericum perforatum*). The herb dissolves obstructions and reduces swelling. It is an alterative, anti-inflammatory, antiseptic, cholagogue, and vulnerary. In rare cases, this herb causes photosensitivity. Do not combine Saint John's wort with monoamine oxidase (MAO) inhibitors (chemical antidepressants) or selective reuptake inhibitors, such as Prozac.

Saw palmetto (*Serenoa repens*). The berry reduces inflammation, lessens pain, and relieves the need to urinate frequently. It also inhibits the conversion of testosterone to dihydrostestosterone (DHT). It enhances blood flow to the prostate and thus lowers the rate of cellular regeneration in the prostate gland. It is often recommended in treatments for prostatic hyperplasia and prostatitis. It is a diuretic, rejuvenative, urinary antiseptic, and tonic.

Uva ursi (*Arctostaphylos uva-ursi*). The leaf contains arbutin, which the body converts to hydroquinone, an antiseptic. It is a genitourinary antiseptic, astringent, bladder tonic, demulcent, diuretic, and vasoconstrictor.

Homeopathic Remedies

There are several homeopathic remedies that can be used to improve prostate problems. If the description matches the symptoms of your prostatic condition, try the suggested homeopathic remedy. The usual dosage is four pellets, or as many liquid drops as the package label recommends, taken under the tongue four times daily. Rather than swallowing the pellets whole, allow them to dissolve slowly.

Aconitum Napellus. The patient is suffering from the initial stage of prostatitis.

Apis Mellifica. The prostate is inflamed.

Argentum Metallicum. The patient is elderly and suffers from chronic prostate enlargement.

Argentum Nitricum. The patient is elderly and suffers from prostate enlargement with burning in the rectal anterior.

Baryta Carbonica. The patient is elderly and suffers from prostatic enlargement. He may experience a frequent urge to urinate and a burning sensation when he does so.

Belladonna. The patient suffers from throbbing prostatitis.

Cannabis Indica. The patient feels that he is sitting on a ball in the anal region.

Chimaphila Umbellata. The patient experiences discomfort and the need to urinate frequently.

Conium. The patient has chronic prostatic enlargement and difficulty urinating, with the flow of urine starting and stopping.

Ferrum Picricum. The patient is elderly and suffers from prostate enlargement and inflammation.

Lycopodium. The patient has an enlarged prostate and feels pressure in the perineum during urination.

Pulsatilla. The patient has prostate inflammation accompanied by increased sex drive and frequent erections.

Sabal Serrulata. The patient has either chronic or acute prostate enlargement accompanied by burning or difficulty in urination.

Solidago Virgaurea. The patient has chronic prostate enlargement and obstructed urine flow.

Spongia Tosta. The patient has prostate enlargement, and his testicles are red and swollen.

Staphysagria. The patient experiences frequent urges to urinate but can produce only small amounts of urine, and it burns.

Sulfur. Prostatic fluid escapes during urination or during bowel movements.

Thuja Occidentalis. The patient feels a constant urge to urinate but can produce only small amounts of urine. There is pain from the rectum to the bladder.

Sitz Baths

To boost circulation and clear stagnation from the genital area, alternate hot and cold sitz baths, as directed in Chapter 12.

Warm baths on their own will also have some benefit, relaxing the pelvic muscles and softening the prostate. In lieu of a bath, apply a hot water bottle to the perineal area (between the anus and scrotum).

Exercise

Various exercises can help improve circulation and clear congestion from the prostate. A slant board or inverted yoga posture such as the shoulder stand can help clear congestions. Kegel exercises are also helpful. (See page 30.)

When you get up in the morning and retire in the evenings, try this simple exercise. Lie on your back and bring the soles of your feet together. Extend the legs as far as you can while keeping the soles together, then bring them as close to your chest as possible, still keeping the soles together. Repeat ten times.

Of most importance, get adequate exercise. There's nothing better for improving circulation and supporting overall health. Try walking, swimming, or dancing, all of which are excellent, nonjarring forms of exercise.

21

Fertility and Infertility

ertility is, in essence, the ability to create and maintain a viable fetus. Although the human body is designed to procreate, conceiving a child is not as easy as it sounds. As we were all taught in our younger years, fertilization takes place only when a female egg (the ovum) fuses with a male sperm cell. The fertilized egg then finds its way into the uterus, where it is nurtured for approximately nine months, until birth. But there are a lot of very complicated processes that have to transpire correctly to set the stage for the meeting of ovum and sperm. And there are plenty of things that can knock the rendezvous off course.

> Among the many reasons why a couple might have difficulty conceiving are the esoteric, which are no less powerful for being intangible. Consider this: The attempt to conceive a child is an invitation to a being, a soul, to come spend its life with you. If you were a child, is your house where you would want to live? If you spend all your time in front of the television, if you argue constantly with your spouse, if you have no regard for the health and beauty of the world, then the answer is probably no. Ask the being that you are trying to attract, "What qualities are you looking for in parents and a home?" Then be still. Listen. Create that reality.

WHY CAN'T WE CONCEIVE?

True infertility (or sterility, as it is technically defined for men) is an uncommon, though not rare, condition in which it is physically impossible to conceive a child. Most cases of what we call "infertility" are, instead, situations in which a person or couple is having difficulty conceiving. There's a rather large difference between the two. Fertility can be nurtured, after all, in numerous ways, ranging from pharmaceutical medications to surgery to (and preferably) natural therapies. If you're not infertile but just having trouble conceiving, you will, in most cases, be able to overcome the challenges presented to you and eventually achieve a full-term pregnancy.

For some people, fertility dysfunctions are biological in nature. Sometimes, but not always, it is possible to resolve them. Other people are living with, intentionally or unintentionally, environmental factors that interfere with their ability to conceive. In most cases, these detrimental factors can be eliminated and will not have lasting effects.

Biological Dysfunctions

The many biological dysfunctions that could interfere with fertility are too numerous to count, much less describe in this overview. Some of these problems are present from birth; they may even be insignificant enough, generally speaking, that the dysfunction is not noticed until the time comes when procreation is desired. Other problems result from damage to any of a number of reproduction-linked systems and organs.

Here we will focus on those biological dysfunctions that are most common and that can possibly be overcome or reversed.

Antibodies

A woman can develop antibodies that act against a man's sperm; equally, a man can develop antibodies to his own sperm. If a woman is producing antibodies to a man's sperm, the man should wear a condom. When the woman is ovulating, discontinue use of the condom.

Blockages

Complete or partial blockage anywhere in the reproductive system can contribute to difficulty in conceiving. Blockages may be due to structural malformations, scarring, fibroids, endometriosis, blocked arteries, or even excess mucus. With proper diagnosis, many blockages can be cleared through the use of natural therapies or surgery.

Hormonal Imbalances

Hormones are like spark plugs, providing stimulus to drive both body and mind. Proper hormone function plays a major role in the reproductive cycle.

If the endocrine (hormone-producing) system is not operating properly, ova may release sporadically or not at all, sperm count may be diminished, libido may disappear, and so on. In most cases, hormone production can be normalized through the use of natural therapies or pharmaceutical medications. (For more information, see "Sexual Chemistry" on page 15.)

Hostile Cervical Mucus

If vaginal mucus is too acidic or too alkaline, it can be destructive to sperm. The pH of the vagina can largely be controlled through diet. Cutting back on sugars and carbohydrates can help.

> Peak fertility in women arrives in their early twenties and begins to diminish thereafter, most rapidly from the mid-thirties. One in four women over the age of thirty will have some difficulty in conceiving. Men's fertility drops radically during their mid-forties.

Menstrual Irregularity

Metrorrhagia (irregular menses) or amenorrhea (lack of menses) are symptoms of an imbalanced reproductive system. They also make it difficult to predict when or if ovulation is occurring.

Chapter 18 describes natural therapies that can help normalize menses.

Thyroid Dysfunction

The thyroid is an endocrine gland that secretes a number of hormones, including thyroxin, without which ovulation cannot occur. A healthy thyroid gland is essential for egg development and sperm production. To support the health of the thyroid, add plenty of sea vegetables to your diet, and drink pure water instead of fluoridated tap water.

Weight Problems

For women, being extremely overweight or underweight can inhibit ovulation. (Not much is known about the effects of weight on reproduction for men.) When weight levels normalize, menstrual cycles and ovulation often become more regular. Obesity, in particular, is linked to elevated levels of estrogen, which can interfere with menstruation. However, some body fat—between 17 and 21 percent—is necessary for hormonal production.

If you suffer from weight problems, consult with your health care provider, who may be able to recommend a nutritionist. In general, to gain weight, eat more nuts and seeds. To lose weight, eat more fruits and vegetables.

Environmental Stressors

Environmental factors that can contribute to difficulty in conceiving are all those toxins and physiologically active substances that we ingest or absorb—purposefully or unknowingly—in our daily lives. Most do not have lasting effects; once exposure to them is eliminated, their effects quickly or gradually disappear.

Alcohol

Excessive alcohol depresses testosterone levels in men, which can lead to erectile dysfunction, reduced testicle size, and decreased libido. For women, studies show that even moderate alcohol intake can be a factor in ovulatory infertility.

Contraception

Birth control pills can cause blood stagnation in the reproductive organs, which can impede conception. Some women experience amenorrhea after they discontinue use of birth control pills; menses begin to normalize over time.

Environmental Toxins

Low sperm count is a progressive trend in modern times. Today's average sperm count is almost 40 percent lower than it was in the 1920s. Although biological problems could be a factor, I'm inclined to believe that the radical decrease in average sperm count is primarily linked to environmental causes. Some experts believe that herbicide and pesticide residues in the food we eat, the water we drink, and the land we live on may be factors. This theory makes sense to me—these substances are, after all, designed to destroy life. According to traditional Oriental medicine, low sperm count can be caused by a yin deficiency in the kidneys. The Western and Oriental theories complement each other; the kidneys and liver serve as filters for metabolic wastes, and the toxic residues we absorb eventually pass through them, which could contribute to kidney and liver dysfunctions.

To lessen your exposure to environmental toxins, live organically. Use nontoxic cleaning products, wear organic-fiber clothing, and stop using pesticides and herbicides on your landscape. Eat low on the food chain, focusing the diet on organic vegetables, fruits, nuts, seeds, and whole grains.

Electromagnetic Energy

Fields of electromagnetic energy surround the flow of electric current. Excessive exposure to electromagnetic energy is associated with an increased risk of cancer, a weakened immune system, and hormonal dysfunctions, including fertility problems.

Sixty to two hundred million sperm per cubic centimeter is considered a healthy sperm count. A moderately low sperm count can still be effective; according to the American Fertility Society, there must be twenty to forty million sperm per cubic centimeter of ejaculate for fertilization to occur.

However, a very low sperm count (less than twenty million sperm per cubic centimeter of ejaculate) can negate the possibility of fertilization. Of the millions of sperm in a "normal" ejaculation, only about forty sperm actually reach the egg, and those lucky little ones still have quite a bit of risky work cut out for them. Imagine the odds when sperm count is only half of what it should be.

Electromagnetic energy can be difficult to avoid. Try to minimize contact with household electrical appliances, microwaves, electric blankets, water beds (which are warmed by electric heaters), computer monitors without protective screens, x-rays, and power lines. Most important, minimize their proximity to your sleeping area.

Excessive Exercise

Though exercise is wonderful for overall health and vigor, too much of it can tax the body to the point that conception is impossible. Instead of running, biking, or weight lifting to exhaustion, practice—in moderation—exercises that facilitate fertility. See Chapter 3 for suggestions.

"Professional" Gear

Toxic residues and yin deficiencies aren't the only modern-day causes of low sperm count. For optimal sperm production, the testes must be at a temperature between ninety-four and ninety-six degrees Fahrenheit, which is just less than body temperature. Therefore, the testicles are suspended from the body in the scrotum; being slightly removed from the torso allows them to exist at a slightly cooler state. However, the amenities of civilization that are part and parcel of having a professional life, including synthetic-fiber clothing and office jobs that require men to sit all day long, can raise the temperature of the testes and reduce sperm production.

If you're having trouble with low sperm count, take cool showers instead of hot baths. Wear boxer shorts instead of briefs. Avoid synthetic-fiber fabrics. And do your best to get up and move around as much as possible.

Pharmaceutical Medications

Many drugs, particularly those prescribed for ulcers, can lower sperm count, diminish libido, contribute to erectile dysfunction, and negatively effect fertility in countless other ways.

If you're taking a pharmaceutical medication that has an adverse effect on fertility, ask your health care provider if there are alternatives. However, do not stop taking medication without first consulting with your health care provider. If you must continue to take these drugs, also undertake some of the natural, fertility-supporting therapies such as those suggested later in this chapter; with luck, they will counteract the side effects of your medication.

Smoking

Smoking has a tremendously potent effect on fertility. Unfortunately, that effect is strictly negative. Female smokers have a 40 percent higher rate of infertility than nonsmokers, and 33 percent of male smokers have reduced sperm motility. Cigarettes also diminish the production of testosterone, leading to a wide range of erectile and sperm production dysfunctions.

TIPS FOR FERTILE LOVEMAKING

There are a thousand and one sure-fire, guaranteed-to-work, folkloric "cures" for conceiving. Some of them are quite insightful; others are just plain strange. I prefer to stick with common sense.

- **Build up sexual chi.** A man should avoid ejaculation for a week before ovulation to "save up" sexual energy.

- **Make sure you're both ready.** Traditional Oriental medicine suggests that having intercourse when you are extremely angry, grieved, frightened, or intoxicated can increase the risk of a stillborn child.

- **Urinate before, not after.** The woman should urinate before intercourse so that she won't need to urinate immediately afterward. Urinating afterward can wash away some sperm and disrupt the movement of sperm toward the ovum.

- **Avoid artificial lubricants.** Lubricants can interfere with sperm motility, lessening chances of conception.

- **Take time for foreplay.** It is not imperative for a woman to have an orgasm for conception to occur, yet she should be stimulated enough to produce some vaginal mucus. Take some time with foreplay to ensure that the woman is aroused.

- **Stick with the classic position.** The best position for conception is the missionary position.

- **Elevate.** After union, the woman should lie on her back with her knees elevated to her chest for at least twenty minutes. Use a pillow or two to elevate her hips. (The very adept yogini is able to stand on her head after intercourse, but unless you're an expert at yoga, I wouldn't recommend trying it.)

What is most important is that you're making love at the right time. If the woman is not ovulating, the odds of fertilization plummet. To find out how to monitor your ovulation cycle, turn to "Fertility Awareness" on page 218.

NATURAL THERAPIES FOR NURTURING FERTILITY

Natural therapies for nurturing fertility focus on supporting overall health, strengthening the reproductive system, normalizing hormone production, dissolving blockages, clearing heat and congestion, encouraging libido, and nourishing the liver and kidneys.

Diet

I am always delighted to see a couple hoping to conceive that wants first to build their own bodies with good nutrition. Nutrition is the foremost contributor to a healthy baby, as well as a powerful factor in fertility.

The foods that support fertility also support overall good health and vigorous libido. A diet that focuses on the "sex tonic" foods would work wonders for supporting fertility. See Chapter 5 for details.

FERTILITY SHAKE

This is a super shake for a couple trying to conceive to share.
It boosts energy and is rich in protein, zinc, and vitamin E.

1 ½ cups fresh raw almond milk

1 ripe banana

2 tablespoons raw pumpkin seeds

1 tablespoon raw honey

1 tablespoon raw tahini

Combine all the ingredients in a blender and process. Share the mixture with your beloved, first making a toast to each other and to new life.

Nutritional Therapy

Although real food should be the main source of nutrients, various supplements may be of service in supporting fertility.

Arginine. This amino acid enhances blood flow to the genitals and is essential for the production of sperm; it promotes normal sperm count and motility. Arginine may aggravate existing herpes conditions and should be used only after other nutritional approaches have been tried. Take 500–2,000 mg daily.

Beta-carotene. The precursor to vitamin A, beta-carotene supports the production of estrogens and androgens. A beta-carotene deficiency can be a factor in low sperm production. Take 15,000 IU daily.

Carnitine. This amino acid can help improve sperm motility and a man's endurance. Take 1,000–2,000 mg daily.

Chlorophyll. Chlorophyll, the "green blood of plants," helps detoxify the liver, build the blood, and regulate the menses. It is available at health food stores in capsule form or as a liquid. Use as directed on the package label. And remember that raw, dark green, leafy vegetables are a great source of chlorophyll in all-natural packaging. Eat at least one serving a day, and drink a fresh green vegetable juice several times a week.

Vitamin B complex. The B vitamins can raise progesterone levels, relieve erectile dysfunction, and remedy estrogen-related biochemical problems. Folic acid, in particular, helps prevent some types of birth defects. Vitamin B_{12} may elevate sperm count and help correct anemia. Look for a 50–100 mg B-complex supplement that contains about 300 mcg of vitamin B_{12}.

Vitamin C. Vitamin C helps prevent sperm from clumping together and can increase sperm count. It also helps protect sperm against free-radical damage. Excessive amounts of vitamin C have been known to bring on menses, so avoid exceeding the recommended dosage during pregnancy. Take 3,000 mg daily.

Vitamin E. Tocopherol, the scientific name for vitamin E, comes from the Greek *tokos* and *phero,* meaning "to bear offspring." A vitamin E deficiency can cause infertility in both men and women and may be a factor in the tendency to miscarry in women. According to various studies, vitamin E enhances sperm's ability to penetrate an egg; a deficiency can contribute to sluggish sperm. This antioxidant vitamin is deficient in many Western diets. Selenium improves the activity of vitamin E and is often combined with it in supplement formulas. Take 400–600 IU of vitamin E daily, in combination with 50–200 mcg of selenium.

Zinc. Zinc is a component of sperm, seminal fluid, and vaginal mucus. It is essential for the growth and maturation of the gonads and can help increase the number and motility of sperm. Men with azoospermia (absence of living sperm) and oligospermia (low sperm count) have benefited from supplementation with zinc. Zinc helps protect the prostate gland and is needed for testosterone production. Take 50 mg of chelated zinc daily.

> Once you are pregnant and rejoicing for sure, you should begin taking a good natural prenatal vitamin. And actually, prenatal vitamins often contain all the nutrients that are helpful in the pre-pregnancy state, too, so you might consider taking them before you try to conceive.

Herbal Therapy

The herbs generally recommended for boosting fertility are among the most potent activators of whole-body health. Once you choose and undertake an herbal regimen, you'll find that both your energy and health improve.

> **Herbal Dosages**
> Unless stated otherwise, the therapeutic adult dosage for a recommended herb is:
>
> - 1 cup of tea three times daily;
> - 1 or 2 capsules three times daily; or
> - 1 dropperful of tincture three times daily.
>
> If you become pregnant, discontinue using herbs, except under the guidance of your health care provider.

Alfalfa (*Medicago sativa*). The herb is one of the most nutrient-rich herbs on Earth. It is a nutritive, phytoestrogenic, and tonic.

Alisma (*Alisma orientale*). The rhizome is a kidney tonic and benefits libido and fertility for both sexes.

Angelica (*Angelica archangelica, A. atropurpurea*). The root helps regulate the menstrual cycle. It is usually taken from the time of ovulation to the time of menses. It is a tonic and a uterine stimulant. Avoid during pregnancy and in cases of heavy bleeding or diabetes. In rare cases, the root causes photosensitivity.

Ashwagandha (*Withania somnifera*). The root helps increase sperm count and is an excellent reproductive tonic for men. It is an adaptogen, aphrodisiac, hormonal regulator, nutritive, rejuvenative, and uterine sedative.

Asparagus (*Asparagus officinalis, A. cochinchinensis*). The root is an ovarian tonic that supports estrogen activity. It is also an aphrodisiac, cardiotonic, demulcent, galactagogue, nutritive, rejuvenative, and kidney tonic.

Astragalus (*Astragalus membranaceus*). The root helps increase sperm motility and count. It is an adaptogen, adrenal tonic, blood tonic, and chi tonic.

Damiana (*Turnera aphrodisiaca, T. diffusa*). The leaf improves sexual vitality by allowing nerve messages to spread more expansively through the body. It is an aphrodisiac and yang tonic. Avoid in cases of high blood pressure, urinary tract infections, kidney disease, or liver disease. Damiana is not recommended for use by pregnant women or nursing mothers, so discontinue when you know you are pregnant.

Dandelion (*Taraxacum officinale*). The root helps decongest the liver, aiding the breakdown of hormones.

Dong quai (*Angelica sinensis*). The root helps normalize menses. As a blood tonic, it builds the blood and improves circulation in the pelvic region. It is also a uterine tonic and a yin tonic. Avoid during pregnancy, except under the guidance of your health care provider. Do not use in cases of diarrhea, heavy menstrual flow, poor digestion, or bloating. Do not use in conjunction with blood-thinning medications such as ibuprofen.

False unicorn (*Chamaelirium luteum*). The root is an alkaline uterine, ovarian tonic, and reproductive tonic. As one of my teachers once said, "It's the next best thing to sperm for getting you pregnant." The bitter taste of this herb can cause vomiting. Excessive amounts may cause kidney and stomach irritation, blurred vision, and hot flashes. Do not use without employing birth control during sex unless pregnancy is desired. Discontinue use during pregnancy. False unicorn is endangered in the wild; do not use wildcrafted supplies.

Fenugreek (*Trigonella foenum-graecum*). The seed tonifies the uterus and the kidneys. It is an aphrodisiac, rejuvenative, restorative, and yang tonic. Avoid during pregnancy. If you have diabetes, consult with your health care provider before use.

Ginkgo (*Ginkgo biloba*). The leaf has long been used to increase sperm count. It is an antioxidant, cerebral tonic, circulatory stimulant, kidney tonic, and rejuvenative.

Ginseng, Chinese (*Panax ginseng*). The root nourishes the entire being. It is often recommended as a treatment for erectile dysfunction and low sperm count. It is an adaptogen, aphrodisiac, chi tonic, rejuvenative, restorative, and tonic. Avoid in cases of excess heat, such as inflammation, fever, and high blood pressure. Since ginseng can be energizing, avoid taking it within four hours of bedtime. Avoid once pregnancy is confirmed.

Ho shou wu (*Polygonum multiflorum*). The root is used to increase sperm count in men and fertility in women. It is an aphrodisiac, chi tonic, liver tonic, rejuvenative, and yin tonic.

Licorice (*Glycyrrhiza glabra, U. uralensis*). The root helps normalize the ovulation cycle. It contains phytosterols, the raw material for hormone production. It is an adrenal tonic, chi tonic, nutritive, and rejuvenative. Avoid once pregnancy is confirmed and in cases of edema, high blood pressure, or diabetes. Do not use in combination with digoxin drugs. Excessive use can cause sodium retention and potassium depletion.

Nettle (*Urtica dioica, U. urens*). The leaf strengthens the kidneys and the adrenals. It is rich in both minerals and chlorophyll. It is a thyroid tonic and a cholagogue. This is a great herb for use during pregnancy; talk with your health care provider about its benefits. Contact with the fresh plant will irritate the skin. Use only dried herb. Wear gloves when collecting.

Oat (*Avena sativa, A. fatua*). The herb and spikelets help relieve exhaustion and stress, nourish the nerves, and make tactile sensations more pleasurable. They are aphrodisiacs, endocrine tonics, nutritives, rejuvenatives, and uterine tonics.

Poria (*Poria cocos*). The fungus strengthens the kidneys. It is a chi tonic, restorative, and tonic.

Red clover (*Trifolium pratense*). The blossom is very alkaline and can help correct overly acidic vaginal conditions that prevent sperm from reaching the uterus. It is nutritive and phytoestrogenic.

Red raspberry (*Rubus idaeus*). The leaf helps regulate hormones. It is a kidney tonic, nutritive, prostate tonic, uterine tonic, and yin tonic. This is a great herb for use during pregnancy; talk with your health care provider about its benefits.

Rehmannia (*Rehmannia glutinosa*). The root strengthens the kidneys and liver. It is a blood tonic, rejuvenative, and yin tonic. Avoid in cases of loose stools, poor appetite, bloating, or a coated tongue.

Sarsaparilla (*Smilax* spp.). The root contains phytosterols, the raw material of hormone production. It helps cleanse toxins from the reproductive system, and it is often recommended in treatments for erectile dysfunction, infertility, and ovarian cysts. It is an aphrodisiac, rejuvenative, and tonic.

Saw palmetto (*Serenoa repens*). The berry relieves inflammation and blockage in the genitourinary tract. It helps increase sperm count and is often recommended in treatments for erectile dysfunction, infertility, premature ejaculation, and prostatitis. It is an aphrodisiac, nutritive, rejuvenative, and tonic.

Schizandra (*Schisandra chinensis*). The berry is a whole body tonic and is often recommended in treatments for sexual debility. It is also an adaptogen, aphrodisiac, kidney and liver tonic, rejuvenative, and restorative.

Siberian ginseng (*Eleutherococcus senticosus*). The root is an anti-stress tonic for men and women. It is an adaptogen, aphrodisiac, and chi tonic.

Vitex (*Vitex agnus-castus*). The berry helps normalize hormone production and stimulates ovulation. Vitex can be used the first trimester of pregnancy to maintain the corpus luteum in women with a history of miscarriage before the twelfth week.

Wild yam (*Dioscorea opposita, D. villosa*). The root helps clear congested chi. It is an aphrodisiac and nutritive. Avoid therapeutic doses once pregnancy is confirmed, except under the guidance of your health care provider. The *Dioscorea villosa* species is endangered in the wild; do not use wildcrafted supplies.

Chinese Patent Remedies

There are a number of patent formulas from traditional Chinese medicine that can be used to nurture fertility.

Jin Kui Shen Qi Wan (Goldenbook Tea Pills). Use to counteract low sexual vitality accompanied by lower back pain and cold extremities.

Nu Ke Ba Zhen Wan (Eight Precious Herbs). This chi and blood tonic works equally well for men and women. It is often recommended to regulate menses and to relieve fatigue.

Zhong Guo Shou Wu Zhi. Use this formula to nourish the liver, support the kidneys, and invigorate the blood.

There are many other Chinese patent formulas available for many specific conditions. Consult with a practitioner of Oriental medicine to find a formula best suited to your needs.

Homeopathic Remedies

When an inability to conceive is accompanied by the conditions described, use the suggested homeopathic remedy. The usual dosage is four pellets, or as many liquid drops as the package label recommends, taken under the tongue four times daily. Rather than swallowing the pellets whole, allow them to dissolve slowly.

Agnus Castus. The patient experiences general weakness, low sex drive, and vaginal discharge.

Aletris Farinosa. The uterus is weak.

Aurum Muriaticum Natronatum. The patient experiences ovarian swelling or has undescended testicles.

Baryta Carbonica. The patient experiences general weakness, accompanied by premature ejaculation and immature ovarian function. He or she might also suffer from low hormonal output and lymphatic blockage.

Borax. Sexual desire and vitality are diminished.

Chininum Sulphuricum. Sexual desire is diminished and the patient is not able to produce sperm.

Conium. If the patient is a woman, the breasts feel hard and tender. If the patient is a man, he suffers from erectile dysfunction and is not able to produce sperm.

Ferrum Metallicum. The patient experiences low sex drive, amenorrhea, and pain or decreased sensitivity during intercourse.

Graphites. The patient has an aversion to sex and a history of sexual abuse. If the patient is male, he is unable to ejaculate.

Iodum. The patient feels pain and tenderness in the right ovary or the testicles.

Kali Bromatum. There is atrophy in the ovaries.

Lycopodium. If the patient is male, he experiences impotence or premature ejaculation. If the patient is female, the right ovary was previously inflamed.

Nux Vomica. The patient has a history of painful, irregular periods. She experiences leukorrhea, constipation, and irritability.

Phosphoricum Acidum. Fertility is diminished after an extended illness. If the patient is male, he experiences impotence, weak testicular function, and weak erections.

Phosphorus. The patient feels no desire for sex and tends to overuse salt.

Pituitrinum. The patient experiences vertigo, an inability to concentrate, and feelings of confusion.

Platina. The genital region is extremely sensitive. The left ovary may be tender. The patient is often prideful. He or she has a high sex drive but is unable to conceive.

Sabal Serrulata. The genitals are atrophied.

Sabina. The patient experiences recurrent miscarriage at eleven weeks.

Sepia. In men, sex drive is diminished. Intercourse is painful, and there is yellowish leukorrhea. The patient experiences abdominal pain, constipation, painful intercourse, and irregular menses.

Silicea. The uterus and fallopian tubes are weak and the patient lacks physical stamina.

Flower Essences

Flower essences to improve fertility include the following. The usual dosage is 7 drops under the tongue or taken with a glass of water three or four times daily.

Bells of Ireland. This flower essences encourages fertility in men and women.

Blackberry. Blackberry can counteract barrenness in women; it stimulates body rhythms.

Fig. Couples will find that Fig flower essence helps them develop trust.

Jasmine. This essences has a moderate effect on male fertility by stimulating sperm production.

Mallow. Mallow improves virility.

Mugwort. Mugwort is recommended as a treatment for male infertility.

Pomegranate. This essences can help women develop a sense of nurturing and can increase fertility.

Squash. Squash improves hormonal balance and helps rejuvenate sexual organs.

Watermelon. Watermelon encourages fertility in women and potency in men.

Aromatherapy

Essential oils that can be used to nurture fertility in massage, bathing, and inhalations include angelica, anise, basil, clary sage, cumin, fennel, geranium, jasmine, lemon balm, neroli, and rose. See Chapter 7 for more information on these oils and their applications. Avoid these essential oils once you are pregnant.

Reflexology

To stimulate fertility, try rubbing the kidney point (see illustration below) in a circular motion for three minutes a day. This reflexology point is located at the center of the ball of the foot. Also work on the area of the Achilles heel, which correlates to the reproductive organs.

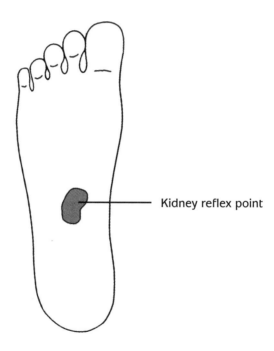

Kidney reflex point

22

Sexually Transmitted Diseases

exually transmitted diseases are the number one scourge of humankind. They have most likely been around since humans first started having sex—that is, as long as we have been in existence. They should not be taken lightly. They must be guarded against (see Chapter 17), watched for, and treated appropriately.

In the United States alone, there are more than twelve million new cases of sexually transmitted diseases (STDs) diagnosed every year. They range from crabs, a type of pubic lice that causes no more harm than a terrible itchiness, to chlamydia, which can cause serious reproductive dysfunctions, to AIDS, which can be fatal. Some STDs can be treated effectively with natural therapies, but others require the strength and aggressiveness of allopathic medicine. When allopathic medicine is used, natural therapies can serve as a complement, helping the body rebound from the effects of the treatment and supporting overall good health.

You cannot tell from outward appearance whether a potential lover is likely to have an STD. STDs occur in persons of both genders, all ethnicities, all sexual orientations, and all social classes. Even those seemingly clean-cut, carefully groomed, vibrantly healthy heartthrobs decked out in the latest chic clothing may be carriers of disease. You never know, and for that reason, it's important to ask a potential new lover whether he or she has been tested for STDs. You, too, must be tested on a regular basis for as long as you are engaging in sexual activity with multiple partners.

If you have an STD, it takes courage to talk to a potential sexual partner about it. However, it's important that you do. Keeping silent about an STD can lead to a situation in which your partner unknowingly puts himself or herself at risk of contracting the disease. If you're not responsible about discussing an STD, you may be responsible for giving it to a lover.

Having an STD does not equate to the end of your sex life; it does mean that you and your partner will have to take extra precautions to avoid sharing the disease. Tell your partner how you contracted the disease, how you felt, and how you are now dealing with it. Offer support literature (available from Planned Parenthood Federation of America and the STD and AIDS Hotline; see Resources), and ask for understanding.

Transmission of an STD is usually dependent on skin contact or the exchange of bodily fluids. Some STDs are borne only in the blood; others can be transmitted through mucus and saliva in addition to blood. Some, like crabs, can get around on their own, though these organisms generally cannot travel more than a few inches. It's important to know how the different types of STDs can be transmitted. While you need to be careful not to put yourself at risk, you don't want to wear a Level 4 biohazard suit, so to speak, if you're going to come in contact with an infected person. That sort of paranoia shows ignorance, and it makes the infected person feel like a social pariah, which doesn't do much to help him or her adjust to new parameters for sexual activity.

As the old saying goes, the path to wisdom is knowledge. I hope this chapter will start you off in the right direction.

> "*STD* can stand for 'savor the disease,' as catching one is a major wake-up call. The soul's messages through STDs is to invite you to investigate sexuality—what it truly means for you. 'Savor the disease' means to embrace it as an opportunity to know yourself more deeply by honoring the message. STDs are a souvenir of love—rather than trying to 'get over it,' go 'through it.'"
>
> —PERSONAL COMMUNICATION WITH JEANNINE PARVATI BAKER, AUTHOR OF *HYGIEIA: A WOMAN'S HERBAL, CONSCIOUS CONCEPTION,* AND *PRENATAL YOGA AND NATURAL CHILDBIRTH.*

Herbal Dosages

You'll find many recommendations for herbal therapy in this chapter. Unless stated otherwise, the therapeutic adult dosage for a recommended herb is:

- 1 cup of tea three times daily;
- 1 or 2 capsules three times daily; or
- 1 dropperful of tincture three times daily.

AIDS

Acquired immune deficiency syndrome (AIDS) is caused by a virus known as HIV, which stands for *h*uman *i*mmunodeficiency *v*irus. The virus destroys white blood cells, the warriors of the body's immune system, and makes the body susceptible to disease. Infection with the HIV virus does not equate to having AIDS. Most people experience at least three years of symptom-free living after being infected with the virus.

AIDS itself doesn't kill; instead, it compromises the body's immune system, allowing serious illness, as well as what should be innocuous illness, to take hold. Common killers for AIDS-infected persons include candidiasis, pneumonia, and a type of skin cancer called Kaposi's sarcoma.

Transmission

The virus is spread through blood, semen, vaginal fluids, and mother's milk. It is not an airborne virus, nor can it be spread through casual contact. Contrary to common opinion, AIDS is not a disease of homosexuals or drug users. In fact, children and straight women are among the fastest growing groups in the population of people infected with HIV.

Treatment

AIDS is still a relative medical mystery. There is no vaccine against the virus; there is no guaranteed method of preventing HIV infection from becoming AIDS; there is no known cure. We have learned how the disease is spread, but we haven't been able to stop its spread across North America and the global community. We have discovered formulations of various chemical cocktails that prolong the lives of those infected with the virus, but we haven't learned how to cure them.

What we do know is that eating and living right contributes to better health and longevity for those with HIV. There have been cases of HIV-positive people becoming HIV-negative (although many still carry the inactive virus) by following a raw foods or macrobiotic diet. Others have been able to maintain health by using herbal and vitamin therapies.

Following are what I have found, through my own experience and that of my peers in the herbalist community, to be among the most effective herbs and supplements for supporting the immune system of a person infected with HIV. They are best used under the supervision of a health care provider.

Nutritional Therapy

A person with AIDS must take great care to nurture the body with good nutrition. Avoid refined sugar, which can contribute to suppressed immune system activity, as well as caffeine and alcohol, which can deplete the body of nutrients, especially calcium and B vitamins. Cooked fats can interfere with the efficiency of the immune system and should also be avoided.

Focus on including the following foods, nutrients, and supplements in the diet.

Antioxidants. Antioxidants can strengthen mucous membranes and help the body resist infections. Antioxidants are best absorbed through natural sources of the nutrients beta-carotene, vitamin C, vitamin E, selenium, and superoxide dismutase. Good sources of each are listed in Chapter 5.

Chlorophyll. Chlorophyll builds the blood, speeds up the healing of wounds, and supports immune system health. Easy-to-digest natural sources include green juices, such as wheat grass, barley grass, and kamut grass.

Coenzyme Q_{10}. Coenzyme Q_{10} is another excellent nutrient for maintaining health with HIV infection. It facilitates the production of energy at a cellular level. Take 40 mg daily. Also consider incorporating into your diet natural sources of coenzyme Q_{10}, including broccoli, spinach, and whole grains.

Protein. Protein is necessary for the production of white blood cells. Natural sources that are easy to digest include soaked nuts and seeds and avocados.

Sea vegetables. Seaweeds such as kelp, dulse, hiziki, and nori provide a wide range of minerals that nourish the kidneys, bones, and teeth. They contain compounds that bind with toxins and carry them from the body. They also exhibit antibiotic, antiviral, and antifungal properties.

Herbal Therapy

Herbal therapy for treating HIV focuses mainly on supporting the immune system, improving the body's ability to absorb nutrients from food, and strengthening the lungs, liver, and kidneys. Persons with AIDS exhibit varying symptoms and will benefit most from herbal therapy by working with a trained herbalist to tailor treatment to their needs.

Astragalus (*Astragalus membranaceus*). The root stimulates immune system activity and diminishes the production of white blood cells in bone marrow. It also improves the body's digestion and assimilation of nutrients. It is an adaptogen, antiviral, blood tonic, chi tonic, immune tonic, and lung tonic.

Atractylodes (*Atractylodes lancea, A. macrocephala*). The rhizome strengthens the body's digestive system. It also increases white blood cell counts and immunoglobulin activity, both of which are essential to immune system function. It is a chi tonic, immunostimulant, and restorative.

Bitter melon (*Momordica charantia*). The fruit, also known as bitter melon, has strong antiviral properties. It also can improve mood and energy. It is an antitussive and lymphatic cleanser.

Cleavers (*Galium aparine*). The herb improves lymphatic function and clears heat. It is an alterative.

Codonopsis (*Codonopsis pilosula*). The root boosts energy levels and increases T-cell production in the immune system. It is an adaptogen, chi tonic, nutritive, and yin tonic.

Epimedium (*Epimedium aceranthus, E. grandiflorum*). The leaf is considered to be a restorative and is often recommended in treatments for respiratory infection. It is also an antiviral and a kidney tonic. Large doses may cause vertigo, vomiting, dry mouth, and nosebleed. Do not use for longer than one month, except under the guidance of your health care provider. Men who have overactive sex drives and wet dreams should avoid epimedium.

Garlic (*Allium sativum*). Compounds in the bulb help the body resist a wide range of pathogens and improve lung function. Garlic is an alterative, antioxidant, antiseptic, and immunostimulant. Some people are allergic to garlic. Excessive use can cause emotional irritability and irritation of the stomach and kidneys. Avoid therapeutic doses during pregnancy, and avoid during the first three months of nursing, as it can cause breast milk to become unpalatable for infants. Avoid use the week before having surgery.

Ginseng, Chinese (*Panax ginseng*). The root strengthens the body against stress and can speed recovery time during convalescence. It also improves physical and mental energy. It is an adaptogen, chi tonic, digestive tonic, immunostimulant, and restorative. Avoid in cases of excess heat, such as inflammation, fever, and high blood pressure. Since ginseng can be energizing, avoid taking it within four hours of bedtime. Avoid during pregnancy.

Ho shou wu (*Polygonum multiflorum*). The root is considered a tonic for the blood and the kidneys. It is an anti-inflammatory, antiseptic, and chi tonic. Avoid in cases of diarrhea.

Isatis (*Isatis tinctoria*). The root is antiviral and can inhibit secondary infection.

Licorice (*Glycyrrhiza glabra, G. uralensis*). The root boosts natural immunity and helps prevent secondary infection. It is an adrenal tonic, anti-inflammatory, antiviral, chi tonic, and nutritive. Avoid during pregnancy and in cases of edema, high blood pressure, or diabetes. Do not use in combination with digoxin drugs. Excessive use can cause sodium retention and potassium depletion.

Ligustrum (*Ligustrum lucidum*). The fruit helps restore normal immune function and increases the production of red and white blood cells. It is an alterative, kidney tonic, rejuvenative, and yin tonic.

Lomatium (*Lomatium dissectum*). The root protects the body against pathogens that cause respiratory infection. It is an anti-inflammatory, antiviral, and immunostimulant. In rare cases, it can cause skin reactions. This herb is endangered in the wild; do not use wildcrafted products.

Milk thistle (*Silybum marianum*). The seed helps protect the liver from free radicals while the body is clearing itself of drugs and chemicals. It is an antioxidant and digestive tonic.

Ophiopogon (*Ophiopogon japonicus*). The root lubricates the lungs and intestines. It is an antibiotic, antitussive, aphrodisiac, demulcent, febrifuge, nutritive, restorative, sedative, and yin tonic. Avoid in cases of respiratory congestion or diarrhea.

Pokeweed (*Phytolacca americana*). The root of the herb is a strong lymphatic cleanser. It also stimulates macrophage activity in the immune system. It is alterative, antifungal, anti-inflammatory, antirheumatic, antitumor, emetic, an immunostimulant, a lymphatic decongestant, and spermicidal. In large amounts, pokeweed root can be toxic. Take only 2 or 3 drops of the tincture daily; after one week, increase the dosage to 5 drops (2 drops in the morning, 3 drops at night). Drink copious amounts of water while you are taking pokeweed root. Consult with your health care provider before use.

Redroot (*Ceanothus americanus*). The root is a strong lymphatic cleanser. It can break up engorgements, cysts, and tumors. It is also antiviral.

Rehmannia (*Rehmannia glutinosa*). The root is a blood, liver, and kidney tonic as well as an alterative and rejuvenative. The raw root is used to quiet inflammation and heat. The cooked root is more of a building tonic, strengthening bones, marrow, and tendons. Avoid in cases of loose stools, poor appetite, bloating, or a coated tongue.

Reishi (*Ganoderma lucidum*). This mushroom promotes blood circulation, improves immune system function, and stimulates phagocytosis. It is an adaptogen, antidepressant, anti-inflammatory, antiseptic, antitussive, and rejuvenative. There have been reports of dry mouth, digestive distress, nosebleed, and bloody stools when reishi is used for extended periods of time (at least three to six months).

Saint John's wort (*Hypericum perforatum*). The herb has alterative, antiviral, antibacterial, antidepressant, and sedative properties. In rare cases, this herb causes photosensitivity. Do not combine Saint John's wort with monoamine oxidase (MAO) inhibitors (chemical antidepressants) or selective reuptake inhibitors, such as Prozac.

Schizandra (*Schisandra chinensis*). The berry is a kidney and liver tonic. It can stimulate immune system function and improve bone marrow production. It also has adaptogen and rejuvenative properties.

Shiitake (*Lentinus edodes*). The mushroom is rich in immunostimulating polysaccharides and can help the user resist infection. It is antiviral and rejuvenative.

Siberian ginseng (*Eleutherococcus senticosus*). The root is a strong adaptogen and helps the body acclimate to physical and emotional stress. It tonifies the lymph system and adrenals and increases macrophage activity in the immune system. It is also a chi tonic.

Trichosanthes (*Tricosanthes kirilowii*). The fruit clears phlegm and stimulates interferon production in the immune system. It is an antitussive, antiviral, and febrifuge. Avoid during pregnancy.

Turmeric (*Curcuma longa, C. aromatica*). The root inhibits the replication of viral proteins and the overgrowth of yeast. It is an alterative, antifungal, and cholagogue.

Usnea (*Usnea barbata*). The lichen is often recommended in treatments for streptococcal infection and pneumonia. It is an antifungal, antiseptic, and immunostimulant.

Acidophilus

Because AIDS compromises the immune system, a person with AIDS is at great risk of yeast overgrowth. Acidophilus supplements colonize the body with friendly bacteria that help combat unfriendly microorganisms, preventing yeast, fungal, and other pathogenic proliferations. Acidophilus can also help improve digestion, immune system strength, and bowel function. Take one or two capsules three times daily, or as recommended on the package label.

CHLAMYDIA AND NONGONOCOCCAL URETHRITIS

Chlamydia is an infection caused by the parasitic bacterium *Chlamydia tra-*

chomatis; in men, a chlamydial infection causes nongonococcal urethritis (infection of the urethra). Chlamydial infection is currently the most common sexually transmitted disease in the United States.

Most infected women and about half of infected men are asymptomatic; that is, they don't exhibit any symptoms of chlamydial infection. For this reason, the disease often goes undetected—and untreated—for years.

When symptoms do make an appearance, they manifest in men as a yellowish or whitish penile discharge, tenderness in the genitals, a need to urinate frequently, burning or painful urination, and redness at the tip of the penis. Women may notice a need to urinate frequently, yellow or greenish vaginal discharge, cramping, and occasional bleeding after intercourse. These symptoms are similar to those of gonorrhea, and chlamydia is often misdiagnosed as gonorrhea. Unfortunately, the treatment for gonorrhea does not have any effect on the *Chlamydia* bacteria.

A chlamydial infection can have very serious consequences. In women, it can cause inflammation of the cervix (cervicitis) and pelvic inflammatory disease, which can lead to fertility dysfunctions. Pregnant women with chlamydia have an increased risk of miscarriage; their babies often suffer from a chlamydial eye infection, which can lead to blindness, as well as ear, lung, and genital infections. In men, it can cause inflammation of the epididymis (epididymitis), which also can lead to fertility dysfunctions.

Given that most cases of chlamydial infection do not exhibit symptoms, it is wise to get tested for the disease whenever you've engaged in at-risk behavior—unprotected sexual activity with a new partner or in a nonmonogamous relationship. Your gynecologist can perform the test.

Transmission

Chlamydia can be spread through sexual contact involving the genitals, anus, or mouth. Taking birth control pills, which can deplete friendly vaginal bacteria, cause vitamin and mineral deficiencies, and unbalance hormone levels, can make women more susceptible to the infection.

Treatment

Given the severity of the possible consequences, chlamydial infection demands aggressive treatment. The most effective treatment is antibiotics. If you are committed to natural therapies, try one of the herbs described below, then get retested. If the infection has not disappeared, I strongly recommend that you begin a course of antibiotics. Otherwise, you risk compromising your fertility.

Herbal Therapy

Three herbs have particularly potent antibiotic activity against the *Chlamydia* bacteria.

Echinacea (*Echinacea purpurea, E. angustifolia*). The root has a power-fully stimulating effect on the immune system, activating T cells, interferons, and macrophages. It is also an alterative, antifungal, and antiseptic.

Goldenseal (*Hydrastis canadensis*). The root is active against a wide range of pathogens and is especially effective for relieving inflammation of the mucous membranes. It is an alterative and antibiotic. Goldenseal is very bitter, and most people find it easiest to ingest in capsule form. Avoid during preg-nancy. This herb is endangered in the wild; do not use wildcrafted products.

Usnea (*Usnea barbata*). Like goldenseal root, usnea lichen is active against a wide range of pathogens. It is an antibiotic, antifungal, and immunostimulant.

Probiotics

When you must take antibiotics, add to your diet fermented foods such as plain yogurt and unpasteurized sauerkraut, apple cider vinegar, miso, and tamari. These foods support and replenish the friendly bacteria in the body.

After a course of antibiotic therapy, begin a course of acidophilus therapy to restore the friendly bacteria that are necessary for digestion, elimination, and healthy reproductive organs. Take one or two capsules three times daily for three to four months.

CRABS

Crabs, also known as pubic lice, are creepy-crawly creatures (*Pthirus pubis*) that live in pubic hair and feed on human blood. They multiply rapidly by lay-ing eggs (nits) at the roots of the pubic hair. They cause intense itching and irritation in the pubic area. They are not a serious health risk, but they can be an indicator that your sexual activity has put you at risk of contracting STDs.

Crabs are difficult to see; you'll most likely notice the itching first. Adult lice appear as very small black or rust-colored flecks; the nits look like tiny, shiny ovals clinging to the base of the hairs. A magnifying glass can help you identify what you're looking at.

Transmission

Crabs are usually spread from intimate contact. Intercourse can allow crabs to wander from one pubis to another; oral sex can allow them to infest the scalp, eyebrows, and chest hair. Like head lice, they can also infest clothing and bedsheets; sleeping in a lice-infested bed puts you at risk of waking up with crabs.

Treatment

Natural therapies can be as effective as allopathic medicine for ridding the body of these parasites. The therapies focus on killing the lice, getting rid of nits, and making the body an inhospitable environment for lice. Note that the telltale itching can persist for several days, even after lice are dead.

The Shampoo Treatment

Find a lice-treatment shampoo, which is formulated to kill crabs and other types of lice, at your local herb shop or health food store. (If you can't find the right shampoo at these outlets, you can find a medicated version at your local pharmacy.) Follow the instructions on the product label. After the shampoo treatment, work through your pubic hair with a fine-toothed comb to remove dead crabs and eggs. Then disinfect the combs by placing them in boiling water for ten minutes.

The lice shampoo will kill lice but not nits. Repeat the treatment in seven to ten days to get rid of any lice that may have hatched from eggs that survived the washing and combing.

Wash all clothing, bedding, and towels in hot water followed by a full hot cycle in a dryer. Dry clean all clothes and bedding that can't be washed, or pack them away in a plastic trash bag for two weeks; without access to human blood, the lice will starve and die. Vacuum all furniture. Scrub the house from top to bottom. Practice obsessive hygiene!

Diet

Garlic deters not only vampires but crabs, as well. Take two 500 mg garlic capsules three times daily for a month. Seaweed can have a similar effect on your blood, imbuing it with a salty flavor that seems to repel crabs.

Crabs, like other parasites, seem to prey on weakness. A healthy liver and healthy blood are key to making your body inhospitable to critters looking for an easy ride. Consume plenty of liver-cleansing foods such as carrots, beets, burdock, dandelion greens, and barley, and drink teas made from blood-purifying plants, such as cleavers herb, dandelion root, echinacea root, and red clover blossoms.

Salt Rub

Dampen your pubic hair, then apply a handful of salt mixed with just enough water that it will stick. Leave on for thirty minutes. Then shower.

Aromatherapy Heat Treatment

Heat tends to discourage crabs from sticking around; they'll leave a person overheated by fever or exercise. To replicate that effect, spend some time in a sauna. Crabs won't survive 120 degrees Fahrenheit for more than five minutes. After this heat treatment, apply a few drops of undiluted tea tree or lavender essential oil to the infested areas of the skin. (Both tea tree and lavender have a potent antiparasitic effect.)

Avoid this treatment if you are pregnant.

Homeopathic Staphysagria

The homeopathic remedy *Staphysagria* deters both crabs and head lice. Take four pellets, or as many liquid drops as the package label recommends, under the tongue four times daily for ten days. Take ten days off, then repeat the treatment for ten more days.

Crab Apple

The flower essence Crab Apple can help you recover emotionally from the lice infestation. It restores feelings of beauty in a person who feels physically and mentally unclean. Take 7 drops under the tongue or with a glass of water three or four times daily.

GENITAL WARTS

Warts are caused by human papillomavirus (HPV), a group of over seventy viruses. The viruses are contagious, and the warts can be spread via sexual contact. On women, the warts appear on the vulva, on the labia, inside the vagina, and on the cervix. On men, they appear on the shaft of the penis, under the foreskin, and on the scrotum. They also can appear on the anus and in the mouth and throat.

External genital warts manifest as small, hard bumps; they are similar in appearance to regular warts. If left untreated, they grow, taking on a cauliflower-like appearance. Warts on the cervix are more properly called lesions. Cervical lesions have been linked to cervical cancer; likewise, rectal warts have been linked to rectal cancer. Cervical lesions are not visible to the naked eye and are usually discovered by Pap smear.

External warts may be too small to see with the untrained eye. They are generally painless, but if irritated, they can burn or itch. If you suspect that you have warts, try soaking the genitals in a 5 to 10 percent vinegar solution. After about six minutes, any warts will turn white, making them easily visible.

Genital warts take from one to nine months after exposure to appear.

They may go away on their own or grow aggressively. They can be especially aggressive during pregnancy.

Transmission

Genital warts can be contracted through oral, vaginal, or anal contact with an infected person. Condoms can offer some protection against the spread of the disease. People with a suppressed immune system—such as HIV-infected persons—are at a higher risk for contracting the infection. Taking birth control pills, which can deplete friendly vaginal bacteria, cause vitamin and mineral deficiencies, and unbalance hormone levels, can make women more susceptible to the infection.

Treatment

There is no known cure for HPV. Upon diagnosis, it is important to remove existing warts to prevent the growth and transmission of the disease. Try the natural therapies described below. If the natural therapies do not cause the warts to disappear, then the more aggressive allopathic treatment is necessary. In allopathic medicine, genital warts are usually painted with a caustic chemical that burns them away. The most common wart-removing chemical treatment is podophyllin, which is made from the root of mayapple (*Podophyllum peltatum*). Podophyllin can irritate the skin; you can protect the surrounding tissue by applying a calendula-comfrey salve. (You can often find calendula-comfrey salve in natural food stores and herb shops, or you can make your own following Cascade Anderson Geller's instructions on page 111.) Your gynecologist or urologist may also recommend cryotherapy (freezing them off), laser surgery, or surgical excision.

Removing the warts will not eliminate the infection. New warts may appear at some point in the future, and they, too, will have to be removed. The following natural therapies can deter the growth and occurrence of warts.

Topical Applications

Topical applications for removing genital warts include the following:

- Papaya sap
- Milky white sap from dandelion stems
- Garlic-infused oil
- Celandine juice
- Fresh elderberry juice

- Juice from the inner side of the pods of fresh broad beans

- Lemon juice

- Thuja (cedar leaf) essential oil

Be persistent. Apply these compounds three times daily for as long as it takes.

Herbal Therapy

Herbal therapy for genital warts focuses on attacking the virus, stimulating the immune system, strengthening the liver, and reducing inflammation. Many of the herbs are also thought to have antitumor properties, which can help prevent the warts from progressing to cancerous growths.

Burdock (*Arctium lappa*). The root is an alterative, antiseptic, antifungal, anti-inflammatory, and antitumor.

Cleavers (*Galium aparine*). The herb is an alterative, anti-inflammatory, antitumor, and lymphatic cleanser.

Dandelion (*Taraxacum officinale*). The root is an antifungal and cholagogue.

Echinacea (*Echinacea purpurea, E. angustifolia*). The root strengthens the immune system. It is an alterative, antiseptic, antifungal, anti-inflammatory, antitumor, and antiviral.

Nettle (*Urtica dioica, U. urens*). The herb is an alterative, cholagogue, and circulatory stimulant. Contact with the fresh plant will irritate the skin. Use only dried herb. Wear gloves when collecting.

Peppermint (*Mentha piperita*). The herb is an antiseptic, antiviral, and cholagogue.

Nutritional Therapy

Supplements that can be useful for eliminating warts and preventing them from returning include the following.

Antioxidants. Antioxidants support the body's immune system. They are best absorbed through natural sources of the nutrients beta-carotene, vitamin C, vitamin E, selenium, and superoxide dismutase. Good sources of each are listed in Chapter 5.

Lysine. The amino acid lysine can inhibit viral replication and seems to have a strong effect on HPV. Try taking 500 mg daily.

Homeopathic Remedies

When the development of genital warts matches one of the descriptions below, try the suggested homeopathic remedy. The usual dosage is four pellets, or as many liquid drops as the package label recommends, taken under the tongue four times daily. Rather than swallowing the pellets whole, allow them to dissolve slowly.

Calcarea Carbonica. The warts are smooth, soft, and round; they may be inflamed.

Calendula Officinalis. The warts occur in the vaginal membranes, outside the uterus.

Lycopodium. The warts are split and surrounded by an areola.

Natrum Muriaticum. The warts are old and cause a cutting pain.

Nitricum Acidum. The warts are jagged, large, and in the genitoanal area. They may ooze, emit a fetid odor, or bleed upon washing.

Phosphoricum Acidum. The warts are on the glans. They are indented and rugged.

Sabina. The warts are on the prepuce. They bleed easily and may produce feelings of numbness or a burning sensation.

Sepia. The warts are on the margin of the prepuce. They feel horny in the center and are accompanied by a burning pain and inflammation.

Staphysagria. The warts are figlike in appearance.

Sulfur. The warts are horny.

Thuja Occidentalis. This is the most common homeopathic remedy for genital warts. It is especially beneficial in cases where the warts are broad and conical, split easily, and appear in the genitoanal area and, in men, on the glans.

Essential Oil Treatments

A variety of essential oils with antimicrobial properties can be applied topically to warts to shrink or eliminate them. These oils include bergamot, cedar leaf, cinnamon, eucalyptus, lemon, niaouli, patchouli, tea tree, or a combination thereof. Combine these oils with an equal measure of olive oil and apply with a cotton swab to the wart. Take care to keep the solution on the wart; avoid painting the skin around the area as best you can.

Sitz Baths

Hot and cold sitz baths increase circulation to the pelvic region, thereby helping the immune system combat the warts. See Chapter 12 for instructions. Spend three minutes in the hot water and one minute in the cold water. Alternate, always commencing with hot and ending with cold.

GONORRHEA

Commonly known as "clap," gonorrhea is caused by the bacterium *Neisseria gonorrhoeae*. It is the second most common sexually transmitted disease in the United States.

It is not uncommon for a gonorrheal infection to exhibit no symptoms. When symptoms do manifest, they show up about a week after exposure in men and about two weeks after exposure in women. Symptoms in men include frequent and painful urination, lower abdominal pain, and a greenish or gray discharge from the penis. Women may also suffer from painful urination, as well as a greenish yellow discharge, inflammation of the cervix, and bleeding between menstrual periods.

If left untreated, gonorrhea can lead to chronic pain, tubal pregnancy, pelvic inflammatory disease, and damage to the testicles and the prostate. In rare cases, gonorrhea can spread to the heart, brain, and joints.

If you suspect that you have gonorrhea, visit your gynecologist or urologist for a complete examination.

Transmission

The bacteria cannot survive outside the body for more than a few seconds. It is transmitted via direct contact with an infected person during vaginal, anal, or oral sex.

Pregnant women can pass the disease to their newborns, where it can manifest as an acute eye inflammation known as gonococcal conjunctivitis, an ear infection, or a lung infection.

Treatment

Antibiotics are the standard treatment; different strains of the disease have become resistant to different antibiotics, so you may not find relief with the first prescription.

While you are taking antibiotics, add to your diet fermented foods such as plain yogurt and unpasteurized sauerkraut, apple cider vinegar, miso, and tamari. These foods support and replenish the friendly bacteria in the body.

After a course of antibiotic therapy, begin a course of acidophilus therapy to restore the friendly bacteria that are necessary for digestion, elimination, and healthy reproductive organs. Take one or two capsules three times daily for three to four months.

Gonorrhea is infamous for its high rate of recurrence, so follow-up visits are essential to be sure the infection has cleared.

HEPATITIS

Hepatitis is a virus that uses liver and immune cells as its hosts, destroying them in the process. There are many different strains, of which Hepatitis A, Hepatitis B, and Hepatitis C are most common.

Hepatitis A is most often transmitted through infected water, food, or shellfish. In very rare cases, it may be sexually transmitted. Its symptoms include jaundice, vomiting, diarrhea, and lethargy. Hepatitis A is a short-term illness; it usually resolves on its own and is considered dangerous only for infants, elders, and people with hepatitis C.

Hepatitis B can be transmitted through blood, sperm, vaginal secretions, and saliva. It can also be transmitted from mother to child in utero. Hepatitis B is usually a short-term illness that resolves on its own; only about 7 percent of infected persons become chronic carriers. Although it is rarely fatal, it is widespread; according to the World Health Organization, one to two million people die every year from complications caused by hepatitis B.

Hepatitis C is most often transmitted through blood. The infection can lie dormant for years before erupting; most infected persons do not know that they carry the virus. Symptoms include nausea, unexplained fatigue, dark urine, general malaise, short-term memory problems, depression, mood swings, liver pain, and sometimes jaundice. More than 50 percent of infected persons become chronic carriers. Hepatitis C causes a multitude of potentially serious liver problems and is fatal for about 5 percent of infected persons.

Treatment

Using natural therapies to treat hepatitis gives the body an opportunity to regenerate without overloading the weakened liver with compounds and toxins from synthetic drugs. The treatments focus on strengthening the liver, reducing inflammation, supporting the immune system, and controlling the virus.

Herbal Therapy

Herbs that can be used to control hepatitis include the following.

Bupleurum (*Bupleurum chinense, B. falcatum*). The root promotes blood circulation to the liver. It is an alterative, anti-inflammatory, antiviral, and hepatoprotective (liver-protecting) agent. Avoid in cases of fever, headache, or high blood pressure.

Burdock (*Arctium lappa*). The root improves the ability of the liver to remove toxins. It is alterative, anti-inflammatory, nutritive, and rejuvenative.

Dandelion (*Taraxacum officinale*). The root helps the liver purify blood. It is a cholagogue.

Fringe tree (*Chionanthus virginicus*). The bark reduces symptoms of liver toxicity, aids in digestion, and relieves pain and bloating. It is often recommended for people recovering from long-term illness, especially conditions originating in the liver. It clears heat and reduces inflammation. It is an alterative, cholagogue, and liver stimulant.

Licorice (*Glycyrrhiza glabra, G. uralensis*). The root is anti-inflammatory, antiviral, nutritive, and rejuvenative. Avoid during pregnancy and in cases of edema, high blood pressure, or diabetes. Do not use in combination with digoxin drugs. Excessive use can cause sodium retention and potassium depletion.

Milk thistle (*Silybum marianum*). The seed stimulates protein synthesis in the liver, helping it to rebuild. It is an antioxidant, a cholagogue, and a hepatoprotective agent.

Oregon grape (*Mahonia aquifolium*). The root has a broad range of antimicrobial activities and is often recommended in treatments for chronic liver infection. It contains the alkaloid berberine, which is a potent antiviral agent. It is also an alterative, cholagogue, and immunostimulant. Avoid during pregnancy, and do not exceed the recommended dosage.

Reishi (*Ganoderma lucidum*). The mushroom has a broad range of immunostimulating activities. It is also an adaptogen, anti-inflammatory, and rejuvenative. There have been reports of dry mouth, digestive distress, nosebleed, and bloody stools when reishi is used for extended periods of time (at least three to six months).

Schizandra (*Schisandra chinensis*). The berry is among the most potent hepatitis remedies. Studies have shown 76 percent of persons infected with hepatitis experience some relief from symptoms, without negative side effects, when treated with schizandra. It is an adaptogen, immunostimulant, and rejuvenative. The tincture and capsules tend to be more effective than the tea.

Turmeric (*Curcuma longa, C. aromatica*). The root helps protect the liver from chemical exposure. It is an alterative, antiseptic, anti-inflammatory, cholagogue, and vulnerary.

Yellow dock (*Rumex crispus*). The root improves liver function and aids in the elimination of contaminating agents. It is an alterative, antiseptic, blood tonic, and cholagogue.

Compresses and Poultices

A castor oil compress applied to the stomach on the area over the liver can be helpful. The mechanism that makes castor oil compresses beneficial has not yet been determined; however, but the theory is that when the oil is absorbed into the body, it stimulates prostaglandin activity, which helps regulate both the division of cells and the production of B and T cells, which are lymphocytes of the immune system. Just soak a flannel cloth in castor oil and apply over the liver area. Cover with a sheet of plastic and a hot water bottle.

Clay poultices can help draw toxins from the body. Use only dry, cosmetic-quality clay. In a glass bowl, mix together about ½ cup of clay powder with enough water to make a paste. Apply over the liver area. Leave on until it dries thoroughly, then rinse off.

A cabbage poultice is a traditional folk remedy for drawing out infection. Simply grate raw cabbage finely, then apply over the liver area. Remove the poultice when it begins to feel hot. (Compost the cabbage.)

Apply your poultice or compress of choice daily for at least ten consecutive days.

Acidophilus

Acidophilus supplements colonize the body with friendly bacteria that help combat unfriendly microorganisms, preventing yeast, fungus, and other pathogenic proliferations. Acidophilus can also help improve digestion, immune system strength, and bowel function. Take one or two capsules three times daily for three or four months.

Homeopathic Remedies

When the development of hepatitis matches one of the descriptions below, try the suggested homeopathic remedy. The usual dosage is four pellets, or as many liquid drops as the package label recommends, taken under the tongue four times daily. Rather than swallowing the pellets whole, allow them to dissolve slowly.

Byronia. The patient craves cold water and feels weak while sitting in bed. Symptoms are worse if the patient arises before noon.

Chelidonium Majus. The face, the sclera of the eyes, and the palms of the hands are yellowish. Symptoms improve after eating.

Chionanthus. The liver is enlarged and painful.

Cinchona Officinalis. The abdomen is bloated. Symptoms worsen from light touch and improve with strong touch and after passing gas.

Lycopodium. The patient is very flatulent. Symptoms feel worse first thing in the morning and when the right side is touched.

Mercurius. The patient exhibits profuse sweat and salivation. Symptoms worsen when the patient is lying on his or her right side.

Natrum Sulphuricum. The patient is noisily flatulent. Symptoms improve after bowel movements. Symptoms worsen when the patient is lying on his or her left side and in the morning.

Phosphorus. The patient is unable to lie on his or her right side, craves cold drinks, and fears death.

HERPES

Herpes is a relative of chicken pox, Epstein-Barr virus, mononucleosis, and shingles. There are more than five types of herpesviruses; yet only herpes simplex I and herpes simplex II are considered sexually transmitted diseases. Herpes simplex I, or oral herpes, occurs usually on or around the lips and nose. It's sometimes referred to as cold sores or fever blisters. Herpes simplex II, or genital herpes, occurs usually on the labia, vulva, vaginal membranes, cervix, prepuce, glans, shaft of the penis, anus, rectum, buttocks, and thighs. There is a growing lack of distinction between the symptoms of these two types of viruses, however, because oral-genital contact has allowed some crossover.

Many people infected with herpes do not know that they have it, because the disease is often asymptomatic, meaning it produces no symptoms. The virus is highly contagious; it is estimated that one-sixth to one-third of the population in the United States aged fifteen to seventy-five is infected with genital herpes.

When symptoms do occur, they manifest as blisters on and around the genitals. The blisters may be accompanied by itching, pain, and fever. The blisters then burst and become oozing ulcers or lesions. The lesions will eventually crust over and heal.

It usually takes from two to twenty-eight days after exposure to the virus for an initial outbreak to occur. Stage I, called the prodromal or early-warning stage, can produce a localized numbing, tingling, burning, or itching sensation. Some infected persons also experience flulike symptoms, including fatigue and swelling of the lymph nodes in the neck or groin area, which indicates that the body is working hard to deal with an infection. During stage II, a single blister or a cluster of blisters will appear. These blisters, also called vesicles, are small and grayish. Eventually they burst, leaving red, raw ulcerations. During stage III, the blisters may develop a yellowish crust before drying up and disappearing. The total attack may last anywhere from four days to a month.

After the symptoms of primary infection fade, the virus retreats to nerve cells deep within the body, where it lies dormant. When reactivated (see "Herpes Triggers," following in this section), it initiates a new outbreak of herpes lesions.

There are now sensitive and accurate blood tests available to diagnose herpes. To confirm a diagnosis of herpes topically, the blisters must be present. Your health care provider will use a cotton swab to collect serum from a lesion. The serum is examined for viral infection under a microscope. Other lesion-producing conditions that are sometimes confused with herpes include impetigo, fungal infections, syphilis, abrasions, boils, and some allergic reactions. The microscopic examination of the serum is necessary to distinguish one from the other.

Transmission

Herpes is most contagious during its active stages. The rate of transmission when no symptoms are present is less than 1 percent.

The virus can enter the body when an existing lesion comes in contact with the mucous membranes of the mouth or genitals. The transference may take place between an infected person and an uninfected person or between different sites on an infected person.

Direct contact is the most common means of transmission, but the herpesvirus can survive for brief periods of time outside the body. That means that towels, cigarettes, sex toys, eating utensils, and other items that may pick up fluid from an oozing herpes lesion can carry the disease.

To avoid transmitting the disease, practice safe sex using barrier methods. (See Chapter 17.) Do not engage in sexual contact during an outbreak of herpes lesions.

Wash your hands after touching the lesions and also first thing in the morning, in case you inadvertently touch them during the night. Wear cotton underwear and pajamas while sleeping to help prevent yourself from touching the lesions.

Never touch your eyes after touching a lesion. If the cornea becomes infected with the herpesvirus, scarring and blindness may result. If you wear contact lenses, wash your hands before placing them in your eyes.

Herpes and Pregnancy

If the virus is contracted during the first twenty weeks of pregnancy, there is an increased risk of abortion. If genital herpes lesions are present during the actual birth, the virus can be transmitted to the newborn; for one in four herpes-infected infants, the virus can have fatal complications. Depending on the location of the sores, doctors and midwives will recommend a cesarean section or will cover the lesions for vaginal delivery.

Fortunately, women seem to develop a resistance to herpes toward the end of a pregnancy; only 1 out of every 250 herpes-infected women has an active outbreak at the time of delivery. Interestingly, some babies born to mothers with herpes are endowed with an immunity to the disease.

Herpes Triggers

The first outbreak of herpes lesions is usually the worst. Most people find that outbreaks diminish in occurrence and severity over time. Most people also find that their bodies produce unique symptoms that signal an imminent herpes outbreak. These include tingling, burning, or tenderness in the area of the first outbreak.

New eruptions are most likely to occur when an infected person is experiencing physical, emotional, or immune system stress. These types of stress can be triggered by fatigue, illness, fever, overexposure to sun and wind, an imbalanced diet, poor thyroid function, liver congestion, having multiple sexual partners, or even wearing tight, chafing clothes.

Treatment

There is no cure for herpes. Those who have it must learn to live with it. Natural therapies can be of benefit in preventing new outbreaks and minimizing the severity and duration of outbreaks. They focus on promoting overall good health, strengthening the body's immune system, supporting the nervous system, and expediting the healing of an outbreak.

Diet

Proper diet is essential for minimizing the occurrence of herpes outbreaks. Of particular interest is the amino acid lysine, which has been shown to inhibit replication of the virus. Foods rich in lysine include:

- Beans (especially lima, mung, and soy)

- Cultured foods, such as cheese (preferably made from unhomogenized milk), kefir, nutritional yeast, sauerkraut, and yogurt

- Fish (especially flounder, halibut, salmon, shark, shrimp, and tuna)
- Poultry
- Quinoa and millet
- Red meat (but be sure that it comes from animals that were raised using organic methods and without hormone treatments)

The amino acid arginine has been shown to promote the activity of the herpesvirus. Arginine-rich foods to avoid include barley, chocolate, coconut, coffee, nuts, oats, peanuts, and wheat. If you do consume arginine-rich foods, balance their effect by also eating lysine-rich foods. Lysine tends to inhibit the body's absorption of arginine.

Be sure to consume plenty of immune-strengthening foods such as apples, carrots, garlic, green, leafy vegetables (kale, collards, mustard greens, and spinach), onions, and winter squashes. Sea vegetables such as kelp, dulse, wakame, and hiziki also offer excellent support for the immune system, and they improve thyroid function, as well. Minimize your intake of high-fat foods, especially those containing hydrogenated oils, which can make the immune system sluggish.

Herbs to include in the diet include basil, cilantro, coriander, and parsley. These green wonders are rich in antioxidants and have strong antimicrobial activity.

An alkaline diet will improve the quality of the blood and make you less susceptible to a herpes outbreak. Wild greens, such as dandelion and lamb's-quarter, can be of great help in alkalinizing the blood. Avoid acidic foods such as alcohol, citrus fruits, coffee, hot spices, sugar, and tomatoes.

Topical Applications

A multitude of topical treatments have been reported to give relief, fight infection, or speed up the healing process when an outbreak occurs. Most experts agree that a moist herpes lesion should be kept dry and a dry herpes lesion kept moist, so choose from the list below accordingly.

- Aloe vera gel—soothes and dries the lesions.
- Chaparral extract or powder—dries the lesions.
- Comfrey salve—moistens the lesions and promotes wound healing.
- Echinacea extract—dries the lesions and has antiviral activity.
- Geranium essential oil—dries the lesions and has antiviral activity.
- Hyssop essential oil—dries the lesions and has antiviral activity.

- Ice—reduces inflammation, particularly in the early stages.

- Melissa (lemon balm) essential oil—dries the lesions and has antiviral activity.

- Myrrh tincture—dries the lesions and has antiviral activity.

- Osha tincture—dries the lesions and has antiviral activity.

- Propolis—dries the lesions and promotes wound healing.

- Saint-John's-wort oil—dries the lesions and relieves pain.

- Spirits of camphor—dries the lesions and has antiviral activity.

- Tea tree oil—dries the lesions and has antiviral activity.

- Vitamin E oil—moistens the lesions, promotes wound healing, and helps prevent scarring.

- Wine—promotes wound healing.

- Witch hazel—dries the lesions.

Herbal Therapy

Herbs that can help heal herpes lesions and prevent future outbreaks include the following.

Black walnut (*Juglans nigra*). One theory holds that the herpesvirus blocks electromagnetic energy from flowing through the nervous system. The leaf and green nut of black walnut, which are high in ellagic acid and manganese, improve energy flow through the nervous system. They are alterative, anti-inflammatory, and antiseptic.

Burdock (*Arctium lappa*). The root improves the function of the organs of elimination and helps purify the blood and lymphatic system. It has an overall cooling effect and is alterative, anti-inflammatory, antiseptic, astringent, demulcent, febrifuge, and nutritive.

Chaparral (*Larrea tridentata*). Take 1 teaspoon of chaparral leaf tincture in 1 ounce of water first thing in the morning for twenty-one days to inactivate the virus at the first sign of an outbreak. The leaf is an alterative, antiseptic, antioxidant, antiviral, bitter tonic, and immunostimulant. Avoid in cases of liver or kidney disease, cirrhosis, or hepatitis and during pregnancy. Discontinue use if nausea, fatigue, fever, or jaundice occur. Do not use for more than one month at a time. Consult with your health care provider before use.

Echinacea (*Echinacea purpurea, E. angustifolia*). The root stimulates macrophage and interferon activity, making cells less susceptible to viral takeover. It is an alterative, antiseptic, anti-inflammatory, antiviral, astringent, immunostimulant, and vulnerary.

Goldenseal (*Hydrastis canadensis*). The root clears heat and dries dampness. It soothes irritated mucous membranes and stimulates macrophage activity in the immune system. It is an alterative, anti-inflammatory, antiseptic, and astringent. Goldenseal is very bitter, and most people find it easiest to ingest in capsule form. Topical applications of goldenseal tincture or powder can help dry the lesions, but they will stain clothing. Avoid during pregnancy. This herb is endangered in the wild; do not use wildcrafted supplies.

Lemon balm (*Melissa officinalis*). The herb has an overall cooling effect and strengthens the nervous system. It is an antipyretic, antiviral, and nervine.

Licorice (*Glycyrrhiza glabra, G. uralensis*). The root supports the body's production of interferon and soothes irritated mucous membranes. It also helps calm the emotions. It is anti-inflammatory, antiviral, demulcent, and emollient. Avoid during pregnancy and in cases of edema, high blood pressure, or diabetes. Do not use in combination with digoxin drugs. Excessive use can cause sodium retention and potassium depletion.

Oregon grape (*Mahonia aquifolium*). The root contains the alkaloid berberine, which has strong antiseptic properties. It is also an alterative, antipyretic, antiseptic, and immunostimulant.

Peppermint (*Mentha piperita*). The herb is cooling and calming and improves circulation. It is an analgesic, anodyne, antiseptic, and antiviral.

Sarsaparilla (*Smilax* spp.). The root has an affinity for the genitourinary tract, which it helps purify and clear of eruptions. It is an alterative and a tonic.

Tea (*Camellia sinensis*). The leaf is high in tannins that coat the virus cells and can neutralize them. Because this herb also contains caffeine, its use should be limited to an occasional cup of tea. It is an analgesic, antioxidant, antiseptic, astringent, immunostimulant, and nervine.

Yellow dock (*Rumex crispus*). The root is cooling and detoxifying. Like tea, it is high in virus-neutralizing tannins. It is an alterative, antipyretic, antiseptic, antiviral, and astringent.

Nutritional Therapy

Nutritional supplements can play an important role in supporting overall good health and making the body resistant to activation of the herpesvirus.

Acidophilus. Acidophilus boosts immune system activity; as a happy side effect, it destroys harmful bacteria. Take two capsules three times daily.

Beta-carotene. Beta-carotene is the precursor to vitamin A, which stimulates the production of antibodies and strengthens mucous membranes. Take 25,000–500,000 IU daily.

Calcium and magnesium. These two nutrients, which are often combined in a single supplement, nourish the nervous system. Take 1,000 mg of calcium and 500 mg of magnesium daily.

Essential fatty acids. EFAs, strengthen cells, making them more resistant to viral infiltration. Fresh ground flaxseed, hempseed, and evening primrose oils are excellent sources of EFAs. Take 3 tablespoons daily.

Lysine. As previously explained, lysine is a potent ally against the herpesvirus. Take 500 mg daily as a preventive. When symptoms of an imminent herpes outbreak appear, increase that dosage to 500 mg three to six times daily for no more than ten days.

Vitamin B complex. Like vitamin A, the B vitamins support the production of antibodies; they also nourish the nervous system. Take 50 mg daily.

Vitamin C plus bioflavonoids. This formula can speed the healing of oral sores and strengthen capillaries. Quercetin, a component of bioflavonoids, has demonstrated antiherpes activity. Take 1,000 mg of vitamin C with 500 mg of bioflavonoids three times daily.

Vitamin E. Vitamin E helps the body make better use of oxygen, thereby supporting immune system function and promoting the healing of herpes sores. Take 400 IU daily.

Lung Tan Xie Gan Pill

According to traditional Oriental medicine, herpes infection is a condition of damp heat. The Chinese patent formula Lung Tan Xie Gan Pill, or Gentiana Purge Liver Pills, helps clear damp heat from the body.

Homeopathic Remedies

When the development of herpes matches one of the descriptions below, try the suggested homeopathic remedy. The usual dosage is four pellets, or as many liquid drops as the package label recommends, taken under the tongue four times daily. Rather than swallowing the pellets whole, allow them to dissolve slowly.

Apis Mellifica. The lesions cause a stinging pain.

Arsenicum Album. The lesions are deep and bleed when the crusts are removed; they cause a shooting, burning pain. Symptoms are worse at night.

Borax. The patient is a child.

Calcarea Carbonica. The skin ulcerates easily. Symptoms are worse in open air and better in a warm room.

Carbo Vegetabilis. The lesions are evident on the chin, lips, and face. Glands swell; lesions itch, then burn when scratched.

Dulcamara. Ulcerations are oozing and moist; they have thick brown crusts with reddish borders and occur in clusters. Symptoms are more likely to be evident during cold and wet weather, during changes in temperature, or around the time of menses.

Graphites. There is a painful or clear oozing from the lesion.

Hepar Sulphuris Calcareum. This remedy can help control infection and prevent the need for antibiotics. It is particularly helpful for the patient who has tender oral sores located in the center of the lower lip and across the face toward or in the eyes, making them moist and weepy. There may be swelling in the upper lip. The lesions are sensitive to cold air.

Mercurius Solubilis. The lesions bleed easily and burn when touched.

Natrum Muriaticum. The sores occur in the middle of the upper or lower lip (or both), as well as on the chin and the sides of the nose. The eruptions are moist and itchy. The infection may be stress related; the patient may be a stoic who doesn't express emotions, bears burdens silently, and rejects sympathy even though he or she craves it. This remedy is excellent when used in the early stages of infection, while the upper lip is swollen but vesicles have not yet formed. It is best used in a 200C potency, which can be obtained from a homeopathic practitioner.

Nitricum Acidum. The lesions are in the corners of the mouth and may crack or feel tender. This remedy can also be used for genital outbreaks.

Psorinum. The patient feels chilled and weak. Application of heat brings relief. Use for chronic cases that cause itching.

Rhus Toxicodendron. The outbreak is sudden and includes intense itching and burning. Red, irritated tissue surrounds the sore, from which acrid, crusty, yellow fluid may emerge. The cold sores erupt around the nose, lips, and chin. The patient may be sensitive to cold and dampness. If the herpes is preceded by fever and diarrhea, heat helps relieve the symptoms.

Sepia. The patient experiences feelings of pressure, itching, constipation, and irritability. In other cases, the lesions may appear inside the nasal cavities, on the lips, and in the corners of the mouth. The face may swell, there may be dark circles under the eyes, and the patient may experience chills, exhaustion, and depression. This remedy is suitable for sores that occur during pregnancy, before menses, or during menopause.

Silicea. The skin is very sensitive and ulcerates easily.

Sulfur. The patient experiences burning discomfort, often with a secondary infection. Heat may increase the discomfort.

Therapeutic Baths

To bring relief to a painful outbreak of genital herpes, add one of the following therapeutic formulas to the bath:

- 1 to 2 pounds of sea salt

- 1 to 2 pounds of Epsom salts

- 2 cups of apple cider vinegar

- 10 black tea bags

- 4 or 5 drops of an antiviral essential oil, such as geranium, hyssop, melissa, tea tree, wintergreen, or wormwood

   Soak, relax in the warmth, and enjoy.

Acupressure

The acupressure point known as Bladder Meridian Point #63 can help relieve pain and even curtail an outbreak of genital herpes, if used at the first sign. The point is located three thumbs' width forward of the crown of the outer ankle bulge, moving toward the little toe. Apply deep pressure with the thumb. You should feel a twinge of sensitivity. Press this point for twenty seconds, on both feet, four or five times daily.

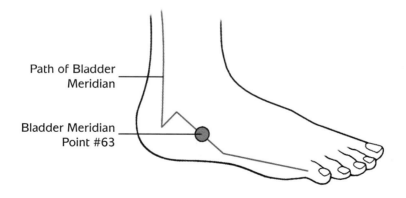

Path of Bladder Meridian

Bladder Meridian Point #63

SYPHILIS

Syphilis is caused by the spiral-shaped bacterium *Treponema pallidum*. The disease progresses through four stages: primary, secondary, latent, and tertiary. The primary stage occurs ten days to twelve weeks after exposure and includes the development of a small, hard lesion, known as a chancre. The chancre usually appears on the penis, vagina, or rectum but may also appear on the face or hands. It is painless and may secrete a clear fluid.

The secondary stage sets in several weeks later. Some infected persons do not experience any symptoms at this stage, but if symptoms do appear, they manifest as fever, swollen glands, fatigue, headache, joint pain, and a rash on the hands and feet. Multiple lesions may form in the mucous membranes, such as those of the mouth, throat, rectum, and vagina. The infection is highly contagious during this stage, because secretions from the lesions carry the bacteria.

During the latent stage, the disease seems to disappear. For many infected persons, the infection does not progress any further. For others, it resurfaces years later, in the tertiary stage. In this stage, the bacteria spreads throughout the body, causing irreversible damage to the brain, spine, heart, eyes, and other organs. It can be fatal.

Until the discovery of penicillin, syphilis was a major killer, causing dementia and a slow, agonizing decline of health in infected persons. It does respond readily to antibiotic treatment, and its spread has been controlled in most developed countries. *Control,* however, does not equate to *elimination.* Syphilis is still present in the population of the United States.

Transmission

Syphilis is spread through direct contact with mucous membranes. It can be transmitted through vaginal, anal, and oral sex, and even kissing. If you spot a genital lesion, suspect that you have syphilis, or have been exposed to syphilis, cease all sexual activity until you have been properly diagnosed and treated. Proper diagnosis can be made only through a blood test or microscopic examination of fluid from a sore.

Treatment

When detected early, syphilis is treatable. Antibiotic therapy—penicillin is most effective against the bacteria—is called for.

While you are taking antibiotics, add to your diet fermented foods such as plain yogurt and unpasteurized sauerkraut, apple cider vinegar, miso, and tamari. These foods support and replenish the friendly bacteria in the body.

After a course of antibiotic therapy, begin a course of acidophilus therapy to restore the friendly bacteria that are necessary for digestion, elimination, and healthy reproductive organs. Take one or two capsules three times daily for three to four months.

TRICHOMONIASIS

Trichomonas vaginalis is a parasitic single-celled protozoan. Infection with "trich," as it's called, can lead to trichomoniasis. In women, trichomoniasis infects the vagina and cervix and can cause painful urination, genital itching, a green or yellow vaginal discharge that smells unpleasant (like dirty sneakers), and small reddish spots. In men, trichomoniasis infects the urethra and can cause painful urination and a whitish discharge. It is often asymptomatic in men and sometimes asymptomatic in women. It frequently occurs in combination with other STDs.

Left untreated, trichomoniasis can result in cervicitis, fertility dysfunctions, urethritis, and prostatitis.

Transmission

Though trichomoniasis is usually transmitted through sexual contact, the parasite can survive for several hours outside the body and be transmitted through sharing of towels, washcloths, underclothing, sex toys, and similar items.

Treatment

Trichomoniasis can be treated successfully with natural therapies. The therapies focus on strengthening the body's immune system and making the vagina or urethra an inhospitable environment for the protozoans.

Men who suspect they have trichomoniasis should avoid ejaculating, because semen nourishes the protozoans. If the diagnosis is confirmed, continue to avoid ejaculating for a total of ten days.

Women who suspect they have contracted trichomoniasis should begin using an antiseptic suppository until diagnosed. Soak a tampon in a mixture of 2 tablespoons of apple cider vinegar, 1 drop of tea tree essential oil, and 2 cups of warm water. Insert the tampon; do not remove for at least four hours. Skip the suppository treatment on the day you're going to be tested, as it can affect the test results.

Herbal Therapy

Herbs that support the immune system, nurture overall health, and fight off infection are especially helpful for treating trichomoniasis.

Calendula (*Calendula officinalis*). The flower increases peripheral circulation and helps dispel infections that are trapped in the body. It is an alterative, antifungal, anti-inflammatory, antiseptic, and vulnerary.

Chaparral (*Larrea tridentata*). The leaf is an alterative, antiseptic, antioxidant, antiviral, bitter tonic, and immunostimulant. Avoid in cases of liver or kidney disease, cirrhosis, or hepatitis and during pregnancy. Discontinue use if nausea, fatigue, fever, or jaundice occur. Do not use for more than a month at a time. Consult with your health care provider before use.

Echinacea (*Echinacea purpurea, E. angustifolia*). The root has a powerfully stimulating effect on the immune system. It is also an alterative, antifungal, and antiseptic.

Garlic (*Allium sativum*). The bulb contains compounds that help the body resist a wide range of pathogens. It is an alterative, antibiotic, antioxidant, antiseptic, immunostimulant, and vasodilator. Try eating a clove of raw garlic daily. Some people are allergic to garlic. Excessive use can cause emotional irritability and irritation of the stomach and kidneys. Avoid therapeutic doses during pregnancy; also avoid during the first three months of nursing, as it can cause breast milk to become unpalatable for infants. Avoid use the week before having surgery.

Goldenseal (*Hydrastis canadensis*). The root is active against a wide range of pathogens and is especially effective for relieving inflammation of the mucous membranes. It is an alterative and an antibiotic. Goldenseal is very bitter, and most people find it easiest to ingest in capsule form. Avoid during pregnancy. This herb is endangered in the wild; do not use wildcrafted supplies.

Licorice (*Glycyrrhiza glabra, G. uralensis*). The root boosts immune system function and soothes irritated tissues. It is an antibiotic, anti-inflammatory, antiviral, and nutritive. Avoid during pregnancy and in cases of edema, high blood pressure, or diabetes. Do not use in combination with digoxin drugs. Excessive use can cause sodium retention and potassium depletion.

Nettle (*Urtica dioica, U. urens*). The leaf is rich in chlorophyll. It builds overall health, inhibits infection, and speeds healing. It is an alterative, circulatory stimulant, and antiparasitic. Contact with the fresh plant will irritate the skin. Use only dried herb. Wear gloves when collecting.

Usnea (*Usnea barbata*). The lichen helps rid the body of infection without killing friendly intestinal flora. It is an antibiotic, antifungal, and immunostimulant.

Vinegar Douche

A douche made from 2 tablespoons of apple cider vinegar and 4 cups of warm water can help clear the infection. Douche just twice daily; getting overzealous with this treatment can wash away friendly vaginal flora.

Suppositories

A garlic clove or two capsules of acidophilus can be used as vaginal suppositories to eliminate the infection. See page 277 for instructions. The garlic has an antiparasitic effect; acidophilus supports friendly vaginal flora that compete with *Trichomonas vaginalis*.

Sitz Baths

Sitz baths increase circulation to the pelvic area, which can bring great relief to people suffering trichomoniasis symptoms. See Chapter 12 for instructions. Add to the tub 1 cup of apple cider vinegar and the juice from 7 cloves of garlic.

Part 5

Love and Relationships

23

Healing the Spirit from a Broken Heart

t is a rare person who lives without having experienced grief. In fact, I might go so far as to say that a life cannot be truly full without the experience of grief. It is a strong and terrible emotion, breaking us open, drilling deep into the nerves of our soul, often unleashing a torrent of emotion that seems impossible to contain.

But without the capacity to express grief, we cannot express love. Grief is the flip side of the coin, the risk we take when we open our hearts to another. It is the cleanser of the broken heart, the cool ocean streaming over the hot and angry sands, the salt that stings the open wound and purifies it.

Experiencing grief is a part of being human. Too often we try to contain it, a study in impassivity, feeling that it shows stronger character to wade through without wincing or crying. In fact, when we don't allow ourselves to experience grief, the sadness is never realized and becomes buried like a sticky burr in the soul. We become emotionally numb, distant from friends, family, and other loved ones, never able to fully enter into life.

To live fully, we must love fully and, hence, grieve fully. I hope this chapter will help.

EXPRESSING GRIEF

It is healthier to express grief than to repress it. The force of grief is contractive. Crying provides emotional release that lowers blood pressure and muscular tension. Crying can also help relieve stress on the central nervous system. The more you grieve, the sooner the heartache will pass.

If tears won't come even though you feel crying would help, here is a technique you can try. Find a safe, quiet space where you will not be disturbed. Place one hand in the middle of your upper chest, on your collarbone. Breath down only as far as your hand. Then begin to breathe more rapidly. Make a sound of some sort. Hear the feeling in your voice. Go ahead and sound like a crying baby. Give yourself the space to feel the sadness. Think about what's causing the grief, and let the tears flow.

Groaning is another sound that can help dissipate sadness and pain. While groaning, think of your reasons for suffering. When you exhale, visualize sorrow being exhaled from your system.

These breathing exercises are lent extra power when performed in concert with sunrise. Stand facing the rising sun, and let its rays beam on your heart. Visualize the sun healing your grief. Breathe!

> "What soap is for the body, tears are for the soul."
> —ANONYMOUS

AFTER A BREAKUP

Breaking up with a loved one can cause feelings similar to the grief we feel after the death of a loved one. It's also often mixed with anger, frustration, and tremendous disappointment.

When someone breaks up with you, do your best to stay calm; save the freaking out for later. Screaming and throwing things tends to make the person who is departing feel that he or she is justified in leaving, because you're acting like a lunatic. When things simmer down, try writing a letter to your ex, for your eyes only. Use the letter-writing as an opportunity to collect your thoughts and express your feelings, getting everything off your chest. Vent venomously! Eventually you may want to send a modified version (without the bad language) to your ex, or you may want to burn the letter. The important thing is to clear your feelings.

Encourage the physical separation; without it, the emotional separation will take longer and be more painful. Put your ex's belongings in a box and return them to him or her with a minimum of drama. If there are mementos you wish to keep, put them in a box and put the box in storage. Clean everything. Feng shui your home. Burn some sage or artemesia to clear the air.

Don't call your ex when you are sad, scared, or depressed. Minimize calling just to "check in." Tell your friends not to give you constant gossip reports about where they saw your ex and who he or she was with. Ask friends who invite you to gatherings to let you know whether your ex will be there, so that you can avoid surprises.

Have a closure ritual. Place a photo of your ex and a sprig of rosemary (for remembrance) in a bowl filled with sand or dirt. Etch a candle with your ex's name, and anoint it with a fragrance that reminds you of him or her. Then place the candle in the bowl with the photo and the rosemary, and light it. Offer a prayer of thanks for the lessons you learned in the relationship. As the candle burns down, reflect upon your relationship, perhaps writing down your thoughts in a journal. It can be therapeutic to remember your "love story." Include memorable dates and events, how you met, and what your feeling and expectations were. Make note of clues that, in retrospect, signaled that the relationship wasn't going to last. Make a list of all the reasons the relationship could not have survived, as well as a list of things you learned from the relationship. Write about what you will look for in a new partner. Be willing to look at any aspect of yourself that may have contributed to the ending, and then let go of it. Give your story a title. Allow the candle to burn itself out. Play "your song" one last time.

OVERCOMING GRIEF

Therapy for grief focuses on three aspects:

- Rest
- Positive energy
- Health

Of greatest importance, take care of yourself, and indulge in pampering. The loving support of friends and family members can be a blessing. Ask them to visit; allow them to try to cheer you up. Seek out those who want to see you happy, and avoid people with negative attitudes.

Channeling positive energy into different aspects of your life, such as your career, your children, and your personal growth, can help diffuse grief. Put energy into your career. Develop new talents. Take a class. Read self-help books. Learn a new language. Exercise. Practice yoga. Quit bad habits; overdoing alcohol, drugs, and junk food will only make this time more difficult.

Aromatherapy Baths

Soaking in a bath can encourage muscles and mind to relax and healing tears to flow. Light a candle, blue for calming the emotions or violet for easing grief and raising consciousness. Add 7 drops of a grief-dispelling essential oil, such as cedarwood, clary sage, cypress, geranium, grapefruit, hyssop, lavender, lemon balm, jasmine, marjoram, neroli, orange, rose, rosemary, rosewood, sage, sandalwood, tangerine, or ylang ylang.

When you are done bathing, let out the water, and visualize sorrow passing down the drain with the water and being healed by the earth. Then towel dry and apply a massage oil made from one or more of the essential oils mentioned above (8 ounces of coconut oil mixed with 30 drops of the essential oil) over your heart and lungs.

Gem Therapy

Rose quartz can calm anger, promote love, and help heal grief and emotional wounds. If you sleep with a rose quartz in your hand, your dreams may have a healing effect on your heart. You might also consider wearing rose quartz jewelry.

Color Therapy

The color violet, worn and visualized, is good for healing grief. Visualize yourself breathing in a healing violet light. As you exhale, see the somber colors of your sadness departing with your breath.

Nutritional Therapy

According to traditional Oriental medicine, grief corresponds to the metal element and the lungs and large intestine. Eat green- and orange-colored foods, such as violet leaf, dandelion, kale, collards, carrots, and sweet potatoes, which support the liver. Eat celery to help comfort the pangs of a broken heart. Use pungent condiments such as clove, coriander, and ginger, which move lung energy. Vitamin B complex, which promotes both calmness and vitality, is always a great ally during times of emotional distress.

Herbal Therapy

Herbs can be a great comforter during times of grief.

Hawthorn (*Crataegus* spp.). The leaf, flower, and berry are generally used in herbal medicine to strengthen and improve the physical heart, but they also benefit the emotional heart. They can aid sleep and establish a feeling of serenity.

Hops (*Humulus lupulus*). The strobile quiets the nerves, calms anxiety, and promotes rest. It is an anodyne, muscle relaxant, nervine, and sedative.

Lemon balm (*Melissa officinalis*). The herb, according to some German studies, acts upon the part of the brain governing the autonomic nervous system. It is a nervine and a sedative.

Motherwort (*Leonurus cardiaca*). The herb calms anxiety and hysteria and relieves depression. It can help open the mind to joy after a loss. It is a cardiotonic, hypotensive, nervine, sedative, and vasodilator.

Mullein (*Verbascum thapsus*). The leaf protects the lungs from harm during periods of sadness.

Passion flower (*Passiflora incarnata*). The herb provides precursors to the neurotransmitter serotonin and reduces the rate at which the body breaks down serotonin and norepinephrine. It can induce a mild euphoria and quiet mental chatter. It is especially helpful for those who are weak and exhausted with anxiety, irritability, nervous breakdown, stress, or suicidal tendencies. It is an anodyne and a nervine.

Saint John's wort (*Hypericum perforatum*). The herb has antidepressant properties and can help heal physically damaged nerves. It relieves anxiety, fear, irritability, melancholy, and suicidal tendencies. It is a mild sedative and can be especially helpful for someone who is worn out from sobbing.

Violet (*Viola odorata*). Violet also goes by the name "heartsease"—a good indicator of its use in healing grief. The leaf and flower calm the physical and emotional heart. They are also demulcents.

Homeopathic Remedies

When grief is accompanied by the conditions that are described, try the suggested homeopathic remedy. The usual dosage is four pellets, or as many liquid drops as the package label recommends, taken under the tongue four times daily. Rather than swallowing the pellets whole, allow them to dissolve slowly.

Ignatia. The patient experiences hysteria. He or she sighs frequently and has difficulty sleeping.

Natrum Muriaticum. The patient dwells in the past, holds grudges, and rejects sympathy.

Pulsatilla. The patient feels extreme anxiety. He or she is sad, yielding, indecisive, and weepy and needs to be with others.

Flower Essences

Flower essences, which have a strong connection to the emotions, can be used in a variety of ways to help heal a broken heart. The usual dosage is

7 drops under the tongue or taken with a glass of water three or four times daily. You can also add flower essences to bathwater, massage oils, and body lotions. Try applying them to the sensitive skin on the inside of the wrists and the "third eye" at the center of the forehead.

Bleeding Heart. This essence helps foster peace and detachment.

Borage. Borage helps lift the spirits.

Hawthorn. Hawthorn protects the spirit, reminding us of our resiliency during periods of intense grief and stress. It washes negativity from the heart and soothes the pain of emotional separation.

Honeysuckle. For the person who finds it difficult to adjust after the loss of a loved one, honeysuckle can help him or her move out of the past and reintegrate into present life.

Mustard. Mustard helps to dispel deep gloom that comes on strong, then suddenly leaves.

Pear. Pear helps relieve extreme grief that arises from unbalancing emergency situations.

Rescue Remedy. This remedy can be taken to calm the mind in moments of extreme crisis. Take 2 drops under the tongue, as often as necessary.

Star of Bethlehem. Star of Bethlehem soothes the mind when you are having a difficult time coping with the death of a loved one. Dr. Edward Bach called this essence "the comforter and soother of pains and sorrows."

24

The Twenty-Five Principles of a Strong Relationship

elationships are like plants. They thrive when cared for; they wither when neglected. To maintain a commitment to a lover, we must learn to tend our relationships as if they were gardens, cultivating the flowers of spiritual fulfillment and the fruits of earthly nourishment. How? By following these twenty-five principles:

1. Understand that relationships take work.
2. Make a commitment to daily appreciation.
3. Be kind.
4. Practice romance.
5. Respect each other's sexual energy.
6. Make your relationship a priority.
7. Make time for sex.
8. Allow spiritual energy to imbue your relationship with higher meaning.
9. Keep your voice pleasant.
10. Develop mutual interests. Allow space for individual interests.
11. Spend time with couples who are positive role models.
12. Evolve together.
13. Make room for quiet time with each other.
14. Communicate.

15. Praise in public; criticize in private.

16. Express, rather than accuse.

17. When having an argument, stick with the issue at hand.

18. Argue from both sides.

19. Be affectionate.

20. Greet each other warmly.

21. If you have children, find a babysitter whom you trust implicitly.

22. If you have children, maintain a united front.

23. Give gifts.

24. Be open to therapy.

25. Be responsible for your own happiness.

1. UNDERSTAND THAT RELATIONSHIPS TAKE WORK.

The marriage cliché "This match was made in heaven" is both erroneous and potentially harmful. There are no perfect relationships or even perfect mates. A marriage or committed relationship is made and continually remade by two people who work very hard at it.

Fuel your love with daily expressions of affection, appreciation, and attention. Upon waking each morning, turn to face your partner and remind yourself why you are in love with this person. Be willing to nourish love, and to repair it when necessary. Celebrate love! Celebrate life! Keep the magic alive.

2. MAKE A COMMITMENT TO DAILY APPRECIATION.

Never take the love, presence, or daily contributions of a lover for granted. Express appreciation not only for acts that go above and beyond what you might expect but also for the mundane—meals prepared, lawn mowed, car fixed, and so on. Let each other know *every day* that you appreciate each other.

Be generous with compliments, not only about the way a partner looks but also about what he or she says or does. Appreciate each other's strengths. Accept each other's weaknesses.

3. BE KIND.

Simple acts of kindness can go a long way toward strengthening a relationship. You and your partner should each try to perform at least one act of selfless kindness each day. When your beloved is stressed out, offer to give him or her a back massage or to run a tub so that he or she can take a relaxing bath. If he or she will be out late, leave a light on when you retire to bed. Surprise your mate occasionally by taking care of some of his or her usual chores. You get the picture, right?

Practice politeness. Being polite to each other, day in and day out, helps you build, support, and express a measure of respect for each other. And when politeness becomes a habit, it can help you maintain civility and remind you of your connection in times of marital strife.

Some conflict is normal in relationships. Everyone is entitled to an occasional bad mood. How you treat each other during these times of difficulty is a gauge of the strength of your relationship.

4. PRACTICE ROMANCE.

Find ways to be romantic every day. Remember all those "silly" things you used to do to try to make a good impression when you were courting? Don't stop doing them now, just because you're in a committed relationship. Long-term relations should be given more, not less, effort than courtship.

Go on regular dates, taking turns planning them. Plan for special times and surprises. Dress up for each other. Take walks after dinner. Hold hands. Enjoy nature together. Go on elegant picnics, even in your own backyard. Eat in romantic places—by the shore, fireplace, overlooking the city. Have teatime. Work on a project together, such as starting a garden and eating the food you grow. Make your home beautiful with candles, art, and music. Obtain a guidebook for your region or town, and explore together the local sights and scenes you've never visited.

Leave love notes for each other. Write poems together. If you have to be away for a few days, leave your beloved a farewell note. While you're away, send home a postcard, even if you'll end up beating it back.

5. RESPECT EACH OTHER'S SEXUAL ENERGY.

Sexual energy is like the changing moon. Sometimes we are filled with desire; other times, we would rather lie quietly next to our beloved, enjoying intimacy without sex. No matter how great a relationship is, there will be times of mismatched libido.

However, if lovers always waited to have sex until they were both in a high state of arousal, sex would be a rare occurrence. Be patient. You didn't choose to be with each other just so you'd always have someone to have sex with. Give yourselves the space to say no when you're not in the mood. Make masturbation a part of your sexual repertoire; if you don't feel sexual but your partner does, he or she could masturbate while you hold and kiss him or her. You might also offer to please him or her orally or manually. And recognize that it is perfectly acceptable for your partner to simply "go for it" once in a while, meeting his or her own needs.

Most important, communicate. It's better to say "no" than to say "yes" and make love with a "no" attitude.

6. MAKE YOUR RELATIONSHIP A PRIORITY.

Your lover should always feel that he or she is more important to you than your job, your parents, your hobby, the television, or anything else. You would never start a business, putting tremendous energy into it for the first few years, and then expect it to thrive without any effort. Should you do less for love?

In the same vein, your lover may occasionally find himself or herself involved in a project that requires all of his or her attention for a short span of time. During this time, recognize that supporting the relationship is more important than allowing yourself to feel neglected. Find ways to keep yourself occupied rather than adding to the burden by making your lover feel guilty for not paying attention to you. Remind yourself that your job is to keep your relationship strong so that, when the project is finished, your lover can return to you with joy and gratefulness for your support.

7. MAKE TIME FOR SEX.

Making time for sex is essential for a healthy relationship. Too often sex happens late at night, when you're exhausted, or first thing in the morning, when you have to be at work in an hour. Though these quickies can be lovely expressions of pure physical lust (not every sexual experience has to be long and romantic), in general, leftover time makes for leftover sex. Saving sex for last indicates that it's your last priority.

Schedule sacred times for making love, such as sunset, evenings of the full moon (open the windows), sunrise (set your alarm clock for an early hour, and leave enough time for a nap afterward), solstices, equinoxes, and Sunday afternoons. Build sexual connection into your celebration of the holidays. For example, on New Year's Eve, instead of toasting at midnight, be making love.

> Wait two or three hours after eating before having sex. It's difficult for the body to supply chi and blood to both the sexual organs and the digestive system at the same time. Instead of eating before bed, save some hunger for your beloved.

8. ALLOW SPIRITUAL ENERGY TO IMBUE YOUR RELATIONSHIP WITH HIGHER MEANING.

Spiritual depth in a relationship lends meaning to life. Find a form of faith, organized or not, that allows spiritual energy to flow through your lives. Pray together. Give thanks for your blessings, including your love. Honor the god and goddess in each other. If you are of different faiths, participate occasionally in each other's ceremonies and services.

9. KEEP YOUR VOICE PLEASANT.

Voice can be an important factor in attraction. A high voice indicates lower sexual vitality; a low voice indicates greater sexual vitality. Do your best to modulate your voice, avoiding shrill tones, shrieking, and mumbling. If you're not sure what you sound like, record yourself speaking and then play it back.

When you speak to your lover, inject warmth into your voice. Use your beloved's name often, always allowing the name to come softly and lovingly from your lips.

10. DEVELOP MUTUAL INTERESTS. ALLOW SPACE FOR INDIVIDUAL INTERESTS.

Don't let children, finances, or other conveniences be the glue that keeps you together. Occasionally do something with your partner that he or she enjoys and you could care less about. Do it with good cheer. Make a practice of finding at least three things you like about it, rather than grumbling or being critical. Enjoy your beloved's enjoyment!

Have friends in common, but also have friends on an individual level. Give each other space to spend time alone with friends. (And find goodness in at least a few of your partner's friends.)

11. SPEND TIME WITH COUPLES WHO ARE POSITIVE ROLE MODELS.

If you only spend time with friends who complain constantly about their relationship, watch out. It could rub off. Instead, surround yourself with positive role models that can bring positive energy to your relationship

Of course, you should certainly be there for your friends when they're struggling with relationship problems. But if they're always telling the same story of trouble and grief, without progress, it may be time to remove yourself from the circle of negative energy.

As for yourself, if you find that you are complaining about marital problems to a friend, resolve that you will spend twice as much time discussing the issue with your beloved.

12. EVOLVE TOGETHER.

The only constant in human life is change. Over the course of a long-term relationship, partners will find that they each continue to grow and learn, and not always together or in the same manner. Rather than getting hung up on what's different about each other, partners must learn to appreciate their differences. Recognizing that a person is never the same from one day to the next, see your partner's evolution as an opportunity to learn more about him or her and to grow and evolve yourself.

If your beloved is developing a new passion, learn more about it so that you can support and encourage his or her new dreams. And develop new passions together, such as pottery, yoga, dance, tennis, drawing, massage, and so on. Every once in a while, take a class on enhancing relationship and communication skills.

13. MAKE ROOM FOR QUIET TIME WITH EACH OTHER.

Find at least twenty minutes a day when you and your partner can speak with each other undisturbed, whether to share concerns or just to check in with each other. Do this beyond the reach of the television, the radio, the phone, or the kids. If you find that the only time you have together is in the evening, don't save your twenty minutes for bedtime, when you're exhausted. Instead, put your kids to bed with a lovely story, turn off the television and the computer, and sit down with each other at a reasonable hour.

14. COMMUNICATE.

When you communicate with your beloved, do so honestly, openly, and considerately. Share with each other your feelings, hurts, fears, and disappointments. Be supportive of each other. Thank each other for sharing. Don't dismiss your partner's feelings in an effort to help him or her stop crying. Instead, be a good listener. Allow your beloved to express his or her feelings fully and openly. Don't attempt to problem-solve unless you're sure that your partner wants you to; sometimes, a person who is upset doesn't want a solution to the problem so much as just a quiet space and a willing listener.

15. PRAISE IN PUBLIC; CRITICIZE IN PRIVATE.

In front of others, praise and criticism have significantly greater impact. There-fore, whenever possible, praise in public, building up your beloved in a way that shows your love and support. Reserve criticism for private times, when you can speak kindly and won't embarrass your beloved in front of others.

Above all, be generous with praise and words of love. There will be times when you'll want to criticize your beloved, but make sure that you praise at least three times as much as you criticize.

16. EXPRESS, RATHER THAN ACCUSE.

Avoid speaking in an accusatory manner. Rather than saying "You always . . ." or "You never . . . ," try "I feel . . ." or "I need . . ." For example, rather than saying "You never help with housework," try "I feel that I am doing all the house-work."

Rather than being defensive, the listener should mirror back what he or she heard to make sure that the issue is clear. For example, your lover might say back to you "I hear you saying that the housework is not split evenly between us."

Taping a discussion or argument and listening to it later by yourself or together can be an opportunity to evaluate and improve communication skills.

17. WHEN HAVING AN ARGUMENT, STICK WITH THE ISSUE AT HAND.

The golden rule for a healthy argument is "One issue, one argument." Dis-cussing just one issue at a time keeps negative emotions in check and allows you to focus on finding a solution for a particular problem, instead of just get-ting angry with each other.

When an argument becomes heated, practice the "talking stick." Pick out a special stick, crystal, rock, or other item and designate it as the talking stick. Only when you are holding the talking stick are you are allowed to speak—and, then, without interruption, until you are finished. Pass the stick back and forth until the issue has been cleared.

18. ARGUE FROM BOTH SIDES.

When communication over a problematic issue breaks down, write a letter to your partner, expressing your feelings and point of view. Then write a letter that you believe expresses your partner's feelings and viewpoint. Your partner should do the same. Then trade letters.

19. BE AFFECTIONATE.

Physical affection is important for maintaining and building emotional affection. It can help smooth over negative emotions lingering after an argument. A light caress on the shoulders lets your beloved know that you're thinking about her as she works at the computer. A kiss on the cheek when your lover walks in the door tells him that you are delighted to see him.

Delight in one another's embrace! There doesn't have to be a reason other than maintaining that heart-to-heart connection. Connect in a loving way daily—through eye contact, kissing, hugging, dancing, massage, caresses, and loving words.

Try to go to bed at the same time at least a few times a week to ensure more opportunities for connection. If you need to stay up, at least tuck in your beloved and share some talk and cuddling before going back to the television, the computer, or whatever is keeping you up.

20. GREET EACH OTHER WARMLY.

Let your relationship be a place to retreat to instead of a place to escape from. When you or your beloved returns home, greet each other warmly. Let each other know that you're pleased by the other's presence. If you're engrossed in an activity, no matter what it is, at least pick up your head, smile, and welcome your lover back to you.

If you happen to be at home awaiting the arrival of your partner, take a few minutes to straighten up the house. It can make for a wonderful reception. It's harder to relax when things are messy. Unclutter countertops and rooms. Sweep up. Empty the dishwasher. Light a candle, and turn on some music. When your lover walks in the door, she or he will immediately feel more relaxed, and very much welcome.

21. IF YOU HAVE CHILDREN, FIND A BABYSITTER WHOM YOU TRUST IMPLICITLY.

Having a babysitter you can trust allows you to enjoy time away from your kids—which is vital for a healthy relationship—with total confidence. Occasionally, have the babysitter take the kids out so that you can quietly enjoy the pleasures of your own home.

22. IF YOU HAVE CHILDREN, MAINTAIN A UNITED FRONT.

Do not allow children to divide and conquer. It weakens their respect for you, can demoralize the parent who says "no" when the other parent says "yes," and can lead to parental bickering. Instead, discuss in private how to deal with issues related to the kids. Then keep a united front, no matter what sort of begging and pleading you're subjected to.

23. GIVE GIFTS.

Giving a gift can be as delightful as receiving one, and unexpected gifts help maintain warmth, laughter, and kindness in a relationship. Gifts don't have to be expensive. Try gift certificates, books, music, your beloved's favorite snack, or other small treats. Roses are nice, but also predictable. Have a stash of gifts that you can dip into when the moment calls for one.

A true gift of love is something you make with your own hands. When I first realized that Tom (now my husband) was my true love, I embroidered a beautiful mandala on a T-shirt for him. It was the same mandala he had as a decoration on his Jeep the night we first met, when he gave me a ride home from a rock concert. More than twenty-five years later, he still has that T-shirt.

Do not give a gift with an ulterior motive, such as giving your partner a book because you'd like him to read more or a pair of skis because you love winter sports and you wish she did, too.

When you receive a gift from your beloved, accept it graciously and warmly, even if you're not delighted with it. If your beloved keeps picking out gifts that don't suit you, take him or her window or catalog shopping, pointing out a range of items that would appeal to you. If you have a good relationship, your partner will appreciate the advice.

24. BE OPEN TO THERAPY.

When a relationship devolves into difficult patterns, be willing to see a good marriage therapist, and be willing to find a good therapist before you have reached the point of no return. Therapists aren't just for couples who are on the verge of divorce. They are facilitators of open discussion; sometimes it can be helpful just to talk through difficult issues with them. Sometimes even one or two sessions can be enough to yield a better flow of energy in a relationship.

Refusal on the part of one partner to see a therapist may indicate that he or she is unwilling to work to improve the relationship. On the other hand, it may also indicate that he or she is skeptical of therapy. One way to convince a skeptical person to see a therapist is to affirm your love but insist that you both could develop some communication skills. Volunteer to go see the therapist on your own for the first session, to check it out and return with feedback.

25. BE RESPONSIBLE FOR YOUR OWN HAPPINESS.

True happiness comes from within, not from an outside source. A relationship can be an anchor in your life, allowing you to grow, change, try, succeed, and fail, always with a stable center to come back to. But it cannot and will not be the true source of joy in life. If you are not grounded within yourself, you will find that you cannot fully develop a healthy, strong, joyous relationship.

Your beloved cannot be the sole source of your joy. He or she can support you, comfort you, encourage you, and challenge you to grow. But in the end, only you can be responsible for your own happiness. Take this lesson to heart, and your joy in life will grow and grow.

Resources

HERBS AND NATURAL PRODUCTS

allGoode Organics
P.O. Box 61256
Santa Barbara, CA 93160-1256
1-800-864-8327
www.allgoodeorganics.com
*Maker of fine organic herbal teas
and natural snacks formulated by
Brigitte Mars, including Sensualitea,
Femininitea, and Maternitea.*

BodySlant
P.O. Box 1667
Newport Beach, CA 92663
1-888-243-3279
www.ageeasy.com
*Offers slant boards, body arches, and
other healthful tools.*

Botanica Erotica
P.O. Box 2
Sebastopol, CA 95473
707-829-6474
*Maker of natural lubricants, massage
oils, chocolate body crème, passion
potions, and more.*

Flower Essence Services
P.O. Box 1769
Nevada City, CA 95959
916-265-0258
Purveyor of quality flower essences.

Frontier Herbs
P.O. Box 299
Norway, IA 52318
1-800-669-3275
www.frontiercoop.com
*A great mail-order service for
herbs.*

Gaia Herbs
108 Island Ford Road
Brevard, NC 28712
1-800-831-7780
www.gaiaherbs.com
*Maker of liquid extracts and plant-
based capsules.*

Herbalist and Alchemist
51 South Wandling Avenue
Washington, NJ 07882
1-800-611-8235
www.herbalist-alchemist.com
*Purveyor of Western and Oriental
herbal formulas.*

Herb Pharm
P.O. Box 116
Williams, OR 97544
1-800-348-4372
www.herb-pharm.com
Maker of excellent herbal tinctures.

Homegrown Herbals

P.O. Box 251
Hygiene, CO 80533
303-702-0833
www.homegrownherbals.com
Another source of excellent herbal tinctures.

Horizon Herbs

P.O. Box 69
Williams, OR 97544-0069
541-846-6704
www.chatlink.com/~herbseed
The best source for herb seeds, including many herbs that are endangered in the wild.

Island Herb

1525 Danby Mountain Road
Danby, VT 05739
802-293-5996
www.partnereartheducationcenter.
    com
Seaweeds and excellent wildcrafted organic herbs. Send an SASE for a catalog.

Little Moon Essentials

P.O. Box 771893
Steamboat Springs, CO 80477
1-888-273-0683
www.littlemoonessentials.com
Maker of cosmic aromatherapy, bath, health, and sensual products.

Natural Pleasure

P.O. Box 395
Newton Center, MA 02459
717-633-1850
www.naturalpleasure.com
A good source of transdermal arginine creams.

Star West

11253 Trade Center Drive
Rancho Cordova, CA 95742
1-800-800-4372
www.starwest-botanicals.com
A mail-order source for quality herbs.

Vedic Harmonics Essential Oils

P.O. Box 35284
Sarasota, CA 34242
1-800-370-3220
ayurvedichealers.com
Offers quality essential oils as well as tantric workshops and an aromatherapy and Ayurvedic school.

SEX TOYS, BOOKS, AND VIDEOS

Eve's Garden

119 West 57th Street, Suite 1201
New York, NY 10019
1-800-848-3837
www.evesgarden.com
Videos, books, and sex toys. On-site retail store and a mail-order catalog.

Good Vibrations

938 Howard Street
San Francisco, CA 94103
1-800-289-8423
www.goodvibes.com
Videos, books, and sex toys. On-site retail store and a mail-order catalog.

Xandria Collection
161 Valley Drive
Department UTC
Brisbane, CA 94005
1-800-242-2823
www.xandria.com
Videos, books, and sex toys. Mail-order catalog.

EDUCATIONAL RESOURCE GROUPS

American Association of Oriental Medicine
433 Front St.
Catasauqua, PA 18032
888-500-7999
www.aaom.org
Their website offers an up-to-date listing of certified acupuncturists across the United States.

American Association of Sex Educators, Counselors, and Therapists
P.O. Box 238
Mount Vernon, IA 52314
319-895-8407
Can provide a list of certified sex therapists in your area.

American Botanical Council
P.O. Box 14345
Austin, TX 78714-4345
www.herbalgram.org
1-800-373-7105
A member-supported education and research organization in the field of herbal medicine. Sells herb-education books and publishes Herbalgram magazine.

American Herb Association
P.O. Box 1673
Nevada, CA 95959
530-265-9552
www.ahaherb.com
Complete listing of schools, programs, seminars, and correspondence courses in the herb category. Excellent newsletter.

American Herbalists Guild
1931 Gaddis Road
Canton, GA 30115
770-751-6021
www.americanherbalist.com
The only national organization for professional, peer-reviewed herbal pratitioners. Offers a directory of members.

Annie Sprinkle, PhD.
P.O. Box 396
Sausalito, CA 94966
amsprinkle@aol.com
www.gatesofheck.com/annie/index.
  html
Prostitute/porn star turned artist/sexologist. She offers a variety of women's workshops, including Taoist Erotic Massage, Super Sex Technologies, and Ecstasy Breathing. A one-woman show will bring her performance wherever it is needed.

The Endometriosis Association
8585 North 76th Place
Milwaukee, WI 53223 USA
414-355-2200
www.endometriosisassn.org
This international nonprofit organization provides information

about the causes, symptoms, and treatments of endometriosis. It also offers a physician registry and referrals to holistic health care practitioners.

Herb Research Foundation

1007 Pearl Street, Suite 200
Boulder, CO 80302
303-449-2265
www.herbs.org
A clearinghouse for herb information.

Impotence Information Center

1-800-843-4315
Offers general information on the causes and treatment of erectile dysfunction.

Institute for the Advanced Study of Human Sexuality

1523 Franklin Street
San Francisco, CA 94109
415-928-1133
www.iashs.edu
A graduate-level school for the study of human sexuality.

The National Center for Homeopathy

801 North Fairfax Street,
   Suite 306
Alexandria, VA 22314
703-548-7790
www.homeopathic.org
This organization offers general information about homeopathy, practitioner referrals, and educational programs.

National Gay and Lesbian Task Force

5455 Wilshire Boulevard,
   Suite 1505
Los Angeles, CA 90036
323-954-9597
www.ngltf.org
A nonprofit agency focusing on advocacy, electoral work, and sociological research.

National Organization of Circumcision Information Resource Centers

P.O. Box 2512
San Anselmo, CA 94979
415-488-9883
www.nocirc.org
A nonprofit educational center for those questioning the necessity of circumcising male and female infants and children.

Parents, Family, and Friends of Lesbian and Gays

1726 M Street Northwest,
   Suite 400
Washington, DC 20036
202-467-8180
www.pflag.org
Can provide referrals to local chapters.

Rocky Mountain Center for Botanical Studies

2639 Spruce Street
Boulder, CO 80302
303-442-6861
www.herbschool.com
Great herb school.

Sex Addicts Anonymous
P.O. Box 70949
Houston, TX 77270
1-800-477-8191
www.saa-recovery.org

Sexaholics Anonymous
P.O. Box 111910
Nashville, TN 37222-1910
615-331-6230
www.sa.org
*Provides information on local
support groups and resources
for those with sex addictions.*

Sexuality Information and Education Council of the United States
130 West 42nd Street, Suite 350
New York, NY 10036
212-819-9770
*Resources and information on
sexuality.*

Source School of Tantra
P.O. Box 1451
Wailuku, HI 96793
808-243-9851
www.sourcetantra.com
Offers Tantra workshops.

United Plant Savers
P.O. Box 98
East Barre, VT 05649
802-479-9825
www.plantsavers.org
*Group that promotes awareness
about rare and endangered species
of plants. Great newsletter.*

HOTLINES

Centers for Disease Control STD and AIDS Hotline
1-800-227-8922 and
1-800-242-2437
In Spanish:
   1-800-344-7432
For the hearing impaired:
   1-800-243-7889
www.ashastd.org
*Provides information and helps people
find local resources for emergency
housing and medical care.*

Domestic Violence Hotline
1-800-799-SAFE
*Offers information and referrals for
victims, as well as a database of
shelters, counseling services, and
legal services.*

Emergency Contraception Hotline
1-800-584-9911
*Can provide contact information for
health care providers in your area
who can supply you with emergency
contraception.*

Planned Parenthood Federation of America
1-800-230-7526
*Provides information on contraception
and sexually transmitted diseases.*

PMS/Menopause Hotline
1-800-222-4767
*Provides informational packets on
natural hormone replacement therapy
and other women's health issues.*

Bibliography

Aldred, Caroline. *Divine Sex.* San Francisco, CA: HarperSanFrancisco, 1996.

Allardice, Pamela. *Aphrodisiacs and Love Magic.* Dorset, England: Prism Press, 1989.

Anand, Margo. *The Art of Sexual Ecstasy.* Los Angeles, CA: Jeremy P. Tarcher, 1989.

Barbach, Lonnie, Ph.D., and David Geisinger, Ph.D. *Going the Distance.* New York, NY: Doubleday, 1991.

Baroni, Diane, and Betty Kelly. *How to Get Him Back from the Other Woman.* New York, NY: St. Martin's Press, 1992.

Beattie, Antonia. *Love Magic.* New York, NY: Barnes and Noble Books, 2000.

Bechtel, Stefan, and the editors of *Men's Health* and *Prevention* magazines. *The Practical Encyclopedia of Sex and Health.* Emmaus, PA: Rodale Press, 1993.

Bechtel, Stefan, and Laurence Roy Stains. *Sex: A Man's Guide.* Emmaus, PA: Rodale Press, 1996.

Bishop, Clifford. *Sex and Spirit.* New York, NY: Little, Brown and Company, 1996.

Brauer, Alan P., M.D., and Donna J. Brauer. *The ESO Ecstasy Program.* New York, NY: Warner Books, 1990.

Budapest, Zsuzsanna E. *The Goddess in the Bedroom.* San Francisco, CA: HarperSan-Francisco, 1995.

Burke, Peggy, and Evan Burke. *The Woman's Gourmet Sex Book.* Canoga Park, CA: Malibu Press, 1983.

Cabot, Laurie, and Tom Cowan. *Love Magic.* New York, NY: Delta Publishing, 1992.

Cabot, Tracy, Ph.D. *How to Make a Man Fall in Love with You.* New York, NY: St. Martin's Press, 1984.

Castleman, Michael. *Sexual Solutions.* New York, NY: Simon and Schuster, 1983.

Chang, Jolan. *The Tao of Love and Sex.* New York, NY: E.P. Dutton, 1977.

——. *The Tao of the Loving Couple.* New York, NY: E.P. Dutton, 1983.

Chang, Dr. Stephen T. *The Tao of Sexology.* San Francisco, CA: Tao Publishing, 1988.

Chia, Mantak, and Douglas Abrams Arava. *The Multi-Orgasmic Man.* San Francisco, CA: HarperSanFrancisco, 2000.

Chia, Mantak, and Michael Winn. *Taoist Secrets of Love: Cultivating Female Sexual Energy.* Huntington, NY: Healing Tao Books, 1986.

——. *Taoist Secrets of Love: Cultivating Male Sexual Energy.* New York, NY: Aurora Press, 1984.

Chu, Valentin. *The Yin-Yang Butterfly.* New York, NY: G.P. Putnam's Sons, 1993.

Coleman, Dr. Paul. *The 30 Secrets of Happily Married Couples.* Holbrook, MA: Bob Adams Publishers, 1992.

Corn, Laura. *101 Nights of Grrreat Romance.* Tempe, AZ: Park Avenue Publishers, 1996.

Cox, Tracey. *Hot Relationships.* New York, NY: Bantam Books, 2000.

——. *Hot Sex.* New York, NY: Bantam Books, 1999.

Crawford, Amanda McQuade. *The Herbal Menopause Book.* Freedom, CA: The Crossing Press, 1996.

Crenshaw, Theresa. *The Alchemy of Love and Lust.* New York, NY: G.P. Putnam's Sons, 1996.

DeAngelis, Barbara, Ph.D. *How to Make Love All the Time.* New York, NY: Rawson Associates, 1987.

——. *Real Moments for Lovers.* New York, NY: Delacorte Press, 1995.

De Luca, Diana. *Bella Donna.* Sebastapol, CA: Bella Botanica Press, 2001.

——. *Botanica Erotica.* Rochester, VT: Healing Arts Press, 1998.

Devi, Kamala. *The Eastern Way of Love.* New York, NY: Simon and Schuster, 1985.

Douglas, Nik, and Penny Slinger. *Sexual Secrets.* New York, NY: Destiny Books, 1979.

Dunas, Felice, Ph.D., and Philip Goldberg. *Passion Play.* New York, NY: Riverhead Books, 1997.

Edell, Dr. Ronnie. *The Sexually Satisfied Woman.* New York, NY: Dutton, 1994.

Ellenberg, Daniel, Ph.D., and Judith Bell, M.S., M.F.C.C. *Lovers for Life.* Santa Rosa, CA: Aslan Publishing, 1995.

Fellner, Tara. *Aromatherapy for Lovers.* Boston, MA: Charles E. Tuttle Co., Inc., 1995.

Feng Shui Journal 5, no. 1 (Spring 1999). (This is the self-proclaimed "Love Issue.)

Feuerstein, George. *Sacred Sexuality.* Los Angeles, CA: Jeremy P. Tarcher, 1993.

Fisher, Bruce, and Nina Hart. *Loving Choices: A Growing Experience.* Boulder, CO: Fisher Publishing Company, 2000.

Fisher, Helen, Ph.D. *Anatomy of Love.* New York, NY: Fawcett Columbine, 1992.

Flatto, Edwin, M.D. *Super Potency at Any Age.* New York, NY: Instant Improvement, Inc., 1991.

Gach, Michael Reed, Ph.D. *Acupressure for Lovers.* New York, NY: Bantam Books, 1997.

Garrison, Omar. *Tantra: The Yoga of Sex.* New York, NY: Julian Press, 1964.

Gibbens, Kalyn Wolf. *Marrying Smart: A Practical Guide for Attracting Your Mate.* Eugene, OR: Just Your Type Publishing, 1994.

Gladstar, Rosemary. *Herbal Healing for Women.* New York, NY: Simon and Schuster, 1993.

——. *Rosemary Gladstar's Family Herbal.* North Adams, MA: Storey Books, 2001.

Glanz, Larry, and Robert Phillips. *How to Start a Romantic Encounter.* Garden City Park, NY: Avery Publishing Group, 1994.

——. *1001 Ways to Be Romantic.* Boston, MA: Casablanca Press, Inc., 1994.

Gray, John, Ph.D. *Mars and Venus in the Bedroom.* New York, NY: HarperCollins, 1995.

Green, James. *The Male Herbal.* Freedom, CA: Crossing Press, 1991.

Haffner, Debra W., M.P.H., and Pepper Schwartz, Ph.D. *What I've Learned About Sex.* New York, NY: Berkley Publishing Group, 1998.

Hare, Jenny. *Think Sex: The Seven Secrets of Mind-Blowing Sex.* Boston, MA: Element Books, 2000.

Hayden, Naura. *How to Satisfy a Woman Every Time.* New York, NY: Bibliophile Publishing Company, 1982.

Hendrickson, Robert. *Lewd Food.* Radnor, PA: Chilton Book Company, 1974.

Hendrix, Harville, Ph.D. *Getting the Love You Want.* New York, NY: HarperCollins, 1988.

——. *Keeping the Love You Find.* New York, NY: Pocket Books, 1992.

Heng, Cheng. *The Tao of Love.* New York, NY: Marlowe and Company, 1997.

Hooper, Anne. *Anne Hooper's Kama Sutra.* New York, NY: Dorling Kindersley, 1994.

——. *The Ultimate Sex Book.* New York, NY: Dorling Kindersley, 1992.

Jensen, Dr. Bernard. *Love, Sex & Nutrition.* Garden City Park, NY: Avery Publishing Group, 1988.

Jillson, Joyce. *The Fine Art of Flirting.* New York, NY: Simon and Schuster. 1984.

Joannides, Paul. *The Guide to Getting It On!* Santa Monica, CA: Goofy Foot Press, 1997.

Jonas, Barbara, and Michael Jonas. *The Book of Love, Laughter & Romance.* San Francisco, CA: Games Partnership, Ltd., 1994.

Kelley, Susan. *Why Men Stray, Why Men Stay.* Holbrook, MA: Adams Media Corporation, 1996.

Keville, Kathi, and Mindy Green. *Aromatherapy: A Complete Guide to the Healing Art.* Freedom, CA: Crossing Press, 1995.

Kilham, Christopher Scott. *Stalking the Wild Orgasm.* San Diego, CA: ACS Publications, 1987.

Kingma, Daphne Rose. *Coming Apart: Why Relationships End and How to Live through the Ending of Yours.* New York, NY: Ballantine Books, 1993.

Kirban, Salem. *How to Win Over Impotence/Frigidity.* Huntington Valley, PA: Salem Kirban, 1981.

Kreidman, Ellen. *Light Her Fire.* New York, NY: Villard Books, 1991.

——. *Light His Fire.* New York, NY: Villard Books, 1989.

Lapanja, Margie. *The Goddess Guide to Love: Timeless Secrets to Divine Romance.* Berkeley, CA: Conari Press, 1999.

Lee, William H., D.Sc., R.Ph., and Lynn Lee, C.N. *Herbal Love Potions.* New Canaan, CT: Keats Publishing, 1991.

Lloyd, J. William. *Karezza*. Hollywood, CA: Phoenix House, 1973.

Lozowick, Leo. *The Alchemy of Love and Sex*. Prescott, AZ: Hohm Press, 1996.

Masterson, Graham. *How to Make His Wildest Dreams Come True*. New York, NY: Penguin Group, 1996.

———. *Secrets of the Sexually Irresistible Woman*. New York, NY: Penguin Group, 1998.

Meletis, Chris D., N.D. *Better Sex Naturally*. New York, NY: HarperCollins, 2000.

Miller, Light, N.D., and Brian Miller, N.D. *Ayurveda and Aromatherapy*. Twin Lakes, WI: Lotus Press, 1995.

Miller, Richard Alan. *The Magical and Ritual Use of Aphrodisiacs*. New York, NY: Destiny Books, 1985.

Mitton, Mervyn. *Herbal Remedies/Sexual Problems*. Berkshire, England: Foulsham Publishers, 1992.

Moore, Thomas. *The Soul of Sex*. New York, NY: HarperCollins, 1998.

Muir, Charles and Caroline. *Tantra: The Art of Conscious Loving*. San Francisco, CA: Mercury House, 1989.

Nissim, Rina. *Natural Healing in Gynecology*. New York, NY: Pandora Press, 1986.

O'Hara, Kristen, and Jeffrey O'Hara. *Sex as Nature Intended It*. Hudson, MA: Turning Point Publications, 2001.

Oumano, Elena, Ph.D. *Natural Sex*. New York, NY: Plume, 1999.

Paget, Lou. *How to Be a Great Lover*. New York, NY: Broadway Books, 1999.

Parvati Baker, Jeannine. *Hygieia: A Women's Herbal*. Berkeley, CA: Freestone Publishing, 1978.

Peiper, Dr. Howard, and Nina Anderson. *Natural Solutions for Sexual Dysfunction*. New Canaan, CT: Safe Goods, 1998.

Pelton, Charles, M.D. *The Sex Book*. Aberdeen, SD: Family Health Media, 1982.

Ramsdale, David, and Ellen Ramsdale. *Sexual Energy Ecstasy*. Playa Del Rey, CA: Peak Skill Publishing, 1991.

Rätsch, Christian. *Plants of Love*. Berkeley, CA: Ten Speed Press, 1997.

Reid, Daniel P. *The Tao of Health, Sex, and Longevity*. New York, NY: Simon and Schuster, 1989.

Renshaw, Domeena, M.D. *Seven Weeks to Better Sex*. New York, NY: Random House, 1995.

Rich, Penny. *Pamper Your Partner*. New York, NY: Simon and Schuster, 1990.

Richardson, Diana. *The Love Keys*. Boston, MA: Element Books, 1999.

Rose, Jeanne. *Herbs and Aromatherapy for the Reproductive System*. Berkeley, CA: Frog, Limited, 1994.

Saint Claire, Olivia. *Unleashing the Sex Goddess in Every Woman*. New York, NY: Bantam Books, 1996.

Saraswati, Sunyata, and Bodhi Avinasha. *Jewel in the Lotus*. San Francisco, CA: Kriya Jyoti Tantra Society, 1987.

Saul, David, M.D. *Sex for Life: The Lover's Guide to Male Sexuality.* Vancouver, BC: Apple Publishing Company, Ltd, 1999.

Selden, Gary. *Aphrodisia.* New York, NY: E.P. Dutton, 1979.

Sonntag, Linda. *Great Sex for Life.* USA: Hamlyn Publishing, 1997.

Stiller, Richard. *The Love Bugs.* New York, NY: Thomas Nelson, Inc., 1974.

Stoppard, Miriam, M.D. *The Magic of Sex.* New York, NY: Dorling Kindersley, 1992.

Stubbs, Kenneth Ray, Ph.D. *Women of the Light.* Larkspur, CA: Secret Garden, 1994.

Tisserand, Maggie. *Essence of Love.* San Francisco, CA: HarperSanFrancisco, 1993.

Too, Lillian. *Lillian Too's Easy to Use Feng Shui for Love.* London, England: Collins and Brown, 2000.

Tresidder, Megan. *The Secret Language of Love.* San Francisco, CA: Chronicle Books, 1997.

Tseng, C. Howard, M.D., Ph.D., Guilas Villanueva, M.D., and Alvin Powell, M.D. *Sexually Transmitted Diseases.* Saratoga, CA: R & E Publishers, 1987.

Venus, Brenda. *Secrets of Seduction.* New York, NY: Dutton, 1996.

Walker, Morton, D.P.M. *Foods for Better Sex.* Old Greenwich, CT: Devin-Adair Publishers, 1984.

———. *Sexual Nutrition.* Garden City Park, NY: Avery Publishing Group, 1994.

Warburton, Diana. *A–Z of Aphrodisia.* New York, NY: Quartet Books, 1986.

Watson, Cynthia Mervis, M.D. *Love Potions.* New York, NY: Jeremy P. Tarcher, 1993.

Waylor, Susan, Ph.D. *Sexual Radiance.* New York, NY: Harmony Books, 1998.

Wedeck, H.E. *Dictionary of Aphrodisiacs.* London, England: Bracken Books, 1994.

Weed, Susun S. *New Menopausal Years.* Woodstock, NY: Ash Tree Publishing, 2002.

Westheimer, Dr. Ruth. *Sex for Dummies.* Foster City, CA: International Data Group Books, 1995.

Wildwood, Chrissie. *Erotic Aromatherapy.* New York, NY: Sterling Publishing, 1994.

Wilson, Dr. Glenn. *Exotic Sex.* London, England: Marshall Cavendish Books, 1992.

Wong, Bruce. *TSFR: The Taoist Way to Total Sexual Fitness for Men.* Princeton, NJ: Golden Dragon Publishers, 1982.

Yudelove, Eric Steven. *The Tao and the Tree of Life.* Saint Paul, MN: Llewellyn Publications, 1995.

Index

About the Author

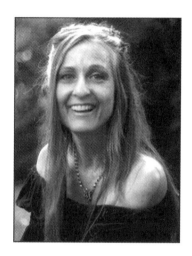

Brigitte Mars is an herbalist and nutritional consultant from Boulder, Colorado, who has been working with natural medicine for more than thirty years. She teaches herbal medicine through the Rocky Mountain Center for Botanical Studies, Boulder College of Massage Therapy, and Naropa University. She is a professional member of the American Herbalist Guild. Brigitte Mars is also available for herbal formulations and consultations. She teaches herb classes from her home. For more information, visit her website at **www.brigittemars.com**.

OTHER PUBLICATIONS BY BRIGITTE MARS

Audiotapes

The Herbal Renaissance: How to Heal with Common Plants and Herbs. Louisville, CO: Sounds True, 1990.

Natural Remedies for a Healthy Immune System. Louisville, CO: Sounds True, 1990.

You can order these tapes directly from Sounds True by calling their mail-order number: 1-800-333-9185.

Books

Addiction-Free Naturally: Liberating Yourself from Sugar, Caffeine, Food Addictions, Tobacco, Alcohol, and Prescription Drugs. Rochester, VT: Healing Arts Press, 2001.

Dandelion Medicine: Remedies and Recipes to Detoxify, Nourish, and Stimulate. North Adams, MA: Storey Books, 1999.

The HempNut Health and Cookbook: Ancient Food for New Millennium, with coauthor Richard Rose. Santa Rosa, CA: HempNut, Inc., 2000.

Herbs for Healthy Skin, Hair & Nails: Banish Eczema, Acne and Psoriasis with Healing Herbs That Cleanse the Body Inside and Out. New Canaan, CT: Keats Publishing, 1998.

Natural First Aid: Herbal Treatments for Ailments and Injuries, Emergency Preparedness, and Wilderness Safety. North Adams, MA: Storey Books, 1999.

Computer Software Program

The Herbal Pharmacy: The Interactive CD-Rom Guide to Medicinal Plants. Boulder, CO: Hale Software, 1998.